Holistic Prayer

A Guide to Jewish Spirituality

מגיד

MAGGID

"The holistic approach to prayer which Rabbi Weiss outlines here... enable[s] us to leave services with an ongoing awareness of God that will last and last."

Rabbi Joseph Telushkin
Author, *Jewish Literacy*

"This is a thoughtful and soulful meditation on Jewish prayer.... An authentic, deeply human exploration."

Dr. Avivah Gottlieb Zornberg
Author, *The Murmuring Deep*

"Rabbi Avi Weiss has an uncanny knack for rendering the complex and sophisticated – simple and understandable. This is not a book which will be relegated to the bookshelf."

Rabbi Dr. Tzvi Hersh Weinreb
Executive Vice President Emeritus, Orthodox Union

"Rabbi Avi Weiss has made a marvelous contribution in helping us all learn how to pray."

Rabbi Shlomo Riskin
Chancellor, Ohr Torah Stone

"A reflective and accessible work on prayer as a central core religious experience... inspiring compassion and fueling our commitments."

Rabbi David Silber
Dean, Drisha Institute for Jewish Education

"[Weiss] gives his reader a... gift by making us privy to the way in which he connects his personal prayer to every aspect of his life – his theology, spirituality, activism, family, profound sense of Jewish history and destiny, and his great love of the Jewish people."

Blu Greenberg
Author, *On Women and Judaism*

"Holistic Prayer... opens the heart of the reader to the deeper meanings of the texts we use to communicate with God and with our own minds, hearts, and souls."

Rabbi Saul J. Berman
Associate Professor, Stern College of Yeshiva University

Avraham Weiss

Holistic Prayer

A Guide to Jewish Spirituality

Maggid Books

Holistic Prayer:
A Guide to Jewish Spirituality

Maggid Edition, 2014

POB 8531, New Milford, CT 06776-8531, USA
& POB 4044, Jerusalem 91040, Israel
www.korenpub.com

The publication of this book was made possible through the generous support of *Torah Education in Israel.*

ISBN 978 159 264 334 9, *hardcover*

A CIP catalogue record for this title is available from the British Library.

Printed and bound in the United States

For Toby

Contents

Preface *ix*

Introduction: What Is Holistic Prayer? *xiii*

PART ONE:

GOALS OF PRAYER

Responsibility 3
Reliance 33
Feeling God's Presence 49

PART TWO:

WHY SET TEFILLA?

Time 73
Place 125
Text 141

PART THREE:

SPIRITUALITY

Kavana 169
Pathway 177
Synagogue 221

Conclusion 257
Role Models & Acknowledgements 261
Judaic Sources 269
Bibliography 275
Prayer Index 283

Preface

I am writing this book because, for a long time, I have lovingly struggled with prayer. It's not that I do not embrace prayer – I do. It's not that I do not love prayer – I do. It's that while prayer is the most exhilarating of spiritual experiences, it is, in the same breath, most daunting.

I am writing this book because, as a rabbi, I know I am not alone. Over the years, I have seen people of all ages, of all backgrounds – students, young adults, middle-aged individuals, seniors, beginners, and the more versed – searching for meaning in *tefilla* (prayer).

Having been involved in this struggle, I feel a need to share ideas, concepts, themes, and approaches that have helped me on my personal journey to realize the infinite depth and power of prayer. My hope is that the teachings offered in this study will help others on their journey. It is an endless one. Precisely when you think you've arrived, there comes recognition that much higher realms can still be reached.

Many brilliant scholarly works have been written on *tefilla*. I pray that this study – without compromising on scholarship – will be a work, not only of cognition, but of emotion; not only of intellect, but of feeling; that it express not only power of the mind, but also softness of the soul and sweetness of the heart. And through the heart, that it inspire fullness of life, spiritual striving, and prayer that is whole – holistic prayer.

The purpose of this book is to help inspire greater meaning in prayer. In the process, fundamental ideas about Jewish spirituality are expounded, as *tefilla* is a microcosm of this larger quest.

For me, the Jewish prayer book – the Siddur – not only reflects varying philosophical approaches to prayer itself, but also serves as a guidebook to Judaism's most fundamental concepts.

With this in mind, commentary on the actual Siddur is found throughout the book. Often a prayer is quoted in its entirety, so the reader can gain a sense of how the full flow of the liturgy relates to the theme being discussed. This is also meant to provide interpretations of the key *tefillot* that make up the prayer service.

The book draws heavily from sources outside the Siddur in an attempt to present themes of *tefilla* in a sophisticated manner while, at the same time, transmitting wisdom in ways that are accessible and uplifting. Hence, biblical and rabbinical passages, contemporary works, personal anecdotes, and stories illustrative of the book's many themes are presented throughout. Indeed, a story begins each chapter. Each one is a tale I've heard, sometimes reshaped through the years. I find great joy in reading and telling stories but often do not know their sources.

The book has been designed with diverse readers in mind. To enhance its usefulness as a guide in learning groups, adult education classes, and private study – in universities, seminaries, high schools across the denominations, and even in non-Jewish classrooms where students may be interested in learning the Jewish approach to prayer – all relevant source materials are quoted. Prayers, biblical texts, and some selected rabbinic passages are quoted in the original Hebrew as well.[1] By quoting texts in their entirety, I hope to allow students the chance to fully study their ideas and encourage discussion of their meaning.

Throughout the book, I have used the new Koren Siddur translation by Rabbi Jonathan Sacks, former chief rabbi of Great Britain, because of its elegance and accuracy.

Well-known translations are used for some of the classical works. Among them are the JPS (Jewish Publication Society) Bible, the Soncino Talmud, the Soncino Midrash Rabba, the Rosenbaum and Silbermann

1. Most of the rabbinic passages quoted are more poetic and spiritual in nature.

translation of Rashi, the Chavel translation of Nahmanides on the Bible, and the Hyamson translation of Maimonides' *Code*. Translations are sometimes tweaked as necessary.

In traditional study halls, authors and Torah scholars are known in different ways. While many are known by their full names, some are known by acronyms (e.g., Rashi), and others are known by the works they have written (e.g., the *Shulḥan Arukh*). Authors quoted in this study are generally referred to by their traditional designations. A complete list of them, together with dates and other biographical information, appears at the end of the book.

A note on pronouns: Obviously, God is neither a He nor a She. God is beyond gender. While I have tried to avoid overusing male pronouns for the Divine, I hope readers will understand that my use of the word "He" to refer to God is merely for the sake of brevity, and in no way reflects a male-centric view of the Divine.

The book includes several parts. In the introduction, I offer an understanding of holistic prayer and how it interfaces with spirituality. This serves as the undercurrent to the entire work, building up to a crescendo in the third section, where these terms are discussed in depth.

The first part of this book discusses the primary goals of prayer. After outlining positions on prayer that deal with our responsibilities in the world, we move on to discuss the natural human reliance upon God. Finally, we suggest that these views converge; their point of commonality is that both emerge from the quest to feel God's presence.[2]

The second part is more conceptual in nature, analyzing why there are specific times, places, and texts for prayer.

The third part covers the theme of spirituality: How does one infuse spirituality into life, into ritual, and, more specifically, into prayer and synagogue?[3]

A conclusion unites the book's many themes.

---

2. This section is a significantly expanded version of my essay "Tefilah: Feeling the Presence of God," which appeared in *Wisdom of Bat Sheva*, ed. Barry S. Wimpfheimer (New Jersey: KTAV Publishing House, 2009), pp. 207–235.
3. The chapter on *kavana*, which serves as the halakhic basis for spiritual *tefilla*, appeared in a slightly abridged version in an earlier work of mine, *Women at Prayer* (New Jersey: KTAV Publishing House, 1990), pp. 101–106.

This book is an outgrowth of classes I have given on prayer throughout my rabbinate, at Yeshiva University's Stern College, at the Bayit – The Hebrew Institute of Riverdale – and, during this last decade, at Yeshivat Chovevei Torah (YCT), Yeshivat Maharat, and the Wexner Heritage Program. I have been inspired by the insights of my students, who in many ways have become my teachers. On many occasions, they pointed me to thoughts and teachings that found their way into the text. Although grateful to them for their input, I take full responsibility for the development and presentation of all aspects of this study. The good is often due to their input; the weaknesses are my own.

Holistic Prayer has become a labor of love. It reflects my conceptual thinking on *tefilla,* even as it includes ingredients that I've incorporated into my personal life and rabbinate to make prayer more meaningful. It is a book I could not have written in my earlier years, as it is a product of my constant evolution as a person, as a rabbi, in search; in search of meaning, in search of my people, in search of all people, in search – constant search – of God.

Avraham Weiss
Winter 5774/2014

Introduction

What Is Holistic Prayer?

The Hebrew word for prayer is *tefilla*. And yet, these two terms are fundamentally different. Prayer is a narrow endeavor, with book in hand, wherein one communicates with God. *Tefilla*, on the other hand, is a broad, all-embracing moment taking into account the mind, body, soul, and heart, in consonance with community and environment. In a world of specialization, *tefilla* represents the opposite of prayer. *Tefilla* is holistic – integrating the whole of the human being with all of creation and with the Creator Himself. *Tefilla* is not prayer, it is holistic prayer.

Prayer literally means petition; it is most associated with request, relief, rescue. *Tefilla* synthesizes a multiplicity of themes to be spelled out in this book.

Synagogues, too, have often become narrow "prayer communities"; a place to pray and not much more. *Tefilla* is broader, its multiple themes inspiring synagogues that are "holistic communities." There, prayer is deeper, wider, and higher, as it is part of a larger, more encompassing synagogue mission.

In Hebrew, *tefilla* (תְּפִלָּה) is an anagram of *petila* (פְּתִלָה), meaning twisting or wrestling. The biblical Rachel uses a form of this word in naming her handmaid's son Naphtali, declaring that נַפְתּוּלֵי אֱלֹהִים נִפְתַּלְתִּי – "I wrestled with God and prevailed" (Gen. 30:8). Onkelos, the Aramaic translator of the Bible, paraphrases:

קַבֵּיל בָּעוּתִי ה׳ בְּאִתְחַנָּנוּתִי בִּצְלוֹתִי.

> The Lord has accepted my request,
> when I supplicated in my prayer.

For Onkelos, prayer is a form of wrestling. The metaphor of wrestling is in sync with holistic prayer, as it involves a complete entanglement of one's whole self with another – with the Other.[1]

Petil (related to *petila*) also means thread. It is most associated with the *petil tekhelet*, the blue thread wrapped around the white strings to form the fringes of the *tzitzit*.[2] The imagery of being bound, twisting round and round, also evokes an embracing holistic sensation.

Tekhelet (תְּכֵלֶת) can be vocalized as *takhlit* (תַּכְלִית), purpose, for the ultimate goal of *tefilla* is to feel the presence of God. As God is the Perfect One, *tefilla* takes different elements of prayer and brings them together in imitation of the Absolute One, of God Himself.

The zenith of holistic prayer is accomplished when all we do becomes an expression of *tefilla*. It is then that *tefilla* is not relegated to a specific place, time, or text, but becomes our very identity. It is that moment in the Bible when Hannah, the paragon of *tefilla*,[3] comes forth with her newly born son, Samuel, and tells Eli the high priest:

> אֲנִי הָאִשָּׁה, הַנִּצֶּבֶת עִמְּכָה בָּזֶה, לְהִתְפַּלֵּל, אֶל ה׳
> אֶל הַנַּעַר הַזֶּה, הִתְפַּלָּלְתִּי; וַיִּתֵּן ה׳ לִי אֶת שְׁאֵלָתִי, אֲשֶׁר שָׁאַלְתִּי מֵעִמּוֹ.
> I am the woman who stood here beside you and prayed to the Lord. It was this boy I prayed for; and the Lord has granted me what I asked of Him. (1 Sam. 1:26–27)

Hannah is declaring not only that she prayed for this child, but that, in fact, this child, Samuel, is *tefilla*. When she proclaims, "It was this boy

1. On the surface it appears that Onkelos is deviating from the literal meaning of the text – prayer is not wrestling. We're suggesting that the two interpretations complement each other. See Israel Drazin and Rabbi Stanley Wagner, *Onkelos on the Torah: Understanding the Bible Text – Genesis* (New York: Gefen Publishing House, 2006).
2. See Num. 15:38, וְנָתְנוּ עַל צִיצִת הַכָּנָף פְּתִיל תְּכֵלֶת – "That they shall attach to the tassel at each corner a thread of blue."
3. See Berakhot 30b, 31a.

I prayed for," she is saying, "This boy is *tefilla,* because I know that he will be the embodiment of the intense relationship between God and humanity." And so it came to be. Samuel became a prophet in Israel, and everything about his life was *tefilla*.

This book is called *Holistic Prayer: A Guide to Jewish Spirituality* because holistic prayer and spirituality intersect. *Tefilla* begins from within but ultimately encompasses all. So, too, spirituality. It is rooted in the *nekuda hapenimit,* the innermost point, the *ḥiyyut,* the life essence of the human being, one's inner godliness. As the *Sefat Emet* posits, "For everything there is a point of essence that comes from the Lord, Blessed Be He" – כִּי בְּכָל דָּבָר יֵשׁ נְקוּדָּה חַיּוּת מֵה' יִתְבָּרֵךְ.[4] He adds that viscerally, "the world is pulled by this single point" – כָּל הָעוֹלָם נִמְשָׁךְ אַחַר נְקוּדָּה אַחַת.[5] That point is ever-evolving. When nurtured, it expands from being infinitesimal to becoming infinite.

In the end, spirituality is endless, it has no borders – it is overflowing; its waves cross the sea, spilling over to the shores and beyond. The Hebrew word for spirit is *ruaḥ* (רוּחַ), which, from a homiletical perspective, can also be vocalized as *revaḥ* (רֶוַח) – width or distance. First we experience the spiritual moment narrowly, intensely, and then it widens, lengthens, comes full circle, and encompasses the whole of our souls, our very beings, our people, the world. The *Sefat Emet* makes this point:

הֲוָיַת כָּל דָּבָר מִמֶּנּוּ
רַק שֶׁהַנְּקוּדָּה סְתוּמָה
וּצְרִיכִין לְהַרְחִיבָהּ....
כְּפִי הַרְחָבָתָהּ בְּנַפְשׁוֹ
כֵּן מִתְגַּלֶּה אֵלָיו בְּכָל מָקוֹם.

The existence of everything comes from God.
But the innermost point is closed,
and requires opening up....
For the more one's soul is expanded,
the more God is revealed to him, in every place.[6]

---

4. *Sefat Emet*, Genesis, *Vayera* 5632, s.v. *VaYera.*
5. Ibid., *Lekh Lekha* 5632, s.v. *Lekh lekha.*
6. Ibid., Deuteronomy, *Re'eh* 5631, s.v. *Bamidrash ki yarḥiv.*

Rabbi Abraham Joshua Heschel purportedly said, "When I was young, I was impressed by clever people. As I grow older, I'm more impressed by kind people." I have experienced a similar transition. When I was in my teens, I was impressed by those who had good feet and hands, those who could run and make long jump shots on the basketball court. As I grew older, I was more impressed by those who had good minds, the thinkers and intellectuals. These days, I am more impressed by people with big hearts.[7]

These elements – the physical, the intellectual, and the spiritual – are all essential in holistic prayer. This is a book that, in part, explicates prayer for physical well-being – the ingredients to thank God for our physical gifts. Hopefully, it adds an intellectual understanding of prayer. But most important, it is a work that comes from the heart. As Rabban Yoḥanan b. Zakkai points out, the heart is holistic – within it lies all else.[8] May these words that emanate from the heart enter into the heart, and into our spirits.

7. I've also heard the heart-mind imagery used in the name of Heschel.
8. See Mishna Avot 2:14, שֶׁבִּכְלָל דְּבָרָיו דִּבְרֵיכֶם.

Part One
Goals of Prayer

In the book of Psalms, King David declares: אַחַת שָׁאַלְתִּי מֵאֵת ה׳, אוֹתָהּ אֲבַקֵּשׁ *– "I ask for one thing of the Lord, this do I request." David could have asked God for help in overcoming his numerous challenges: conflict with his predecessor, King Saul; confronting the Philistines; the anguish of having lost an infant child; the pain of his son Absalom's rebellion. Yet, with all these challenges, what David asks for is* שִׁבְתִּי בְּבֵית ה׳ כָּל יְמֵי חַיַּי; לַחֲזוֹת בְּנֹעַם ה׳ וּלְבַקֵּר בְּהֵיכָלוֹ *– "to live in the House of the Lord all the days of my life, to gaze upon the beauty of the Lord, to frequent His Temple" (Ps. 27:4). The one thing David asks is that he be able to feel the presence of God.*

This yearning constitutes the very essence of prayer.

Chapter One

Responsibility

Two friends were discussing some of the more difficult issues of life. One said, "Sometimes I would like to ask God why He allows poverty, famine, and injustice, when He could do something about it." The other replied, "Well, why don't you ask Him?" The response came quickly: "Because I am afraid that God might ask me the same question."[1]

GOD'S IMAGE – TZELEM E-LOHIM

Citing the biblical phrase וּלְעָבְדוֹ בְּכָל לְבַבְכֶם – "and to serve Him with all your heart" (Deut. 11:13), the Talmud asks and then answers its own question:

אֵיזוֹ הִיא עֲבוֹדָה שֶׁבַּלֵּב? זוֹ תְּפִלָּה.

> What is the service of the heart? This is prayer.[2]

1. The origin of this anecdote is unclear.
2. Ta'anit 2a. See also *Sifrei, Devarim* 41, s.v. *ule'avdo.*

Basing himself on this talmudic statement, Maimonides elaborates:

> מִצְוַת עֲשֵׂה לְהִתְפַּלֵּל בְּכָל יוֹם, שֶׁנֶּאֱמַר: "וַעֲבַדְתֶּם אֵת ה' אֱ־לֹהֵיכֶם." מִפִּי הַשְּׁמוּעָה לָמְדוּ שֶׁעֲבוֹדָה זוֹ הִיא תְּפִלָּה. וְנֶאֱמַר: "וּלְעָבְדוֹ בְּכָל לְבַבְכֶם," אָמְרוּ חֲכָמִים: "אֵי זוֹ הִיא עֲבוֹדָה שֶׁבַּלֵּב? זוֹ תְּפִלָּה."
>
> It is an affirmative commandment to pray every day, as it says, "and you shall serve the Lord your God" [Ex. 23:25]. From tradition, we have learned that "service" is prayer, as it says, "and to serve Him (*ule'ovdo*) with all your heart" [Deut. 11:13]. The sages commented, "What is the service of the heart? This is prayer."[3]

Here, Maimonides reaffirms the Talmud's assertion that prayer is fundamentally a function of *avodat Hashem*, wherein the limited and finite person serves God – the unlimited and infinite Source of all creation. How is this achieved?

In Genesis, the Torah records that God created the human being in His image (*tzelem E-lohim*): **וַיִּבְרָא אֱ־לֹהִים אֶת הָאָדָם בְּצַלְמוֹ, בְּצֶלֶם אֱ־לֹהִים בָּרָא אֹתוֹ זָכָר וּנְקֵבָה בָּרָא אֹתָם** – "And God created Adam in His image, in the image of God He created him, male and female He created them" (Gen. 1:27). This means that when we look at each other, what we see is the surface of a human being. But if we look deeply into each other, we should see a little bit of God – *ḥelek E-loa'h mima'al* – "a portion of God from above" (Job 31:2).

For Ben Azai in the Jerusalem Talmud, this is the most important principle in the Torah:

> וְאָהַבְתָּ לְרֵעֲךָ כָּמוֹךָ ר' עֲקִיבָא אוֹמֵר זֶהוּ כְּלָל גָּדוֹל בַּתּוֹרָה. בֶּן עַזַּאי אוֹמֵר זֶה סֵפֶר תּוֹלְדֹת אָדָם זֶה כְּלָל גָּדוֹל מִזֶּה.
>
> "Love your fellow as yourself" [Lev. 19:18] – R. Akiva says this is

3. Maimonides, *Code*, Laws of Prayer 1:1. *Kesef Mishneh* ad loc., s.v. *mitzvat aseh lehitpallel*, asks why Maimonides quotes "and you shall serve the Lord your God" (Ex. 23:25) as the source of the biblical obligation to pray, and not "and [you shall] serve Him with all your heart" (Deut. 11:13). The *Kesef Mishneh* suggests that the verse from Deuteronomy may be understood as offering advice rather than mandating a requirement, or that it may refer to the "service" of learning Torah as well as the "service" of prayer.

> the great principle of the Torah. Ben Azai says, "This is the record of the descendants of Adam" [Gen. 5:1] is a greater principle.[4]

The verse from Genesis quoted by Ben Azai goes on to mention that the human being was created in the likeness of God. As the Torah states, זֶה סֵפֶר תּוֹלְדֹת אָדָם בְּיוֹם בְּרֹא אֱלֹהִים אָדָם בִּדְמוּת אֱלֹהִים עָשָׂה אֹתוֹ – "This is the record of the descendants of Adam, on the day God created the human being; He made him in the likeness of God" (Gen. 5:1).

We must remember that it was not Abraham, the first Jew, who was created in the image of God, but Adam, the first human being, from whom all peoples are descended. Bearing in mind that all human beings are endowed with a piece of the Divine, it follows that all human beings are of equal value. Just as God is of endless value, every human being is of endless value. Just as God is unique, every human being is unique. No two people have the same fingerprint, the same consciousness, or the same soul.

The Mishna in Sanhedrin asks why the world began with one person. Why did it begin with Adam?[5] The Mishna gives us three reasons:

> לְפִיכָךְ נִבְרָא אָדָם יְחִידִי לְלַמֶּדְךָ שְׁלוֹם הַבְּרִיּוֹת שֶׁלֹּא יֹאמַר אָדָם לַחֲבֵירוֹ אַבָּא גָּדוֹל מֵאָבִיךָ....
>
> וְשֶׁכָּל הַמְאַבֵּד נֶפֶשׁ אַחַת מַעֲלֶה עָלָיו הַכָּתוּב כְּאִילּוּ אִיבֵּד עוֹלָם מָלֵא וְכָל הַמְקַיֵּים נֶפֶשׁ אַחַת מַעֲלֶה עָלָיו הַכָּתוּב כְּאִילּוּ קִיֵּים עוֹלָם מָלֵא....
>
> וּלְהַגִּיד גְּדוּלָּתוֹ שֶׁל הַקָּדוֹשׁ בָּרוּךְ הוּא שֶׁאָדָם טוֹבֵעַ כַּמָּה מַטְבְּעוֹת בְּחוֹתָם אֶחָד וְכוּלָּן דּוֹמִין זֶה לָזֶה וּמֶלֶךְ מַלְכֵי הַמְּלָכִים הַקָּדוֹשׁ בָּרוּךְ הוּא טָבַע כָּל אָדָם בְּחוֹתָמוֹ שֶׁל אָדָם הָרִאשׁוֹן וְאֵין אֶחָד מֵהֶן דּוֹמֶה לַחֲבֵירוֹ לְפִיכָךְ כָּל אֶחָד וְאֶחָד חַיָּב לוֹמַר בִּשְׁבִילִי נִבְרָא הָעוֹלָם.
>
> Therefore, Adam was created as a single entity, to create peace amongst humanity, lest one say, "My ancestor is greater than yours."…

4. Jerusalem Talmud, Nedarim 9:4.
5. The Talmud suggests that Adam was born male and female, with one side being male and the other female. The rib story, according to this opinion, is really the bifurcation of Adam into two distinct people – one male, the other female. See Ketubbot 8a.

> And to demonstrate that if one destroys a single soul, it is as though he has destroyed the entire world. And if one saves a single soul, it is as if he has saved the entire world.... [6]
>
> And to show the greatness of God. For a human being imprints many coins with one mold, and all the coins look the same, while the Ruler of rulers, the Holy One, Blessed Be He, created all of humanity from the mold of Adam, and not one is similar to the other. Therefore, everyone is obligated to say, "The world was created for me."[7]

The world began with Adam to teach us three consequences of the reality of *tzelem E-lohim*. First, because we all come from the same source, we are equal in value. Second, because Adam was of infinite worth (as the only human being, the future of the world depended on him), every human being is of infinite worth. Saving one person, says the Mishna, is tantamount to saving the world; destroying a person means destroying the world. Finally, just as Adam was unique (he was then the only living person), all human beings – Adam's descendants – are unique. In a world of imitation, the Torah emphasizes individual creativity. It teaches us to do our best to tap into our divine spark and find our unique voice.

It must be remembered, however, that *tzelem E-lohim* is potential. When God created Adam, He breathed His spirit into him – וַיִּפַּח בְּאַפָּיו נִשְׁמַת חַיִּים (Gen. 2:7). We, Adam's descendants, have the choice to use or abuse our *tzelem E-lohim*. Like God, the human being has freedom of choice.

6. Some texts in the Mishna read, "a single soul of Israel." Perhaps this is so because the Mishna deals with Jewish jurisprudence, specifically with Jewish capital punishment. The principle, however, that one who saves a single person has saved the world applies to all human beings.

   The flow of the Mishna underscores the text as quoted here, as it deals with why the world started with Adam, who represents the universal human being. See Mishna Sanhedrin 4:5, *Shinuyei Nusḥaot*, s.v. *aḥat miYisrael*.

   See also Ephraim E. Urbach, "'*Kol HaMekayyeim Nefesh Aḥat*...': Development of the Version, Vicissitudes of Censorship, and Business Manipulations of Printers" [Hebrew], *Tarbiz* 40 (1971), pp. 268–284.

7. Sanhedrin 4:5. I've quoted the first two reasons of the Mishna in reverse order to parallel our explanation of the fundamental values derived from *tzelem E-lohim*.

Not coincidentally, after every creation, the Torah records that וַיַּרְא אֱלֹהִים כִּי טוֹב – "And God saw that it was good" (Gen. 1:10, 12, 18, 21, 25). After the creation of the human being, however, this declaration no longer appears. This is because whether a human being is good or not depends on his or her deeds. *Ki tov* – "it was good" – is a more appropriate refrain after the human being has lived a wholesome life, after having made the proper choices.[8] But no matter what we do or how we act, there is a profound Jewish belief that all human beings have the power to return to their inner true self, to the part of God in all of us.

Throughout history, there have been those who have defiled the values of *tzelem E-lohim*. But Judaism insists that goodness will prevail. Rabbi Irving (Yitz) Greenberg elegantly makes this point:

> The central paradigm of Jewish religion is redemption. According to the Bible, the human being is created in the image of God. According to the rabbis, this means that every single person is unique and equal, endowed with the dignity of infinite value. But in history most humans have been degraded or denied their due. Judaism affirms that this condition should never be accepted; it must and will be overcome.[9]

---

8. Nehama Leibowitz, *New Studies in Bereshit (Genesis)* (Jerusalem: Ḥemed Press, 1995), p. 14. She writes: "The phrase 'it was good' was omitted from man's creation, because his good was dependent on his own free choice."

   See Rashi, Genesis 1:26, s.v. *veyirdu vidgat hayam*. Rashi notes that *veyirdu* (וְיִרְדּוּ) may imply dominion as well as descending – this because *veyirdu* comes from one of two roots: ר.ד.ה (R-D-H) or י.ר.ד (Y-R-D). It all depends on human beings making the right choices. In Rashi's words:

   > In the word *veyirdu* there is the language of dominating and descending. If he [man] is worthy he dominates over the beasts and cattle; if he is not worthy he will sink lower than them, and the beast will rule over him.

   Translation from Rev. M. Rosenbaum and Dr. A. M. Silbermann, *Pentateuch with Targum Onkelos, Haphtaroth and Rashi's Commentary* (New York: Hebrew Publishing Company, 1934).
9. Rabbi Irving Greenberg, *The Jewish Way* (New York: Summit Books, 1988), p. 18. While my thoughts on *tzelem E-lohim* have developed over the years, at their core they were inspired by Rabbi Greenberg. I am deeply grateful to him.

The belief that the inner godliness of the human being can always be tapped, as we shall see, is a primary function of prayer in the Jewish tradition.

REACHING IN

The idea of *tzelem E-lohim* is crucial to understanding the Jewish approach to *teshuva* (repentance) and prayer. For Rabbi Abraham Isaac HaKohen Kook, *teshuva* does not deal with a specific wrong. Rather, it has to do with a general feeling of despondency and estrangement from God. *Teshuva* means a return to the self, to the godliness inherent in every human being. Of course, we must assume responsibility for our actions, but on a spiritual level, the human being possesses inner purity. *Teshuva*, whose root is ש.ו.ב (SH-U-V), to return, means to remember that *tzelem E-lohim* makes us who we are.

Rabbi Kook describes *teshuva* this way:

> אֵין חֵטְא אוֹ חֲטָאִים שֶׁל עָבָר עוֹלִים עַל לִבּוֹ, אֲבָל בִּכְלָל הוּא מַרְגִּישׁ בְּקִרְבּוֹ שֶׁהוּא מְדֻכָּא מְאֹד, שֶׁהוּא מָלֵא עָוֹן, שֶׁאֵין אוֹר ה׳ מֵאִיר עָלָיו, אֵין רוּחַ נְדִיבָה בְּקִרְבּוֹ, לִבּוֹ אָטוּם....
>
> הַתְּשׁוּבָה הָרֵאשִׁית, שֶׁהִיא מְאִירָה אֶת הַמַּחֲשַׁכִּים מִיָּד, הִיא שֶׁיָּשׁוּב הָאָדָם אֶל עַצְמוֹ, אֶל שֹׁרֶשׁ נִשְׁמָתוֹ, וּמִיָּד יָשׁוּב אֶל הָאֱ־לוֹהִים.
>
> A person does not conjure up the memory of a past sin or sins, but in a general way he feels terribly depressed. He feels himself pervaded by sin; that the divine light does not shine on him; that there is nothing noble in him; that his heart is unfeeling....[10]
>
> The primary role of penitence, which at once sheds light on the darkened zone, is for the person to return to himself, to the root of his soul and [from there] immediately return to God.[11]

10. Rabbi Abraham Isaac HaKohen Kook, *Orot HaTeshuva* (Jerusalem: Yeshivat Or Etzion, 1992), ch. 3.
11. Ibid., ch. 15, p. 52.

Not coincidentally, the instrument used to rally us to repent is the shofar. The sound of the shofar comes from the inner breath; it is a reversal of the breath God breathed into Adam, וַיִּפַּח בְּאַפָּיו נִשְׁמַת חַיִּים – "and He breathed into his nostrils the breath of life" (Gen. 2:7). The shofar sound releases the breath of God breathed into Adam, breathed into all of us. In the words of the *Sefat Emet*:

> מִצְוַת שׁוֹפָר... וְעַל יְדֵי תְּשׁוּבָה יְכוֹלִין לְעוֹרֵר הַקּוֹל הַפְּנִימִי שֶׁנִּמְצָא בְּנַפְשׁוֹת בְּנֵי יִשְׂרָאֵל.
>
> The mitzva of shofar [is the following]...through *teshuva* we can stir the inner voice found in the souls of the Jewish people.[12]

Our tradition maintains that anybody, no matter who he is or how far she has strayed, can always return to his or her true, incorruptible goodness. The Talmud tells the story of Elisha b. Abuya, a devout and gifted scholar who had gone astray. Elisha's student, Rabbi Meir, implored him to repent. Elisha, who had become known as *Aḥer*, which literally means "other" or "stranger," responded, "I cannot repent, because I heard a *bat kol* (heavenly voice) exclaim, 'Repent, wayward children, except for Aḥer.'"[13] Rabbi Ahron Soloveichik explains that Elisha was called Aḥer, as he was a stranger to his true being. He did not repent because he was "laboring under the erroneous conviction that he was corrupt, basically evil. But this was not true. Aḥer had failed to understand when he heard the *bat kol* that its message was: Aḥer cannot repent, but Elisha b. Abuya can."[14]

---

12. *Sefat Emet*, Rosh HaShana 5651, s.v. *Mitzvat shofar.*
13. The Talmud in Ḥagiga 15a records the story of Elisha b. Abuya:

    Our rabbis taught: Once Aḥer was riding on a horse on Shabbat, and R. Meir was walking behind him to learn Torah at his mouth. Said [Aḥer] to him, "Meir, turn back, for I have already measured by the paces of my horse that thus far extends the Shabbat limit [two thousand cubits in all directions]." He replied, "You, too, go back [do *teshuva*]." [Aḥer] answered, "Have I not already told you that I have already heard from behind the veil: 'Return, you backsliding children' [Jer. 3:22] – except Aḥer (שׁוּבוּ בָּנִים שׁוֹבָבִים – חוּץ מֵאַחֵר)?"
14. Rabbi Ahron Soloveichik, *"Jew and Jew, Jew and Non-Jew,"* in Soloveichik, *Logic of the Heart, Logic of the Mind: Wisdom and Reflections on Topics of Our Times* (Jerusalem:

Rabbi Soloveichik adds that every time the Talmud records an individual who speaks of doing something wrong, the third person singular is used – *hahu gavra,* "that person" – as if the individual had been overtaken by an outer evil force. When the individual recalls having acted righteously, however,the first person singular – *ana* – is used, as righteousness is one's true essence.

Once a person returns to his or her inner godliness, Rabbi Kook explains, **וּמִיָּד יָשׁוּב אֶל הָאֱלוֹקִים** – "one can immediately return to God."[15] The primary role of penitence is return to oneself, to the root of one's soul. It is only from that place that the individual can then return to God.

A beautiful legend reinforces this idea:[16]

A short apple tree grew aside a tall cedar. Every night, the apple tree would look up and sigh, believing that the stars in the sky were hanging from the branches of its tall friend. The little apple tree would lift its branches heavenward and plead, "But where are my stars?"

As time passed, the apple tree grew. Its branches produced leaves, passersby enjoyed its shade, and its apples were delectable. But at night, when it looked to the skies, it still felt discontented, inadequate; other trees had stars, but it did not.

It happened once that a strong wind blew, hurtling apples to the ground. They fell in such a way that they split horizontally instead of vertically (the way apples are normally cut). At the very center of each apple was the outline of a star. The apple tree had possessed stars all along; it just required a different approach to find them. The inner core had always contained the celestial.

If this is true for apples, it is all the more so for human beings, who are created in the image of God. Every person has an inner star, a

---

Genesis Jerusalem Press, 1991), pp. 69–91.

See Rabbi Joseph B. Soloveitchik's analysis of the Aḥer story in *Ḥamesh Derashot* (Jerusalem: Mekhon Tal Orot, 5734), pp. 124–128, and the English translation in Soloveitchik, *The Rav Speaks* (Jerusalem: Tal Orot Institute, 5743), pp. 193–199.

15. Kook, *Orot HaTeshuva*, ch. 15, p. 52.

16. I do not know the author of this legend. I first heard it at a Marriage Encounter seminar that my wife, Toby, and I attended more than thirty years ago. It has been popularized by the gifted storyteller Peninnah Schram. I have reshaped it here in my own way.

nitzotz (inner spark). If we could only find the way to ignite the light, fanning its flames upward, we could reach higher and higher.

Thus, *teshuva* contains two steps: the move inward, the return to one's inner goodness and godliness, which then catapults him or her upward to God, to encounter Him. This idea is based on a passage from Deuteronomy:

> וְהָיָה כִי יָבֹאוּ עָלֶיךָ כָּל הַדְּבָרִים הָאֵלֶּה הַבְּרָכָה וְהַקְּלָלָה אֲשֶׁר נָתַתִּי לְפָנֶיךָ וַהֲשֵׁבֹתָ אֶל לְבָבֶךָ... וְשַׁבְתָּ עַד ה׳ אֱלֹהֶיךָ וְשָׁמַעְתָּ בְקֹלוֹ כְּכֹל אֲשֶׁר אָנֹכִי מְצַוְּךָ הַיּוֹם אַתָּה וּבָנֶיךָ בְּכָל לְבָבְךָ וּבְכָל נַפְשֶׁךָ.
>
> When all these things befall you – the blessing and the curse that I have set before you – and you take them to heart.... And you will return to the Lord your God, and you and your children will heed His voice and all that I command you on this day, with all your heart and soul. (Deut. 30:1, 2)

Note that the first part of the sequence of *teshuva* describes how one returns inward to one's heart. Only then does the Torah speak of returning to God.

Prayer as a function of *ule'ovdo*, of serving God, operates in a similar fashion. The first prayer accepted by God was in the form of a sacrifice that Abel brought to Him.[17] One wonders why Abel's sacrifice, unlike Cain's, was accepted. The *Sefat Emet* suggests an answer based on an insightful reading of the text. After Cain brings his sacrifice, the Torah states, וְהֶבֶל הֵבִיא גַם הוּא – "And Abel also brought [an offering]" (Gen. 4:4). The *Sefat Emet* understands the text this way:

> וְזֶהוּ שֶׁכָּתוּב הֵבִיא גַם הוּא. גַּם אֶת עַצְמוֹ עִם הַקָּרְבָּן. וְלָכֵן נִתְקַבֵּל לִפְנֵי ה׳ יִתְבָּרַךְ.
>
> Abel brought himself [his inner I] with the sacrifice, and therefore it was accepted before the Lord, Blessed Be He.[18]

17. While there are no sacrifices today, many insights concerning prayer can be learned from the sacrificial service.
18. *Sefat Emet*, Genesis, *Bereshit* 5635, s.v. *BeSefer Kol Simḥa*.

Cain's sacrifice was external; it had no inner depth, and was therefore rejected. Abel's sacrifice emanated from his inner purity and was therefore received.

From this perspective, prayer is counterintuitive. It begins not by reaching up, but by reaching in. If prayer is about transcendence, it is first and foremost about inner transcendence. Once the inner soul is revealed, we are in a better position to relate to the infinite God. This idea is expressed in the writing of Shem Tov Ibn Falaquera, who posits that by knowing one's true self, one can come to know God:

> וְאָמְרוּ מִי שֶׁיֵּדַע נַפְשׁוֹ יֵדַע בּוֹרְאוֹ, וְכָל מִי שֶׁהוּא סָכָל בִּידִיעַת נַפְשׁוֹ כָּל שֶׁכֵּן שֶׁהוּא סָכָל בִּידִיעַת בּוֹרְאוֹ. וְאֵיךְ יֵאָמֵן בְּאָדָם שֶׁהוּא חָכָם בְּזוּלָתוֹ וְהוּא סָכָל בְּנַפְשׁוֹ... וְעַל כֵּן אָמְרוּ כִּי יְדִיעַת הַנֶּפֶשׁ קוֹדֶמֶת לִידִיעַת הָאֱלוֹהַּ יִתְבָּרַךְ.
>
> They said that whoever knows his soul knows his Creator, and whoever is ignorant of knowing his soul is ignorant of the knowledge of his Creator. How can one believe that a person is wise concerning something else when he is ignorant concerning himself? ... Therefore, they said that the knowledge of the soul is prior to the knowledge of God.[19]

Joseph Ibn Ṣaddiq echoes this idea:

> וּמִידִיעָתוֹ נַפְשׁוֹ יֵדַע עוֹלָם הָרוּחָנִי וְיַגִּיעַ מִמֶּנָּה לִידִיעַת בּוֹרְאוֹ כְּמוֹ שֶׁכָּתוּב בְּאִיּוֹב "וּמִבְּשָׂרִי אֶחֱזֶה אֱלוֹהַּ."
>
> By man knowing his own soul, he will know the spiritual world from which he can attain some knowledge of the Creator, as it is written, "From my flesh I shall perceive God" [Job 19:26].[20]

This, writes Rabbi Kook, is the gift of prayer:

---

19. Shem Tov Ibn Falaquera, introduction to *Sefer HaNefesh,* in Raphael Jospe, *Torah and Sophia: The Life and Thought of Shem Tov Ibn Falaquera* (Cincinnati: Hebrew Union College Press, 1988), pp. 276, 321.
20. Joseph Ibn Ṣaddiq, *HaOlam HaKatan,* in Saul Horovitz, *The Microcosm of Joseph Ibn Ṣaddiq* (Cranbury, NJ: Associated University Presses, 2003), p. 77.

> הַתְּפִלָּה הִיא מִלְּמַטָּה לְמַעְלָה. כֵּיצַד? מִתּוֹךְ אוֹתוֹ הַמַּעְיָן הַמָּלֵא קְדוּשָּׁה טִבְעִית שֶׁבְּלִבֵּנוּ הֲרֵינוּ דּוֹלִים, מוֹצִיאִים אֶת הַרְגָּשׁוֹתָיו הָעֲדִינוֹת מִן הַכֹּחַ אֶל הַפֹּעַל....
>
> וּכְשֶׁאָנוּ עוֹלִים, עוֹלִים עִמָּנוּ כָּל שָׁרְשֵׁי הֲוָיוֹתֵינוּ, כָּל עַנְפֵי נִשְׁמוֹתֵינוּ, כָּל קַוֵּי הַחַיִּים הַשּׁוֹפְעִים מִמַּהוּתֵנוּ וְכָל מְקוֹרוֹת הַחַיִּים הַמְפַכִּים עָלֵינוּ, עַד הֲבִיאָם אוֹתָנוּ אֶל הַמַּהוּתִיּוּת הַפְּרָטִית שֶׁלָּנוּ. וְהַכֹּל מִתְבָּרֵךְ, הַכֹּל מִתְעַלֶּה, הַכֹּל מִתְקַדֵּשׁ וּמִתְרוֹמֵם, הַכֹּל שָׂמֵחַ שִׂמְחַת יְשָׁרִים, הַכֹּל עָלֵז עֲלִיצוּת קֹודֶשׁ.
>
> Prayer rises up from down below to high above. How does this come about? From that source in our hearts which is filled with natural holiness, we draw out, we transform our refined feelings from potentiality to actuality....
>
> And as we elevate ourselves, all the very sources of our existence – all the ramifications of our soul, all the life that pours out from our inner selves, and all the life sources that gush over us – become elevated with us until they make us reach the level of our own true selves. All becomes blessed; all becomes elevated; all becomes holy and exalted – all rejoices with righteous joy, all exults in holy gladness.[21]

In kabbalistic thought, the goal of humankind is to achieve an all encompassing sense of *tikkun*. According to Lurianic Kabbala, the world is in a state of *shevirat hakelim*, broken vessels. In this state of brokenness, the human being is under stress, often feeling disconnected from all that surrounds him or her. The purpose of Torah, according to this perspective, is *tikkun*, which literally means "fixing" but figuratively refers to "repairing" or "uniting" the world on all levels.[22] The concept of *tikkun* calls on us to unite with our planet in the spirit of ecological peace, to unite with each other in warm camaraderie, and to unite with God in absolute harmony. True *tikkun* occurs when the godly part inside of us

---

21. Rabbi Abraham Isaac HaKohen Kook, "Introduction to the Siddur," in *Seder Tefilla im Peirush Olat Re'iya* (Jerusalem: Aguda LeHotza'at Sifrei HaRa'aya Kook, 5699 [1939]), p. 19. Translation from B. S. Jacobson, *Meditations on the Siddur* (Tel Aviv: Sinai, 1966), p. 27.
22. See Daniel C. Matt, *The Essential Kabbalah* (New York: HarperCollins, 1995); Matt, *Lev HaKabbala* (Jerusalem: Olam Katan, 2011).

unites with the God above. When the soul is kindled, it begins to soar like a flame, leaping to connect to God. Without that rendezvous, the soul feels forlorn, like a lover bereft of his or her beloved. Rabbi Abraham Joshua Heschel poetically captures this encounter:

> As a tree torn from the soil, as a river separated from its source, the human soul wanes when detached from what is greater than itself. Without the holy, the good turns chaotic; without the good, beauty becomes accidental. It is the pattern of the impeccable which makes the average possible. It is the attachment to what is spiritually superior: loyalty to a sacred person or idea, devotion to a noble friend or teacher, love for a people or for mankind, which holds our inner life together. But any ideal, human, social, or artistic, if it forms a roof over all of life, shuts us off from the light. Even the palm of one hand may bar the light of the entire sun. Indeed, we must be open to the remote in order to perceive the near. Unless we aspire to the utmost, we shrink to inferiority.
>
> Prayer is our attachment to the utmost. Without God in sight, we are like the scattered rungs of a broken ladder. To pray is to become a ladder on which thoughts mount to God to join the movement toward Him, which surges unnoticed throughout the entire universe. We do not step out of the world when we pray; we merely see the world in a different setting. The self is not the hub, but the spoke of the revolving wheel. In prayer we shift the center of living from self-consciousness to self-surrender. God is the center toward which all forces tend. He is the source, and we are the flowing of His force, the ebb and flow of His tides.[23]

As the kindled soul soars to connect to God, God comes toward the human being. In the words of Rabbi Heschel, "Our seeking Him is not only man's but His concern and must not be considered an exclusively human affair. His will is involved in our yearnings."[24] For

---

23. Abraham Joshua Heschel, *Man's Quest for God* (New York: Scribner, 1954), pp. 6–7.
24. Abraham Joshua Heschel, *God in Search of Man* (New York: Farrar, Straus and Giroux, 1955), p. 136.

Rabbi Heschel, the human being's inner search for God is reciprocated: "God is in search of man."[25]

The prayer service is punctuated with examples of God reaching out to the human being. The most poignant example is, perhaps, found in the concluding prayer service of Yom Kippur, *Ne'ila*. There, one calls out, אַתָּה נוֹתֵן יָד לַפּוֹשְׁעִים – "You, O Lord, reach out Your hand to transgressors." As Yom Kippur ends, there is concern that perhaps the prayers have not been heard. Precisely then, the petitioner cries out, "O God, please, please take an active step by reaching out to save us." One wonders who takes the first step – God or the human being. In the end, there may be a simultaneous yearning – the human being and God come closer and closer, never "touching," but in their approach toward one another, the encounter takes place.[26]

REACHING OUT

Once kindled, the soul not only soars upward to connect with God, but outward to connect with other souls, other people – all created in God's image. Like lovers longing to embrace, sparks of the Divine seek to rendezvous. In this sense, prayer is not only vertical, but horizontal; it is an encounter not only with God, but with our fellow human being.

25. Ibid.

26. This theme is repeated on Monday and Thursday mornings in the *Taḥanun* prayer as we recite כִּי יְמִינְךָ פְשׁוּטָה לְקַבֵּל שָׁבִים – "Your right hand is outstretched to receive those who return." See chapter 8 and the book's conclusion for further discussion of this mutual encounter.

See Pinchas H. Peli, *On Repentance: The Thought and Oral Discourses of Rabbi Joseph Dov Soloveitchik* (New York: Rowman and Littlefield, 1984), pp. 84–88.

See also *Sefat Emet*, Genesis, *Vayetzeh* 5634, s.v. *BeRashi vayifga*, which argues that as we yearn for God, God reaches for us. The author makes this point in his discussion of Jacob "encountering the place" (*vayifga bamakom*) as he flees from his parents' home (Gen. 28:11).

Vayifga is a term for prayer (Berakhot 26b). The Talmud points out that the Torah uses the word *vayifga* and not *vayitpallel* (and he prayed) to denote that "the place [referring to Mount Moriah] leapt toward him [Jacob]" (Ḥullin 91b).

In the words of the *Sefat Emet*, "Because our forefather Jacob greatly desired to come to Mount Moriah, although it was far away, Mount Moriah leapt to him."

Hence, when commencing prayer, many recite the formula הֲרֵינִי מְקַבֵּל עַל עַצְמִי מִצְוַת עֲשֵׂה שֶׁל וְאָהַבְתָּ לְרֵעֲךָ כָּמוֹךָ – "Behold, I accept upon myself the commandment of 'love your fellow as yourself' [Lev. 19:18]." As the *Magen Avraham* codifies, "Before the morning service, one should accept the affirmative commandment of 'love your fellow as yourself.'"[27]

A Hasid once asked his rebbe (teacher), "When standing before God in prayer, shouldn't one open with the declaration 'I love you, God'? Why begin with a formula that expresses our love for other human beings?"[28] The rebbe responded that the greatest expression of love children can show their parents is the expression of love for their siblings. Similarly, the rebbe explained, the greatest love we can express to God is our expression of love for each other.[29]

Not only does the prayer service begin with a call to love our fellow person, it ends in a similar vein. The conclusion of the *Amida* (Silent Meditation), the central part of the service, is a blessing for peace and loving-kindness:

שִׂים שָׁלוֹם טוֹבָה וּבְרָכָה
חֵן וָחֶסֶד וְרַחֲמִים עָלֵינוּ וְעַל כָּל יִשְׂרָאֵל עַמֶּךָ....
בָּרוּךְ אַתָּה ה׳, הַמְבָרֵךְ אֶת עַמּוֹ יִשְׂרָאֵל בַּשָּׁלוֹם.

Grant peace, goodness, and blessing,
grace, loving-kindness, and compassion
to us and all Israel, Your people….
Blessed are You, Lord,
who blesses His people Israel with peace.[30]

27. *Magen Avraham,* introductory comment on *Shulḥan Arukh, Oraḥ Ḥayyim 46.*
28. There are two major loves in the Torah: love of God, וְאָהַבְתָּ אֵת ה׳ אֱ־לֹהֶיךָ (Deut. 6:5); and love of one's fellow, וְאָהַבְתָּ לְרֵעֲךָ כָּמוֹךָ (Lev. 19:18).
29. It has been noted that the verses "Love the Lord"(וְאָהַבְתָּ אֵת ה׳) and "love your fellow as yourself"(וְאָהַבְתָּ לְרֵעֲךָ כָּמוֹךָ) share the same numerical value.
30. The paragraph is preceded by the Priestly Benediction, which ends with יִשָּׂא ה׳ פָּנָיו אֵלֶיךָ וְיָשֵׂם לְךָ שָׁלוֹם – "May the Lord turn His face toward you and grant you peace."

In between these bookends is a picturesque prayer about angels paying homage to God. But which angel is privileged to speak first? One would expect cut-throat competition for this honor. Yet the liturgy records that each angel steps back, declaring, you go first:

וְכֻלָּם מְקַבְּלִים עֲלֵיהֶם עוֹל מַלְכוּת שָׁמַיִם זֶה מִזֶּה
וְנוֹתְנִים רְשׁוּת זֶה לָזֶה
לְהַקְדִּישׁ לְיוֹצְרָם בְּנַחַת רוּחַ
בְּשָׂפָה בְרוּרָה וּבִנְעִימָה
קְדֻשָּׁה כֻּלָּם כְּאֶחָד
עוֹנִים וְאוֹמְרִים בְּיִרְאָה
קָדוֹשׁ, קָדוֹשׁ, קָדוֹשׁ ה׳ צְבָאוֹת
מְלֹא כָל הָאָרֶץ כְּבוֹדוֹ.

All [the ministering angels] accept upon themselves,
one from another,
the yoke of the Kingdom of Heaven,
granting permission to one another
to sanctify the One who formed them.
In serene spirit,
pure speech, and sweet melody,
all, as one, proclaim His holiness,
saying in awe:
"Holy, holy, holy is the Lord of hosts;
the whole earth is full of His glory" [Is. 6:3].

The formula of קָדוֹשׁ, קָדוֹשׁ, קָדוֹשׁ – "Holy, holy, holy"– is repeated during the repetition of the *Amida*. It is introduced with the words –

In the afternoon and evening services, in some congregations, שִׂים שָׁלוֹם is replaced by שָׁלוֹם רַב עַל יִשְׂרָאֵל עַמְּךָ תָּשִׂים לְעוֹלָם – "Grant great peace to Your people Israel forever."

Kaddish and Grace After Meals (*Birkat HaMazon*) end with a similar call for peace: עֹשֶׂה שָׁלוֹם בִּמְרוֹמָיו הוּא יַעֲשֶׂה שָׁלוֹם עָלֵינוּ וְעַל כָּל יִשְׂרָאֵל וְאִמְרוּ אָמֵן – "May He who makes peace in His high places make peace for us and all Israel, and say: Amen."

נְקַדֵּשׁ אֶת שִׁמְךָ בָּעוֹלָם
כְּשֵׁם שֶׁמַּקְדִּישִׁים אוֹתוֹ בִּשְׁמֵי מָרוֹם
כַּכָּתוּב עַל יַד נְבִיאֶךָ
וְקָרָא זֶה אֶל זֶה וְאָמַר...

We [human beings] will sanctify Your name on earth,
as they sanctify it in the highest heavens,
as it is written by Your prophet,
"And they [the angels] call to one another, saying…" [Is. 6:3].[31]

Here we pray to acknowledge God as the angels do, without competitiveness, reaching out to each other in peaceful, loving coexistence. In a world too often consumed with causeless hatred, this posture of stepping back and making space for others is desperately needed.

Rabbi Shlomo Carlebach tells the story of Rabbi Levi Yitzḥak of Berditchev and the Mitteler Rebbe (the second Lubavitcher Rebbe, Rabbi Dov Ber of Lubavitch) walking to a wedding. They found the doorway leading to the *ḥuppa* (wedding canopy) too narrow. Each implored the other to go first, to no avail. Finally, the Berditchever, a rebbe of fire who was often most assertive, said, "No problem, we'll break through the wall and have room to walk in together." The Mitteler, a much gentler man, responded, "No, that's unnecessary. What we'll do is widen the doorway."

Thus, prayer is not limited to encountering God; it also involves expressing love for our fellow person. And built into love is responsibility to care for the other. For this reason, virtually all our prayers are in the plural. When beseeching God, we speak not only for ourselves, but for the community. Indeed, during the service, there is a custom to give charity to the needy.

The *Keli Yakar*, written by Rabbi Ephraim Lunschitz, illustrates the intersection between laws governing our relationship with God and interpersonal ethics more broadly, by arguing that the Ten Commandments (or, which is probably a better translation, the Ten Declarations) can be divided into corresponding pairs, in which each com-

31. This is from the Ashkenazic text of the *Kedusha,* recited during the repetition.

mandment related to God has a parallel commandment related to one's fellow human being.[32] For example, "You shall not murder" (לֹא תִּרְצַח – Ex. 20:13), the sixth of the Ten Commandments, is found aside the first, "I am the Lord your God" (אָנֹכִי ה' אֱ-לֹהֶיךָ – Ex. 20:2). For the author of the *Keli Yakar*, the two are interconnected: Killing another human being diminishes God, as the *tzelem E-lohim* within the human being has been destroyed. In his words:

> "You shall not murder": After completing the five declarations that concern the connection between God and the human being, the text lists another five corresponding declarations that concern interpersonal relationships, as mentioned in the *Mekhilta*. There, the *Mekhilta* explains the relationship between the parallel commandments. For example, the declaration "You shall not murder" parallels "I am [the Lord your God]," for if anyone sheds blood, it is as though one were diminishing the form and image of God.[33]

Prayer, then, begins by reaching in (to tap into our inner godliness). This involves contemplation of who we can become, and our responsibility to work on ourselves to become that person. Reaching up (toward God Himself) makes us realize we are connected and responsible to a Being far greater than we. Reaching out (to unite with our fellow person's *tzelem E-lohim*) establishes our relationship and our responsibility toward others. These three themes are fundamental motifs of prayer.

Assuming responsibility gives us a deeper insight into the phrase quoted by the Talmud and Maimonides as the source for prayer:

---

32. A good example of this phenomenon in Jewish ritual is Shabbat. On the surface, Shabbat deals exclusively with one's relationship with God. As God rested on the seventh day, we too step back, acknowledging God as the Source of all creation. In Exodus 23:12, however, the Torah states, שֵׁשֶׁת יָמִים תַּעֲשֶׂה מַעֲשֶׂיךָ וּבַיּוֹם הַשְּׁבִיעִי תִּשְׁבֹּת לְמַעַן יָנוּחַ שׁוֹרְךָ וַחֲמֹרֶךָ וְיִנָּפֵשׁ בֶּן אֲמָתְךָ וְהַגֵּר – "Six days you shall do your work, but on the seventh day you shall cease from labor, in order that your ox and your donkey may rest and that your bondman and the stranger may be refreshed." Here, an added dimension of Shabbat is offered – one that is purely interpersonal.
33. *Keli Yakar*, Exodus 20:13. See *Mekhilta DeRabbi Yishmael, Yitro* (*BaḤodesh*) 8.

לְעָבְדוֹ בְּכָל לְבַבְכֶם – *le'ovdo bekhol levavkhem* (Deut. 11:13).[34] *Le* is the prefix "to." *Ovdo* is associated with *avoda,* work. And while *le'ovdo* is commonly viewed as a compound of *la'avod Oto,* "to serve Him," it can also mean *la'avod Ito,* "to work with Him."[35] This does not undercut the standard translation of לְעָבְדוֹ בְּכָל לְבַבְכֶם – "to serve Him with all your heart." Rather, it indicates that if prayer is deeply sincere, serving God can be transformed into a prayerful commitment to work with Him (*la'avod Oto* meshes with *la'avod Ito*). We do this in prayer by committing ourselves wholeheartedly (*bekhol levavkhem*) to establishing a world that follows "the way of the Lord, by doing what is just and right" – וְשָׁמְרוּ דֶּרֶךְ ה׳ לַעֲשׂוֹת צְדָקָה וּמִשְׁפָּט (Gen. 18:19).[36]

Rabbi Samson Raphael Hirsch articulates this understanding of prayer based on a linguistic reading of the word "*tefilla.*" *Tefilla* is derived

---

34. Ta'anit 2a; Maimonides, *Code,* Laws of Prayer 1:1. See the beginning of this chapter.
35. See Rashi, Genesis 37:4, s.v. *dabbero,* who understands *dabbero* as a compound of *ledabber immo* – "to speak with Him."

    Note that *le'ovdo* is found in the flow of the second paragraph of *Shema* ("*Ve-Haya*"), which deals with listening to God's commandments. Loving God is an emotion, while listening to Him is a commitment to action.
36. Rabbi Joseph B. Soloveitchik understands Maimonidean prayer as reflecting the ever present feeling of human inadequacy and inner struggle. In his words:

    > [Maimonides regarded] daily life itself as being existentially in straits, inducing in the sensitive person feelings of despair, a brooding sense of life's meaninglessness, absurdity, lack of fulfillment. It is a persistent *tzara,* which exists *bekhol yom,* daily. The word *tzara* connotes more than external trouble; it suggests an emotional and intellectual condition in which man sees himself as hopelessly trapped in a vast, impersonal universe, desolate, without hope.

    Rabbi Abraham R. Besdin, *Reflections of the Rav* (Jerusalem: World Zionist Organization, 1979), pp. 80–81.

    For Rabbi Soloveitchik, life has no meaning if God is absent; one feels constant despair without God. Hence, one prays daily in constant search of the Lord, without whom life is impersonal, void, empty.

    From Rabbi Soloveitchik's perspective, the need to pray, according to Maimonides, comes from the petitioner as an expression of constant angst when God is not near. In our analysis, the desire to pray emanates from God. I may not feel like praying, yet there is a religious imperative to work with God daily.

    Both approaches are necessary. Prayer from the petitioner expressing individual needs to God can be selfish. On the other hand, praying to God without listening to our soul minimizes our individual worth. The challenge is to find a balance of listening to ourselves and listening to God.

from the word *hitpallel*, whose root is פ.ל.ל (P-L-L) – to engage in a process of self-judgment. Commenting on this relationship between prayer and self-scrutiny, Rabbi Hirsch writes:

> *Hitpallel*, from which "*tefilla*" is derived, originally meant to deliver an opinion about oneself, to judge oneself – or an inner attempt at so doing, such as the *hitpa'el* form of the Hebrew verb frequently denotes. In other words, an attempt to gain a true judgment of oneself. Thus it denotes to step out of active life in order to attempt to gain a true judgment about oneself, that is, about one's ego, about one's relationship to God and the world, and of God and the world to oneself. It strives to infuse mind and heart with the power of such judgment as will direct both anew to active life – purified, sublimated, strengthened. The procedure of arousing such self-judgment is called "*tefilla*"....
>
> Accordingly, you should at times tear yourself loose from this existence which endangers your true life, and strive in *tefilla* to renew your strength for life and regain your right and your will for truth, righteousness and love, as well as the power and the courage for victorious battle.[37]

For Rabbi Hirsch, *tefilla* entails several steps. First, we must take a moment to separate from the humdrum of everyday existence and evaluate our standing in life. Second, we must evaluate our lives in all directions: inward, to examine our ego; upward, to contemplate our relationship to God, and outward, to appraise our relationship with the larger world. Finally, we are called upon to use these insights to spur us to improve our lives. This could include refining our thoughts, being more careful in ritual observance, improving our interpersonal relationships, and doing more to help redeem the Jewish people and the world.

37. See Rabbi Samson Raphael Hirsch, *Horeb* (New York: Soncino Press, 1962), pp. 472–473.

BRIT AND PERSONAL RESPONSIBILITY

Redemption can be achieved only through a joint effort between God and humankind. In creating the world, God intentionally left it incomplete. One can give different rationales for this. Had God created a world of only good, there would be no good, as good is a relative term. Had God created a perfect world, we would be left with no challenges to overcome. Had God created a world where we could only do the right thing, we would be bereft of our freedom of choice, and hence, not be human.[38] Thus, the last word of the creation story in Genesis is *la'asot* – "to do" (Gen. 2:3). God is, in effect, telling us, "I have created the world imperfectly, and I leave it to you to finish that which I have started. In partnership we will redeem the world."

How much the Jewish people and God each contribute to this partnership is part of the core idea of *brit* – the contractual arrangement between God and *Am Yisrael* (the Jewish nation).[39] The degree of input may depend on the historical maturity of the nation. God exercised unilateral authority over Jewish history when *Am Yisrael* was in its infancy. As we grow and develop, however, more is expected of us.

Here, covenant takes a counterintuitive turn. One would suspect that as *Am Yisrael* assumes more responsibility, God is felt to a lesser degree. The opposite is the case. When the Jewish people is first formed, God reveals Himself intensely at Sinai, soon afterward in the *Mishkan* (Tabernacle), and ultimately in the Temple. After the destruction of the Temple, the idea of *Mishkan* evolved into *Shekhina* (Indwelling); in fact, the noun *Shekhina* as a name for God never appears in the Bible. It's a postbiblical idea. The God who particularly appeared in the *Mishkan* manifests as *Shekhina* – the God who is omnipresent. As the Midrash

---

38. Rabbi E. E. Dessler, *Mikhtav MeEliyahu* (Jerusalem: Yotzei LaOr al Yedei Ḥever Talmidav, 5723–5757 [1963–1997]), vol. 1, p. 36.
39. Sometimes *brit* is universal – a contract between God and the whole world. This surfaces in the aftermath of the Deluge in the time of Noah (Gen. 9:8–17). At other times, a *brit* is established with an individual, as it was with Abram, the first Jewish patriarch (Gen. 15:18). Still other times, a *brit* is established with the whole of the Jewish people, as occurred at Sinai (Ex. 24:7).

states, אֵין מָקוֹם פָּנוּי בְּלֹא שְׁכִינָה – "there is no place devoid of God."[40] Thus, at this stage, God is not less present but more so. A parable sheds light on how the post-Temple era is in some ways more conducive to feeling the presence of God:

> מָשָׁל לְמֶלֶךְ שֶׁכְּשֶׁהוּא בְּבֵית מַלְכוּתוֹ קָשֶׁה לָבוֹא אֵלָיו, מָה שֶׁאֵין כֵּן כְּשֶׁהַמֶּלֶךְ נוֹסֵעַ בַּדֶּרֶךְ אָז יְכוֹלִין כָּל בְּנֵי אָדָם אֲפִילוּ אָדָם פָּשׁוּט מְאֹד, לְדַבֵּר אֶל הַמֶּלֶךְ. וְהַיְינוּ כִּי זְמַן זֶה... שֶׁגָּלְתָה הַשְּׁכִינָה מִמְּקוֹמָהּ הֲרֵי הוּא כְּמִי שֶׁהַמֶּלֶךְ מַלְכֵי הַמְּלָכִים הקב"ה הוּא בַּדֶּרֶךְ וְלָכֵן עֵת רָצוֹן הִיא, וכ"א יָכוֹל לְהִתְקָרֵב וְלָבוֹא אֶל הַמֶּלֶךְ.
>
> A parable: When a king is in his palace, it is difficult to approach him. Once he leaves and mingles among his constituents, even the lowest of commoners can interact with him. Similarly in this time… when the *Shekhina* has been exiled from His Temple, it is as if the Ruler of rulers, the Holy One, Blessed Be He, roams among His subjects. This is a more favorable time for the average person to gain access to Him.[41]

Covenant works much like the parent-child relationship. As an infant, the human being is more helpless than any other species at birth. As a child matures, however, he or she becomes more accountable. This is the meaning of the *Barukh ShePetarani* blessing, recited by parents at their child's bar or bat mitzva. It's a statement of parental stepping back, empowering the young adolescent to assume more obligations. In time, the teenager grows to adulthood, taking on more and more commitments.

---

40. Exodus Rabba 2:5.
41. Rabbi Gedaliah Schorr, *Sefer Or Gedalyahu* (Brooklyn, NY, 5745–5746 [1985–1986]), vol. 3, *Matot–Masei*, s.v. *shabbatot*, p. 158. Rabbi Schorr attributes this parable to Reb Ber.

    I have heard Rabbi Yitz Greenberg describe this phenomenon in a kind of populist way. In the Temple, God's "voltage" was high, as it was concentrated in one place (and more diffuse elsewhere), so one could never get close. In the post-Temple era, the voltage is lower, as God's presence is spread out more equally everywhere – making God more accessible, more present.

    It can be suggested that if God – while less "visible" – is more present, then there is greater onus on humans to seek Him where they would least expect to find Him.

In this phase, parents may be less vocal, less visible, but their influence can be greater – in this sense, they are more present.

Rabbi Ahron Soloveichik describes how *Am Yisrael* began to take on increased responsibility for its destiny, even as early as the Splitting of the Sea:

> The word *hatzala* refers to an act of salvation during which the party being saved remains completely passive. *Yeshua*, however, implies a salvation in which the party being saved actively participates. In Egypt, the process through which God redeemed *Benei Yisrael* [the Children of Israel] involved *hatzala* – the people remained totally passive while God, so to speak, did all the work (see Ex. 6:6). At the Red Sea, though, God's salvation was a *yeshua* that required the nation's active participation (see Ex. 14:30).
>
> Thus, the Midrash teaches that God did not split the sea until all the people entered the water.... Thus the *pasuk* [verse] says, ... "And *Benei Yisrael* went into the midst of the sea upon the dry ground" (Ex. 14:22).[42]

At the beginning of Jewish history, God acts unilaterally. As *Am Yisrael* matures, the onus shifts as the Jewish people assumes greater responsibility and acts to help itself. Perhaps for this reason, the Passover Haggada, which recounts the birth of the Jewish nation, contains only a single mention of Moses' name.[43] At the beginning of Jewish peoplehood, God and God alone plays the central role. In the words of the Haggada:

> וַיּוֹצִיאֵנוּ ה׳ מִמִּצְרַיִם: לֹא עַל יְדֵי מַלְאָךְ וְלֹא עַל יְדֵי שָׂרָף וְלֹא עַל יְדֵי שָׁלִיחַ
> אֶלָּא הַקָּדוֹשׁ בָּרוּךְ הוּא בִּכְבוֹדוֹ וּבְעַצְמוֹ.

42. Rabbi Ahron Soloveichik, *The Warmth and the Light: Illuminating Approaches to the Weekly Torah Portion* (Jerusalem: Genesis Jerusalem Press, 1992), pp. 128, 129.

43. The name Moses is found in a relatively minor paragraph quoting R. Yose HaGelili's view that the Egyptians suffered fifty plagues at the Red Sea. Some versions omit Moses' name.

> "The Lord brought us out of Egypt" [Deut. 26:8]: Not by an angel, not by a seraph, not by a messenger, but the Holy One, Blessed Be He, in His own glory, Himself.

Similarly, in the book of Esther, which records the Jewish people's victory over Haman, God's name is not mentioned at all. Having matured, the Jewish nation takes an active role in determining its fate.[44]

Passover, of course, commemorates the Exodus from Egypt, while Purim commemorates the victory over Haman. In general, the biblical holidays (Passover, Shavuot, and Sukkot) celebrate God's intervention in history, while the rabbinical ones (Purim, Hanukka, and Yom HaAtzma'ut), established later, involve greater human initiative. In this sense, the holidays follow the pattern of the *brit*, which demands that over time we become more proactive. The *Sefat Emet* formulates this idea as follows:

> הַג׳ מוֹעֲדוֹת שֶׁנָּתַן לָנוּ הקב״ה הֵם תּוֹרָה שֶׁבִּכְתָב שֶׁמְּפוֹרָשִׁין בַּתּוֹרָה וְהקב״ה נָתַן לָנוּ זְמַנֵּי קוֹדֶשׁ אֲשֶׁר נִתְקַדְּשׁוּ בְּעֵת הַבְּרִיאָה שֶׁהַכֹּל בַּתּוֹרָה נִבְרָא. וְהֵם עֵדוּת שֶׁהקב״ה בָּחַר בְּיִשְׂרָאֵל וְיֵשׁ לוֹ הִתְקָרְבוּת אֲלֵיהֶם שֶׁהֲרֵי מָסַר לָנוּ מוֹעֲדוֹת שֶׁלּוֹ וְזֶהוּ שֵׁם מוֹעֵד מִלְּשׁוֹן עֵדוּת.
>
> וַחֲנוּכָּה וּפוּרִים הֵם מוֹעֲדוֹת שֶׁזָּכוּ לָהֶם בְּנֵי יִשְׂרָאֵל בְּמַעֲשֵׂיהֶן נִקְרָא תּוֹרָה שֶׁבְּעַל פֶּה וְהֵם עֵדוּת שֶׁהֵם בּוֹחֲרִים בְּהקב״ה וּמְיוּחָדִים אֵלָיו וְשֶׁמַּעֲשֵׂיהֶן מְעוֹרְרִין אוֹתוֹ יִתְבָּרַךְ שֶׁהֲרֵי חִידְּשׁוּ בְּמַעֲשֵׂיהֶם זְמַנִּים מְקוּדָּשִׁים.
>
> The three festivals God gave us are commanded expressly in the Written Torah. God gave us those holy times, sanctified since Creation, for all was created through the Torah. They bear witness that the blessed Holy One has chosen Israel and is close to them, giving them His holy testimony. The word *mo'ed* used for these festivals is related to *eidut* (testimony).
>
> But Hanukka and Purim are special times that Israel merited by their own deeds. These are called Oral Torah; they are

---

44. Some suggest that the term *hamelekh* (the king) as found in the Megilla, which on the surface refers to King Ahasuerus, really points to God (*HaMelekh* – the King of kings), who plays a hidden role – working through people and the natural world – to save *Am Yisrael*. While externally God is less manifest, internally God is more present.

testimony that Israel chose the blessed Holy One. Israel are joined to God and their deeds arouse God, for here they are capable of creating new sacred times by their deeds.[45]

EXAMPLES FROM THE PRAYER SERVICE

The prayer service is replete with instances when we recall our responsibility to ourselves, the Jewish people, and the world at large. [46] At the outset of the morning service, we list our interpersonal obligations in the text *Eilu Devarim*. It reads:

אֵלּוּ דְבָרִים שֶׁאָדָם אוֹכֵל פֵּרוֹתֵיהֶם בָּעוֹלָם הַזֶּה
וְהַקֶּרֶן קַיֶּמֶת לוֹ לָעוֹלָם הַבָּא
וְאֵלּוּ הֵן
כִּבּוּד אָב וָאֵם, וּגְמִילוּת חֲסָדִים
וְהַשְׁכָּמַת בֵּית הַמִּדְרָשׁ שַׁחֲרִית וְעַרְבִית
וְהַכְנָסַת אוֹרְחִים, וּבִקּוּר חוֹלִים
וְהַכְנָסַת כַּלָּה, וּלְוָיַת הַמֵּת
וְעִיּוּן תְּפִלָּה
וַהֲבָאַת שָׁלוֹם בֵּין אָדָם לַחֲבֵרוֹ
וְתַלְמוּד תּוֹרָה כְּנֶגֶד כֻּלָּם.

45. See *Sefat Emet*, Hanukka 5636, s.v. *Adoni mori*; translation from Professor Arthur Green, *The Language of Truth: The Torah Commentary of the Sefat Emet* (Philadelphia: Jewish Publication Society, 1998). See also *Sefat Emet*, Ḥanukka 5641, s.v. *Ḥanukka u'Furim*. There, this commentary links Shavuot and Purim. On Shavuot, God revealed the Torah; on Purim the Torah was reaccepted (see Shabbat 88a). The *Sefat Emet* goes on to connect Sukkot and Hanukka. Both are eight days; both focus on *hiddur mitzva*, beautifying the mitzva (see Shabbat 21b and *Sefat Emet*, Ḥanukka 5640, s.v. *Amar avi zekeni*). The *Sefat Emet* then suggests that Passover, the holiday of redemption, will one day have its counterpart. In the author's words, "And we hope that from Passover [a rabbinic holiday] will emerge." Religious Zionists read this point as the *Sefat Emet*'s belief that one day a holiday celebrating the establishment of Israel will be observed.
46. The great basketball player Bill Walton quotes his coach, John Wooden, as having said, "There is no way you can have a perfect day unless you do something to help someone." USA Today, November 4, 2010, p. 36.

> These are the things whose fruits we eat in this world
> but whose full reward awaits us in the World to Come:
> honoring parents; acts of kindness;
> arriving early at the house of study morning and evening;
> hospitality to strangers; visiting the sick; helping the needy bride;
> attending to the dead; devotion in prayer; and bringing peace between people – but the study of Torah is equal to them all.

Moreover, in the introductory psalms (*Pesukei DeZimra*) we say:

> עֹשֶׂה מִשְׁפָּט לָעֲשׁוּקִים, נֹתֵן לֶחֶם לָרְעֵבִים, ה׳ מַתִּיר אֲסוּרִים:
> ה׳ פֹּקֵחַ עִוְרִים, ה׳ זֹקֵף כְּפוּפִים, ה׳ אֹהֵב צַדִּיקִים:
> ה׳ שֹׁמֵר אֶת גֵּרִים, יָתוֹם וְאַלְמָנָה יְעוֹדֵד, וְדֶרֶךְ רְשָׁעִים יְעַוֵּת:
>
> He [the Lord] secures justice for the oppressed; He gives food to the hungry; the Lord sets captives free.
> The Lord gives sight to the blind; the Lord raises those bowed down. The Lord loves the righteous.
> The Lord protects the stranger; He gives courage to the orphan and widow; He thwarts the way of the wicked. (Ps. 146:7–9)

The *Amida* is the classic prayer of standing humbly before God, contrite and subdued as we pour forth our hope for healing and redemption – and much more. It is also the time to ask ourselves whether we are doing our part to realize these goals. Thus, the *Amida* is the classic reverberating prayer.

A story is told of a hasidic rebbe before the establishment of the State of Israel, who – contrary to the sentiments of his community – was a religious Zionist, doing all he could to promote the Zionist cause by encouraging Jews to go to *Eretz Yisrael*. Some of his disciples were critical: "Doesn't the *Amida* say that God and God alone will gather in the exiles?" To make this point, they slowly read him parts of the ingathering request: תְּקַע בְּשׁוֹפָר גָּדוֹל לְחֵרוּתֵנוּ... וְקַבְּצֵנוּ יַחַד מֵאַרְבַּע כַּנְפוֹת הָאָרֶץ – "Sound the great shofar for our liberty... and gather us together from the four corners of the earth."

The rebbe thought for a moment and then replied, "In the *Amida* we seek health, we ask for healing: רְפָאֵנוּ ה׳ וְנֵרָפֵא – 'Heal us, Lord, and we shall be healed.'" Looking at his critics, the rebbe went on, "Even as we ask for God's help, do we totally rely upon Him? Clearly this blessing is not meant to prohibit our seeking out medical advice. Similarly, in the blessing of redemption, when we invoke God's help to redeem Zion, we commit ourselves to actively take part in that process." So too, in all the "request" blessings, as we call out to God for relief we challenge ourselves to assume responsibility to join in this effort.

The theme of responsibility is present throughout the prayer service, particularly toward the end, when we say the second paragraph of *Aleinu – Al Ken Nekaveh*. Note that the prayer is written in the future tense, expressing hope for a time to come:

עַל כֵּן נְקַוֶּה לְךָ ה׳ אֱ־לֹהֵינוּ,
לִרְאוֹת מְהֵרָה בְּתִפְאֶרֶת עֻזֶּךָ....
לְתַקֵּן עוֹלָם בְּמַלְכוּת שַׁ־דַּי.
וְכָל בְּנֵי בָשָׂר יִקְרְאוּ בִשְׁמֶךָ....
וְנֶאֱמַר,
וְהָיָה ה׳ לְמֶלֶךְ עַל כָּל הָאָרֶץ
בַּיּוֹם הַהוּא יִהְיֶה ה׳ אֶחָד
וּשְׁמוֹ אֶחָד.

> Therefore, we place our hope in You, Lord our God,
> that we may soon see the glory of Your power....
> To perfect the world under the reign of the Almighty,
> when all humanity will call on Your name....
> As it is said:
> "Then the Lord shall be King over all the earth;
> on that day the Lord shall be One
> and His name One" [Zech. 14:9].

In this paragraph, when we declare "On that day the Lord shall be One," we are saying that at present, God's rulership, God's Oneness, has not yet been acknowledged by the larger world. Whether this dream will be achieved is dependent upon people assuming responsibility "to perfect the world under the reign of the Almighty."[47]

Kaddish, perhaps more than any other prayer, expresses the mission of Judaism to bring ethical monotheism into the world. It reads:

יִתְגַּדַּל וְיִתְקַדַּשׁ שְׁמֵהּ רַבָּא
בְּעָלְמָא דִּי בְרָא כִרְעוּתֵהּ,
וְיַמְלִיךְ מַלְכוּתֵהּ
בְּחַיֵּיכוֹן וּבְיוֹמֵיכוֹן
וּבְחַיֵּי דְכָל בֵּית יִשְׂרָאֵל
בַּעֲגָלָא וּבִזְמַן קָרִיב, וְאִמְרוּ אָמֵן.

Magnified and sanctified may His great name be,
in the world He created by His will.
May He establish His kingdom
in your lifetime and in your days,
and in the lifetime of all the House of Israel
swiftly and soon – and say: Amen.[48]

יְהֵא שְׁמֵהּ רַבָּא מְבָרַךְ לְעָלַם וּלְעָלְמֵי עָלְמַיָּא

May His great name be blessed for ever and all time.[49]

---

47. See Rashi, Exodus 17:16, s.v. *ki yad*. Note also that *Al Ken Nekaveh* is preceded by the first paragraph of *Aleinu*, which is particularistic: שֶׁלֹּא עָשָׂנוּ כְּגוֹיֵי הָאֲרָצוֹת – "Who has not made us like the nations of the lands." The flow indicates that the goal of the Jewish particularistic mission is universal redemption

48. The opening words of *Kaddish* are taken from God's prophecy through Ezekiel, וְהִתְגַּדִּלְתִּי וְהִתְקַדִּשְׁתִּי וְנוֹדַעְתִּי לְעֵינֵי גּוֹיִם רַבִּים – "Thus will I manifest My greatness and My holiness and make Myself known in the sight of many nations" (Ezek. 38:23). Ezekiel prophesied during the destruction of the First Temple. Although God's presence was diminished, Ezekiel declares that one day God's greatness and holiness will be fully manifest.

49. The central words of *Kaddish* are recorded in Berakhot 3a. There, the prophet Elijah, the harbinger of messianic redemption (Mal. 3:23, 24), is quoted as saying:

    At the time that the people of Israel enter synagogues and houses of study and respond, "May His great name be blessed" (יְהֵא שְׁמֵהּ הַגָּדוֹל מְבוֹרָךְ), the Holy One, Blessed Be He, shakes His head and says, "Blessed be the Ruler who is praised in His house in this way."

יִתְבָּרַךְ וְיִשְׁתַּבַּח וְיִתְפָּאַר וְיִתְרוֹמַם וְיִתְנַשֵּׂא
וְיִתְהַדַּר וְיִתְעַלֶּה וְיִתְהַלַּל
שְׁמֵהּ דְּקֻדְשָׁא בְּרִיךְ הוּא
לְעֵלָּא מִן כָּל בִּרְכָתָא וְשִׁירָתָא, תֻּשְׁבְּחָתָא וְנֶחֱמָתָא
דַּאֲמִירָן בְּעָלְמָא,
וְאִמְרוּ אָמֵן.

Blessed and praised, glorified and exalted, raised
and honored, uplifted and lauded be
the name of the Holy One, Blessed Be He,
beyond any blessing, song, praise, and consolation
uttered in the world –
and say: Amen.

In each paragraph of *Kaddish*, the word *Shmeh* (name) is prominently featured. *Shmeh* can homiletically be read as a compound of the words *Shem Hashem* – "the Name of the Lord," the code term for bringing God and God's system of ethics into the world.[50] The opening words of *Kaddish* – *Yitgadal veyitkadash Shmeh rabba* – can be understood, "May we do our share to magnify and sanctify God's great name by bringing ethical monotheism into the world." When the leader of the service recites *Kaddish* and the congregation responds, "Amen," we declare our intention to partner with God to fulfill this mission. *Kaddish* concludes each section of the service as a refrain, reminding us over and over that

---

Elijah makes this statement after the destruction of the Second Temple. At this time of estrangement, Israel calls out that one day God will rendezvous with His nation, and His name will return to its full greatness. The words יְהֵא שְׁמֵהּ הַגָּדוֹל מְבוֹרָךְ – "May His great name be blessed" became the centerpiece of the *Kaddish* prayer.

See *Arukh HaShulḥan, Oraḥ Ḥayyim* 55:1, which quotes Elijah in Berakhot as saying, יְהֵא שְׁמֵהּ רַבָּה מְבוֹרָךְ – an alternate formulation of "May His great name be blessed." See also *Tosafot,* Berakhot 3a, s.v. *ve'onin*. The words יְהֵא שְׁמֵהּ רַבָּה מְבוֹרָךְ first appear in the book of Daniel, where Daniel says, לֶהֱוֵא שְׁמֵהּ דִּי אֱלָהָא מְבָרַךְ מִן עָלְמָא וְעַד עָלְמָא – "Let the name of God be blessed for ever and ever" (Dan. 2:20).

50. Literally, *Shmeh* means His Name. *Shem Hashem* echoes that historic moment when Abram and Sarai arrive in Canaan, build an altar, and "call out in the name of the Lord" – וַיִּקְרָא שָׁם בְּשֵׁם ה׳ (Gen. 12:8).

prayer is about the assumption of this responsibility.[51] The words of the *Kaddish* are cast in the future tense, indicating that this responsibility continues into the future.[52]

While many people associate prayer with what God does for us, prayer is also a way to access our inherent goodness and increase our personal commitment to God, our people, and humankind. In this way, prayer is multidimensional. As much as we seek God in prayer, God, through prayer, seeks us, encouraging us to partner with Him in redeeming Israel and the world.

Thus, prayer includes aspects of commitment. This is "prayer as responsibility."

---

51. The Half Kaddish is recited after each sub-section. The Whole Kaddish is said after the completion of the entire service. It ends with a prayer for peace:

תִּתְקַבַּל צְלוֹתְהוֹן וּבָעוּתְהוֹן דְּכָל יִשְׂרָאֵל קֳדָם אֲבוּהוֹן דִּי בִשְׁמַיָּא, וְאִמְרוּ אָמֵן.
יְהֵא שְׁלָמָא רַבָּא מִן שְׁמַיָּא וְחַיִּים, עָלֵינוּ וְעַל כָּל יִשְׂרָאֵל, וְאִמְרוּ אָמֵן.
עֹשֶׂה שָׁלוֹם בִּמְרוֹמָיו הוּא יַעֲשֶׂה שָׁלוֹם עָלֵינוּ וְעַל כָּל יִשְׂרָאֵל וְאִמְרוּ אָמֵן.

May there be acceptance of the prayers and supplications of all Israel before their Father in heaven – and say: Amen.
May there be great peace from Heaven and life for us and all Israel – and say: Amen.
May He who makes peace in His high places make peace for us and all Israel – and say: Amen.

In this section, too, we allude to the name of God when saying, "May there be great peace from Heaven (*Shemaya*)." The word *Shemaya* (literally, "heaven," the symbolic abode of God) sounds like *Shmeh* (שְׁמֵהּ). Ultimately, great peace comes when we integrate God into our lives.

52. In time, *Kaddish* was also said by mourners (*Kaddish Yatom*), perhaps as a means of declaring that their beloved helped make life more meaningful by bringing the principles of ethical monotheism into the world. The *Kaddish* is in the future tense, as the influence of the deceased is still felt, and mourners commit themselves to act on his or her teachings. Its text is the same as the Whole Kaddish without the paragraph of תִּתְקַבַּל צְלוֹתְהוֹן – "May there be acceptance of the prayers."

For an analysis of the Rabbis' Kaddish (*Kaddish DeRabbanan*), see chapter 9.

Chapter Two

Reliance

The rabbi was standing before his congregation. Yom Kippur was ending. Over and over he mumbled the *Aleph-Beit*. His disciples were stunned. The rabbi knew Torah by heart, he knew every prayer by rote – why was he reciting the Hebrew alphabet? Later that evening he explained: "There are times when the words of prayer are enough. But then there are times when one does not know the words. All we can do is express feelings. And then there are times, like now, when the situation is so dreadful, we don't even know what to feel. All we can do is turn to God, fully reliant upon Him, and humbly declare, 'I don't know the words. I'm not even sure what to feel. All I can do is recite the *Aleph-Beit* and beg You: Lord our God, you know the letters – please, please, rearrange them so they clearly spell out what I should be asking for.'"[1]

FATE AND SELF-TRANSFORMATION

As we discussed in the previous chapter, prayer involves working with God by assuming responsibility for helping to redeem the Jewish people

---

1. This story is a reformulation of classic legends of rabbis or lay persons offering prayers that "open the heavens" at the last moment of Yom Kippur.

and the world. For Nahmanides, however, prayer is a function of human distress so piercing that it leads one to fully rely upon God:

> שֶׁנִּתְפַּלֵּל אֵלָיו בְּעֵת הַצָּרוֹת וְתִהְיֶינָה עֵינֵינוּ וְלִבֵּנוּ אֵלָיו לְבַדּוֹ כְּעֵינֵי עֲבָדִים אֶל יַד אֲדוֹנֵיהֶם. וְזֶה כְּעִנְיָן שֶׁכָּתוּב וְכִי תָבֹאוּ מִלְחָמָה בְּאַרְצְכֶם עַל הַצַּר הַצּוֹרֵר אֶתְכֶם וַהֲרֵעוֹתֶם בַּחֲצוֹצְרוֹת וְנִזְכַּרְתֶּם לִפְנֵי ה׳ אֱ־לֹהֵיכֶם וְהִיא מִצְוָה עַל כָּל צָרָה וְצָרָה שֶׁתָּבֹא עַל הַצִּבּוּר לִצְעוֹק.
>
> That we pray to Him in times of distress, and that our eyes and hearts be directed toward Him like servants in the hands of their masters. And this is the meaning of the verse, "And when you come to war in your land against an enemy who has besieged you, and you will sound the trumpets and be remembered before the Lord your God" [Num. 10:9]. And it is a commandment to call out (*litzok*) to God for every distress that comes upon the community.[2]

---

2. Nahmanides, *Sefer HaMitzvot*, positive commandment 5. It is unclear whether Nahmanides means that in times of distress we are obligated to pray (*mitzva ḥiyyuvit*), or or that one who prays at such times fulfills a biblical commandment (*mitzva kiyyumit*).

   Maimonides writes:

   > It is a positive commandment to cry out (*lizok*) and sound the trumpets in the event of any difficulty that arises which affects the community, as it states: "[When you go out to war against] an enemy who attacks you, and you sound the trumpets" [Num. 10:9]. [This commandment is not restricted to such a limited scope; rather] the intent is: whenever you are distressed by difficulties – e.g., famine, plague, locusts, or the like – cry out [to God] because of them, and sound the trumpets.... This practice is one of the paths of repentance. (Maimonides, *Code*, Laws of Fasts 1:1–2). Translation from Maimonides, *Code*, ed. and trans. Eliyahu Touger (New York: Moznaim Publishing Corporation, 5752), Laws of Fasts, pp. 12, 14.

   Here, Maimonides quotes the source cited by Nahmanides. Unlike Nahmanides, however, who sees *et hatzarot* as a basis for prayer, Maimonides sees it as an aspect of *teshuva*.

   Note that while Nahmanides uses the term לִצְעוֹק (*litzok*), Maimonides uses the term לִזְעוֹק (*lizok*). *Litzok* is an expression of dependency upon God, as occurred when the Jews left Egypt. Pursued by the Egyptians, they felt helpless and cried out to God – וַיִּצְעֲקוּ בְנֵי יִשְׂרָאֵל אֶל ה׳ – totally reliant upon Him (Ex. 14:10). As we suggest at the conclusion of this chapter, this is the Nahmanidean understanding of prayer.

Joseph Albo, a fifteenth-century Spanish Jewish philosopher, takes it a step further. For Albo, prayer has the power to influence God; that is, it functions as a plea to the omnipotent God to effect change. To explain how prayer works, Albo first discusses *teshuva*:

> וְזֶה יוֹרֶה שֶׁהַגְּזֵרָה הַנִּגְזֶרֶת עַל הָרָשָׁע הוּא בִּהְיוֹתוֹ בַּתּוֹאַר הַהוּא מִן הָרוֹעַ וּכְשֶׁיִּשְׁתַּנֶּה מִן הַתּוֹאַר הַהוּא עַל יְדֵי הַתְּשׁוּבָה הִנֵּה הוּא כְּאִלּוּ נֶהְפַּךְ לְאִישׁ אַחֵר שֶׁלֹּא נִגְזְרָה עָלָיו אוֹתָהּ גְּזֵרָה.
>
> This shows that when a decree is made upon a wicked person, it is conditional upon his maintaining his state of wickedness. But if he changes that state through repentance, he changes into another person, as it were, upon whom that decree was not made.[3]

In other words, explains Albo, God decrees that person X will suffer a certain fate. Once the person does *teshuva*, however, he is purified, and, in effect, becomes person Y. Hence, the decree is inoperative, as person X no longer exists. Albo offers several examples of this phenomenon:

> Take the case of Ahab. The Bible says concerning him, "But there was none like Ahab, who did give himself over to do that which was evil in the sight of the Lord" [I Kings 21:25], and a divine decree was made against him. And then, because he fasted, and

---

It has been suggested that *lizok* means something different: to cry out while resolved to take action, much like Mordecai in the Purim story. After hearing Haman's decree to annihilate the Jews, the Megilla declares, וַיִּזְעַק זְעָקָה גְדוֹלָה וּמָרָה – "and he cried out loudly and bitterly" (Est. 4:1). Here, Mordecai cries out while beginning to devise a plan to save his people. Maimonides' use of *lizok* as a form of *teshuva* is in sync with the approach to prayer outlined in chapter 1 – an expression of assuming responsibility.

3. Joseph Albo, *Sefer HaIkkarim: Book of Principles*, ed. and trans. Isaac Husik (Philadelphia: Jewish Publication Society, 1946), pp. 160–167 (4:18).

See Peli, *On Repentance*, pp. 49–52. There, Rabbi Joseph B. Soloveitchik understands *teshuva* as having two elements: atonement for the sin, and purification of the heart. This is the meaning of the verse recited in the Yom Kippur liturgy, כִּי בַיּוֹם הַזֶּה יְכַפֵּר עֲלֵיכֶם לְטַהֵר אֶתְכֶם מִכֹּל חַטֹּאתֵיכֶם – "On that day God will offer you atonement, purifying you from all your sins" (Lev. 16:30). *Kappara* is atonement for the deed. *Tahara* is purification of the heart.

> covered himself with sackcloth, and humbled himself before God, it was said to Elijah, "Because he humbled himself before Me, I will not bring the evil in his days; but in his son's days will I bring the evil upon his house" [I Kings 21:29].[4]

Prayer, Albo argues, operates in a similar fashion:

> In this way it is clear that prayer and proper conduct prepare a person to receive the good influence or to nullify the evil that has been decreed concerning him, because he changes from the evil state in which he was.[5]

According to Albo, God may have decided a certain fate for a particular individual. But after true, deep prayer, the individual is no longer the person he once was, which by definition alters his fate. Albo concludes:

> That is, if you set your heart to pray and to improve your conduct, there is no doubt that through prayer and correct conduct you will escape from these troubles. From this it is clear that prayer and correct conduct are always helpful in nullifying a divine decree.[6]

---

4. Albo, *Sefer HaIkkarim* 4:18.

   For an analysis of the contradiction between God's omniscience and human freedom of choice (in Ahab's case, the choice to repent/pray, which altered the decree), see Ralbag, Genesis 22:12, and Responsa Rivash 118. Both argue that God's foreknowledge is non-specific. See also Ḥasdai ben Abraham Crescas, cited in Isaac Husik, *Medieval Jewish Philosophy* (Philadelphia: Jewish Publication Society, 1958), p. 397, who posits that freedom of choice is limited. See also Sa'adia Gaon, *Emunot VeDeot* 4:4, who suggests that God's knowledge of the future is reflective. Maimonides, *Code*, Laws of Repentance 5:5, and Ra'avad ad loc., as well as *Tiferet Yisrael,* Mishna Avot 3:99, conclude that God is unknowable.
5. Albo, *Sefer HaIkkarim* 4:18.
6. Ibid. The idea of self-transformation may apply not only when we pray for ourselves, but also when praying for others. Prayer, as we will later point out, operates in a holistic manner. Somehow, through the process of prayer for another, that individual's persona changes.

   Self-transformation may also apply to the communal aspect of prayer in the

THE LIMITS OF PRAYER

Although prayer may have the power to nullify a decree, the Torah includes examples of sincere prayers that were rejected. Consider the passage in the Talmud that posits that the three daily prayer services were introduced by the Patriarchs.[7] Although the Torah does not reveal the content of their prayers, their context points to a request that was not completely fulfilled.

Abraham, for example, prays and pleads with God to save the city of Sodom (Gen. 19:27).[8] The morning after, he sees the city destroyed (Gen. 19:28).[9]

Isaac prays concerning the wife whom his father, Abraham, seeks for him (Gen. 24:63). Although Isaac's prayer seems instantly answered – as he meets Rebecca and marries her – his marriage has its points of serious tension. Isaac and Rebecca disagree about which of their sons, Jacob or Esau, should receive the elder's blessing; and Rebecca deceives her husband by instructing Jacob to take the birthright.

Jacob introduces the evening service. As he leaves home to escape the wrath of his brother for having taken the birthright, Jacob prays for protection (Gen. 28:11). He then dreams of a ladder reaching heavenward, with angels ascending and descending. God promises that Jacob will be protected. The road ahead, however, is not without its struggles. While Jacob manages to flee his home and build a new life for himself, he eventually encounters the trickeries of Laban, his devious father-in-law. Years later, he faces the difficult task of confronting Esau himself.

---

spirit of *arevut*. *Arevut* means that we are inextricably bound to each other. Hence, when one improves oneself through prayer, the other – by virtue of being part of the community – is also elevated.

See Dessler, *Mikhtav MeEliyahu*, vol. 1, pp. 113, 114, who argues that every action affects one's point of choice (*nekudat habeḥira*), impacting one's very nature.

7. See Berakhot 26b. This talmudic passage with its alternative view is discussed at length in chapter 6.
8. Note that the verb associated with morning prayer found here (*amad*) is the same as the one used just prior to Abraham's argument with God that Sodom be saved – *omeid* (Gen. 18:22).
9. Although Abraham's nephew Lot and his daughters were saved, the entire city was destroyed.

The Talmud considers Hannah a model of prayer.[10] Married and unable to conceive, she beseeches God for a child (1 Sam. 1:10–13). Her request is granted, and she gives birth to Samuel. But Samuel's life is filled with struggle; his children Joel and Abijah turn to evil, and the Jewish people rebels against him, demanding that he be replaced by a king (1 Sam. 8).

No biblical prayer is more poignant than that of Moses asking God that he be permitted to enter the Land of Israel:

> דָּרַשׁ רַבִּי שַׂמְלַאי: לְעוֹלָם יְסַדֵּר אָדָם שִׁבְחוֹ שֶׁל הַקָּדוֹשׁ בָּרוּךְ הוּא וְאַחַר כָּךְ יִתְפַּלֵּל. מְנָלַן – מִמֹּשֶׁה דִּכְתִיב וָאֶתְחַנַּן אֶל ה׳ בָּעֵת הַהִיא; וּכְתִיב ה׳ אֱ־לֹהִים אַתָּה הַחִלּוֹתָ לְהַרְאוֹת אֶת עַבְדְּךָ אֶת גָּדְלְךָ וְאֶת יָדְךָ הַחֲזָקָה אֲשֶׁר מִי אֵל בַּשָּׁמַיִם וּבָאָרֶץ אֲשֶׁר יַעֲשֶׂה כְמַעֲשֶׂיךָ וְכִגְבוּרוֹתֶיךָ, וּכְתִיב בָּתְרֵיהּ אֶעְבְּרָה נָּא וְאֶרְאֶה אֶת הָאָרֶץ הַטּוֹבָה.
>
> R. Simlai expounded: A person should always first recount the praise of the Holy One, Blessed Be He, and then pray. From where do we know this? From Moses; for it is written, "And I sought out the Lord at that time," and it goes on, "O Lord God, You have started to show Your servant Your greatness and Your strong hand; for what god is there in heaven and earth who can do according to Your works and according to Your mighty acts?" And afterward it is written, "Let me go over, I pray to You, and see the good land" [Deut. 3:23–25].[11]

In the end, Moses' request is denied. God does not permit him to join the Jewish people in the Land of Israel. עֲלֵה אֶל... הַר נְבוֹ – "Ascend...to Mount Nevo," God tells Moses, from where you will see the land, וְשָׁמָּה לֹא תָבוֹא – "but you shall not enter it" (Deut. 32:49–52). God's answer is final: The people will enter, but you will not.

As the above examples demonstrate, the notion that prayer is characterized primarily by God responding to calls of distress is historically incorrect. The Talmud itself asserts the limitation of prayer – even the purest – in effecting change:

---

10. Berakhot 30b, 31a.
11. Ibid. 32a.

חַיֵּי, בָּנֵי וּמְזוֹנֵי, לָא בִּזְכוּתָא תַּלְיָא מִילְּתָא, אֶלָּא בְּמַזָּלָא תַּלְיָא מִילְּתָא.

Length of days, children, and prosperity depend not on merit, but on *mazal* (fate).[12]

Here, the Talmud informs us that certain critical matters in life depend on *mazal*, fate, which no amount of prayer can alter.

Still, the Talmud tells us elsewhere that we can influence our *mazal*:

תַּנְיָא: אֶת מִסְפַּר יָמֶיךָ אֲמַלֵּא אֵלּוּ שְׁנֵי דוֹרוֹת, זָכָה – מַשְׁלִימִין לוֹ, לֹא זָכָה – פּוֹחֲתִין לוֹ, דִּבְרֵי ר׳ עֲקִיבָא;

וַחֲכָמִים אוֹמְרִים: זָכָה – מוֹסִיפִים לוֹ, לֹא זָכָה – פּוֹחֲתִין לוֹ.

It was taught, "I will let you enjoy the full count of your days" [Ex. 23:26] refers to the years of the generations [the lifespan allotted to every human being at birth]. If one is worthy, he is allowed to complete the full period; if unworthy, his years are reduced. This is the view of R. Akiva.

But the sages said: If one is worthy, years are added to his life; if unworthy, his years are reduced.[13]

In other words, the Talmud asserts that the *mazal* with which we are born is somewhat elastic. While it cannot be absolutely cancelled, it can be changed to some degree.

In practical terms, we all wonder how long we will live, if we will be prone to depression, whether our children will be healthy. We are all born with predispositions to certain traits – but we have some power to overcome them. How can we improve our physical well-being? By eating healthfully, exercising regularly, and seeking medical attention when necessary. How can we cope with depression? By cultivating emotional and spiritual inner peace and seeking professional help. How can we nurture our children? By spending time with them, showing them love

12. Mo'ed Katan 28b. This passage is said in the name of Rava.
13. Yevamot 49b.

and patience. We must always remember that we have a critical role to play in altering our fate to some extent.

Rabbi Joseph B. Soloveitchik distinguishes between fate (*goral*, in his words) and destiny (*ye'ud*). Fate, according to Rabbi Soloveitchik, refers to the dimensions of life that we cannot control. Destiny, on the other hand, "is an active existence in which one confronts the environment into which he is cast with an understanding of his uniqueness and value, freedom and capacity." According to Rabbi Soloveitchik, "One's mission in this world is to turn fate into destiny, an existence that is passive and influenced to an existence that is active and influential."[14]

Esther Wachsman, whose son, Israeli sergeant Nachshon Wachsman, was kidnapped and murdered by terrorists in Israel in 1994, recalled how she was overwhelmed with grief. She was able to move forward only by reminding herself that she had a choice: She could be a victim of her fate, or initiate a new destiny.[15]

Prayer is one of our primary tools for initiating a new destiny. This may be the meaning of the Rosh HaShana and Yom Kippur prayer וּתְשׁוּבָה וּתְפִלָּה וּצְדָקָה מַעֲבִירִין אֶת רֹעַ הַגְּזֵרָה.[16] This phrase is often translated as "repentance, prayer, and charity cancel the evil of the decree." Were this the case, however, the Hebrew would read, מְבַטְּלִין אֶת הַגְּזֵרָה הָרָעָה. *Mevatlin* (מְבַטְּלִין), from the root ב.ט.ל (B-T-L), is a strong verb meaning "cancel." But the word that actually appears in this text is *ma'avirin* (מַעֲבִירִין), which has a gentler connotation, meaning "cause to pass over" or "get through." Moreover, the word *ro'a* (רֹעַ) is descriptive, meaning that acts of repentance, prayer, and charity temper, or remove, the sting or harshness of the decree. In other words, through prayer (and, for that matter, repentance and good deeds) we can shape our fate, even if we cannot change it entirely.[17]

---

14. See Rabbi Joseph B. Soloveitchik, *Kol Dodi Dofek: Listen, My Beloved Knocks*, ed. Jeffrey R. Woolf, trans. David Z. Gordon (New York: Yeshiva University, 2006), pp. 5–6.
15. Commencement address by Esther Wachsman, Yeshiva University, 1995. The entire address was published by YU.
16. This phrase is found in the *U'Netaneh Tokef* prayer, said by Ashkenazim on Rosh HaShana and Yom Kippur.
17. This is not to say that prayer cannot at times be fully accepted. Sometimes our

As Joseph Albo argued, prayer can be self-transformative. Still, that transformation does not necessarily lead to God's intervention.

DOES GOD HEAR US?

When Nahmanides writes, "it is a commandment to call out to God for every distress that comes upon the community" – וְהִיא מִצְוָה עַל כָּל צָרָה וְצָרָה שֶׁתָּבֹא עַל הַצִּבּוּר לִצְעוֹק,[18] his emphasis is on our calling out to God, not God's response. While the request for God's intervention is an implicit part of prayer, it is not, in Nahmanides' view, its fundamental goal. The foundation of Nahmanidean prayer is the reaching out to God in our times of greatest loneliness and despair. Whatever the outcome, prayer allows us the possibility of forging an intimate relationship with God. Whatever the future brings, we are no longer alone.

While Nahmanides points out that God "hears and answers" our prayers, he does not claim God accepts them:

---

wishes are fully granted, and an evil decree is completely abrogated.

See Leviticus Rabba 10:5:

> From where is the view of R. Yehuda b. Rabbi that prayer effects complete pardon derived? From the case of Hezekiah. The original term of Hezekiah's kingship was only fourteen years, as it is written, "Now it came to pass in the fourteenth year of King Hezekiah" [Is. 36:1]. But after he prayed, fifteen more years were given to him, as it is said, "Then came the word of the Lord … behold I will add to your life fifteen years" [Is. 38:5].
>
> From where is the view of R. Yehoshua b. Levi, who said that prayer effects half atonement, derived? From the case of Aaron. At first a decree was pronounced against him, as it is said, "Moreover the Lord was very angry with Aaron to destroy him (*lehashmido*)" [Deut. 9:20]. Said R. Yehoshua of Siknin in the name of R. Levi: Destruction (*hashmada*) means extinction of offspring, as it says, "And I destroyed his fruit from above, and his roots from beneath" [Amos 2:9]. When Moses prayed on his [Aaron's] behalf, half the decree was annulled: Two sons died, and two remained. It is therefore written, "And the Lord spoke unto Moses, saying: Take Aaron and his sons" [Lev. 8:2].

See also Mo'ed Katan 16b: "The God of Israel said… I rule Man. Who rules Me? The righteous one. For I make a decree and he [may] annul it."

18. Nahmanides, *Sefer HaMitzvot*, positive commandment 5.

> אֶלָּא וַדַּאי כָּל עִנְיַן הַתְּפִילָּה אֵינוֹ חוֹבָה כְּלָל, אֲבָל הוּא מִמִּדַּת הַחֶסֶד הַבּוֹרֵא יִתְבָּרֵךְ, שֶׁשּׁוֹמֵעַ וְעוֹנֶה בְּכָל קָרְאֵנוּ אֵלָיו.
>
> But certainly [daily] prayer is not obligatory, but it is a kindly trait of the blessed Creator, who hears and answers whenever we call out to Him.[19]

Rabbi Joseph B. Soloveitchik expounds on this idea, emphasizing God's role as listener:

> Prayer finds its full exoteric expression in the spiritual act of lifting up one's eyes – the inner cry of dependence upon God, the experience of complete, absolute dependence portrayed by the psalmist: "I lift my eyes towards the mountain, from where will come my aid?" (Ps. 121:1).
>
> When man is in need and prays, God listens. One of God's attributes is *Shome'a Tefilla* – "He who listens to prayer." Let us note that Judaism has never promised that God accepts all prayer.
>
> Acceptance of prayer is a hope, a vision, a wish, a petition, but not a principle or a premise. The foundation of prayer is not the conviction of its effectiveness, but the belief that, through it, we approach God intimately, and the miraculous community embracing finite man and his Creator is born.
>
> The basic function of prayer is not its practical consequences but the metaphysical formation of a fellowship consisting of God and man.[20]

---

19. Ibid.
20. Rabbi Joseph B. Soloveitchik, *Worship of the Heart* (New York; KTAV Publishing House, 2003), p. 35.

Interestingly, in the Bible, God is viewed as a saving God. An example of this is the psalmist's petition יִקְרָאֵנִי וְאֶעֱנֵהוּ עִמּוֹ אָנֹכִי בְצָרָה אֲחַלְּצֵהוּ וַאֲכַבְּדֵהוּ – "When he calls on Me, I will answer him; I will be with him in distress; I will rescue him and make him honored" (Ps. 91:15). Here, "I will be with him in distress" and "rescue him and make him honored" is redeeming. God is stating that if a person calls out to Him in distress, He will be there to save that individual.

In the Midrash, however, God is portrayed as an empathizing God. Hence one midrashic explanation of why God appears to Moses in the lowly burning bush and

A contemporary story illustrates this point. After Nachshon Wachsman was kidnapped, his parents asked that prayers be said on his behalf. In the end, Nachshon was killed, as was Nir Poraz, the Israeli captain who attempted to rescue him. Journalists asked Nachshon's father, Yehuda, a devoutly religious man, whether this tragedy raised questions about God and, more specifically, about the efficacy of prayer: "You asked that people pray for your son. Sincere, powerful prayers were offered, and yet God left them unanswered." Nachshon's father responded that he believed God did answer the prayer, but His answer was "no." God's answer is not always "yes," but through the prayers recited by millions of people for Nachshon, a deep sense of fellowship with God and community was forged.[21]

The idea that the essence of prayer can be found in the individual's feeling of closeness to God, rather than in God's response, finds expression in the words of Rabbi Dr. Eliezer Berkovits:

> In its original form, prayer is not asking God for anything; it is not a request. It is a cry; an elementary outburst of woe, a spontaneous call in need; a hurt, a sorrow, given voice. It is the call of human helplessness directed to God. It is not asking, but coming with one's burden before God. It is like the child's running to the mother because it hurts. It is not the bandage that the child seeks instinctively but the nearness of the mother, to unburden his heart to the one of whose love he is certain. So the human being brings his sorrow before God: Look, O God, what has been done to me,

---

not in a taller, more elegant tree: "Because 'I will be with him in distress'" (*Midrash Tanḥuma,* Exodus 14, cited by Rashi, Exodus 3:2, s.v. *mitokh hasneh*). In other words, as long as Jews are enslaved, God can appear only in a thornbush; such is His identification with the plight of His people.

21. Sometimes the greatest response to a godly request is for it to be left unanswered. Garth Brooks, the American country musician, makes this point in his song "Unanswered Prayers":

    Sometimes I thank God for unanswered prayers
    Remember when you're talkin' to the Man upstairs
    That just because He doesn't answer doesn't mean He don't care.
    Some of God's greatest gifts are unanswered prayers.

    Brooks wrote this song with Pat Alger and Larry Bastian.

> consider what has become of me. This is the essence of prayer. Only children can pray like this, or *tzaddikim* – the men of great faith, who in the depth of their piety have gained a new childlike trust in God.... To pour out one's heart before God means simply to tell God about one's troubles. To pray means to make God the confidant of one's sorrow and need. The asking and begging are natural enough, but they are of secondary importance. Decisive is the pouring of the heart because one has to; the pouring out of the heart before God because He is the nearest, because He is the closest, because He is the natural confidant of the human soul.[22]

Thus, for Nahmanides, God's chief role in prayer is that of listener. Yes, prayer can impact a decree, but that is not its primary purpose. In the most basic sense, the purpose of prayer, according to Nahmanides, is to establish a "fellowship" with God.[23]

Here again, prayer begins by moving inward (to tap into our inner godliness), contemplating who we are, our shortcomings, our inadequacies. Given these limits, we reach up to God, asking for His support. Reaching out, we recognize how dependent we are on others.[24]

Prayer, according to Nahmanides, is a function of *et tzara*, feelings of distress, inspiring a sense of dependence on God and our fellow person. Nahmanides' formulation, כְּעֵינֵי עֲבָדִים אֶל יַד אֲדוֹנֵיהֶם – "like the eyes of servants toward the hands of their masters," expresses this dependence.[25]

---

22. Eliezer Berkovits, *Studies in Torah Judaism – Prayer* (New York: Yeshiva University Press, KTAV Publishing House, 1969), p. 107. Here, Rabbi Dr. Berkovits uses the expression "*tzaddikim* – the men of great faith" in a generic sense, referring to women as well.
23. Truth be told, on Rosh HaShana and Yom Kippur, days that are so identified with making requests for a better year, there are, in actuality, very few *bakashot* (requests). The three main elements of prayer on Rosh HaShana are *Malkhuyot* (God rules), *Zikhronot* (God remembers), and *Shofarot* (God redeems). The central part of Yom Kippur is the *Avoda*, the service in the *Beit HaMikdash* (Holy Temple). Even the prayer *Zokhreinu leḥayyim*, "Remember us for life," is found in the section of the *Amida* called *shevaḥ* – "praise of God."
24. See chapter 1 for an analysis of the three directions of "prayer as responsibility."
25. In his commentary on the Bible, Nahmanides makes a similar point:

As noted, the word "*tefilla*" may be derived from הִתְפַּלֵּל (*hitpallel*), whose root is פ.ל.ל (P-L-L), to judge oneself.[26] There is, however, an alternative meaning. It can also mean hope, as when Jacob recalls his many years of separation from Joseph, declaring, רְאֹה פָנֶיךָ לֹא פִלָּלְתִּי – "I never even hoped to see your face" (Gen. 48:11).[27] On a homiletical level, the word פָּנֶיךָ (your face) may refer to God. In this reading, Jacob proclaims, "By seeing Your face, by being reliant upon You and certain of Your love, concern, and support, I never lost hope."

EXAMPLES FROM THE PRAYER SERVICE

The intersection of reliance and hope is beautifully expressed in the High Holy Day prayer of אוֹחִילָה לָאֵ־ל.[28] The complete irst line reads, אוֹחִילָה לָאֵ־ל אֲחַלֶּה פָנָיו אֶשְׁאֲלָה מִמֶּנּוּ מַעֲנֵה לָשׁוֹן – "I put my hope in the Almighty, I plead before Him. I request that He give me the gift of language." In other words, we put our trust in God to know what is in our interest and to help us to articulate our needs. The *tefilla* continues: לְאָדָם מַעַרְכֵי לֵב וּמֵה׳ מַעֲנֵה לָשׁוֹן – "A person prepares the thoughts in his mind, but proper speech comes from the Lord." This can be interpreted to mean that a person may believe he or she has planned for life, but ultimately knowing what to ask for, knowing what is best, comes from God. It is nothing less than the constant refrain of my bubbe (grandmother), *a mensch trakht un Got lakht* – "a person plans and God laughs."

> The purpose of raising our voices in prayer and of the service in synagogues, as well as the merit of public prayer, is precisely this: that people should have a place wherein they assemble and express their thankfulness to God for having created them and supported them, and thus proclaim and say before Him, "We are your creations."

See Nahmanides, Exodus 13:16, s.v. *uletotafot*. This translation is from *Nahmanides, Commentary on the Torah – Exodus,* trans. Charles B. Chavel (New York: Shilo Publishing House, 1973). See also Nahmanides, Leviticus 26:11.

26. See chapter 1.
27. Jacob makes this comment to Joseph after he brings his sons, Ephraim and Manasseh – Jacob's grandchildren – before him. See Rabbi Aryeh Kaplan's translation in *The Living Torah* to Genesis 48:11.
28. This prayer is found in the *Musaf* (Additional) prayer service.

Throughout the daily prayer service, we demonstrate our dependence on God, most notably in the *Taḥanun* section, when we literally fall on our faces, recognizing that we are in God's hands. In the Ashkenazic rite, the *Taḥanun* prayer begins with the story of King David, who has sinned and is given a choice of punishments by the prophet Gad. David chooses pestilence, as that punishment comes completely from God. In the words that open *Taḥanun*:

> וַיֹּאמֶר דָּוִד אֶל גָּד צַר לִי מְאֹד נִפְּלָה נָּא בְיַד ה׳ כִּי רַבִּים רַחֲמָיו וּבְיַד אָדָם אַל אֶפֹּלָה.
>
> And David said to Gad, "I am greatly distressed; let us fall into the hand of the Lord, for His mercies are great, but into the hand of a human being let me not fall." (II Sam. 24:14)

Appropriately, the *Taḥanun* prayer is said as our head falls onto our arm, symbolic of placing trust in God. The prayer ends with the words

> שׁוֹמֵר יִשְׂרָאֵל שְׁמוֹר שְׁאֵרִית יִשְׂרָאֵל וְאַל יֹאבַד יִשְׂרָאֵל הָאוֹמְרִים שְׁמַע יִשְׂרָאֵל.
>
> Guardian of Israel, protect the remnant of Israel, and let not Israel perish, who say, "Listen, O Israel."[29]

For me, the prayer that most eloquently describes reliance upon God is *Barukh Shmeh* – "Blessed Is the Name." As the Torah is taken from the Ark, congregants stand as they express their trust in God:

> אֲנָא עַבְדָּא דְקֻדְשָׁא בְּרִיךְ הוּא, דְּסָגִידְנָא קַמֵּהּ וּמִקַּמֵּי דִּיקַר אוֹרַיְתֵהּ בְּכָל עִדָּן וְעִדָּן. לָא עַל אֱנָשׁ רָחִיצְנָא, וְלָא עַל בַּר אֱלָהִין סָמִיכְנָא, אֶלָּא בֶּאֱלָהָא דִשְׁמַיָּא, דְּהוּא אֱלָהָא קְשׁוֹט, וְאוֹרַיְתֵהּ קְשׁוֹט, וּנְבִיאוֹהִי קְשׁוֹט, וּמַסְגֵּא

29. Note the context of David's prayer. Jerusalem is under siege, a sword over its head. Much like in the *Akeda* story (the Binding of Isaac, Genesis 22), God intervenes. In the end, we are not in control; we are dependent upon God, reliant on His benevolence and kindness.

> לְמֶעְבַּד טַבְוָן וּקְשׁוֹט. בֵּהּ אֲנָא רָחִיץ, וְלִשְׁמֵהּ קַדִּישָׁא יַקִּירָא אֲנָא אֵמַר תֻּשְׁבְּחָן.
>
> I am a servant of the Holy One, Blessed Be He, before whom and before whose glorious Torah I bow at all times. Not in man do I trust, nor on any angel do I rely, but on the God of heaven, who is the God of truth, whose Torah is truth, whose prophets speak truth, and who abounds in acts of love and truth. In Him I trust, and to His holy and glorious name I offer praises.

As discussed in the previous chapter, prayer provides the opportunity to remind ourselves of our responsibility to take action; to improve ourselves, our families, our people, and the world. But prayer is also the time to learn a little bit of humility, to recognize that we can't do it all. It is the time to understand God's central role in our lives. Such recognition allows one to feel God's love and protection, as a child feels the love and protection of a parent. This point is beautifully captured in the responsa of Rivash: "Rabbi Shimshon of Kinon, the greatest rabbi of his generation… [would say,] 'I pray as if I were a child.'"[30]

Thus, prayer includes aspects of utter dependence upon God. This is "prayer as reliance."

30. Responsa Rivash 157. Rivash's responsum is a polemic against kabbalistic prayer, which involves praying to *sefirot*, higher emanations of God. Rivash insists that prayer is a direct link to God, much like a child's simple connection to those upon whom he or she is dependent.

Chapter Three

Feeling God's Presence

A town was under siege. The citizenry was frightened and decided to convene an emergency prayer service. To add meaning to the gathering, an actor was hired to dramatically read the twenty-third psalm: "The Lord Is My Shepherd." To avoid embarrassing the elderly rabbi of the town, he was asked to follow the actor's reading with his own recitation.

At the service, the actor read the psalm with perfect pitch and inflection. The crowd was mesmerized. As he finished, the townsfolk rose as one to their feet, giving the actor a standing ovation.

The rabbi then hobbled to the podium. Showing his age and the pain of the moment, he weakly began reading the psalm. As he read, he was overcome with emotion: His voice broke, and tears flowed down his face. The assembled were overwhelmed. Whimpers, even sobs could be heard. As the rabbi finished reading, no one moved or dared to speak.

Later that night, the actor was asked for an explanation. "You read beautifully, but the rabbi's rendering was deeper. Given your training and expertise, how were you outdone?"

The actor responded, "When I was asked to recite the twenty-third psalm, I memorized the entire chapter. I mastered each sentence and came to know it perfectly. I delivered every word of 'The Lord Is My Shepherd.' But the rabbi knows not only the psalm ... he also knows the Shepherd."[1]

1. I heard this story from my father, Rabbi Moshe Weiss.

ASSERTIVE PRAYER

Our teaching presents two models of prayer: "prayer as responsibility" and "prayer as reliance." "Prayer as responsibility" grows out of the command to work with God every day, whether we are in need or not. "Prayer as reliance" originates in human angst and distress.

Yet for both, prayer finds its ultimate goal in reminding us that God is ever-present. On the one hand, feeling God's presence can inspire one to be godlike, to assume responsibility for oneself, for others, and even toward God. This involves self-assertion. On the other hand, feeling God's presence can lead to a recognition of finitude, of dependence on others and utter reliance upon God. This involves self-submission.

These positions operate in tension: Sometimes we are called upon to be assertive, and other times to be submissive. The Jewish tradition affirms both kinds of prayer. The juxtaposition of the *Amida* and *Taḥanun* may reflect a balance between assertion and submission. In the *Amida,* we stand before God, a brazen act on some level, as we display the inner strength – even hutzpa – to make formal requests of Him. The *Amida* is followed by *Taḥanun,* in which we "fall on our faces," resting our heads on our arms. In this manner, we declare our vulnerability and dependency on God, saying, נִפְּלָה נָּא בְיַד ה׳ כִּי רַבִּים רַחֲמָיו וּבְיַד אָדָם אַל אֶפֹּלָה – "let us fall into the hand of the Lord, for His mercies are great, but into the hand of a human being let me not fall" (II Sam. 24:14).[2]

The themes of these prayers may lead to each other. Asserting oneself can be humbling, as achieving all our goals is impossible. Conversely, recognition of limits can inspire one to overcome them.

In fact, reliance on God may itself involve aspects of assertion. As we stand before God, recognizing our limitations and dependency on the Divine, we do so not only from a posture of supplication, but also with the awareness that we are permitted to lovingly make demands of God.[3]

---

2. For an analysis of *Taḥanun,* see the end of chapter 2.
3. Note that the source of prayer for Nahmanides – *be'et hatzarot* – is found in the narrative that deals with preparation for war (Num. 10:9). The context of Nahmanidean

After Abraham demands justice from God concerning the inhabitants of Sodom, God refers to him as a prophet (Gen. 18:25; 20:7). It is important to note that the role of the prophet is not only to bring the message of God to the people, but also to defend the people before the Divine. Similarly, each of us has the right to respectfully let God know what we expect of Him. Making these demands is precisely what God wants from us. Sound relationships are based on openness and honesty, and that includes our relationship with God.

An incident between God and Moses illustrates this point. After the Israelites construct the Golden Calf, God decrees their annihilation. The language of His decree seems to invite challenge: וְעַתָּה הַנִּיחָה לִּי... וַאֲכַלֵּם – "Now leave Me ... to make an end of them" (Ex. 32:10). According to the Midrash, God's bid to let Him be in order that He might unleash His anger was a clear hint to Moses that he should intervene and thereby appease Him: "*Don't* let Me be. *Don't* let Me off the hook. Be open and honest with your feelings, and demand that I, the Ruler of rulers, nullify the decree." In the words of the Midrash:

> "Now leave Me ... to make an end of them" – Was Moses holding Him?
>
> To what can the thing be compared? To a king who was angry with his son, and when the son was brought into the chamber and about to be beaten, the king cried from the chamber, "Let me alone, that I may smite him!" Now, the instructor [of the son] happened to be standing outside, and he thought to himself, "If both the king and the son are within the chamber, why does he [the king] say, 'Let me alone'? It must be because the king is desirous that I should entreat him on his son's behalf, and for this reason does he say, 'Let me alone.'"
>
> Similarly, God said to Moses, "Now leave Me," and from this Moses inferred, "God is desirous that I should intercede with Him on Israel's behalf, and hence is He saying, 'Now leave Me.'" Forthwith Moses began to plead for mercy on [Israel's] behalf.[4]

prayer – war – lends itself to a petition that is more forceful in nature.

4. Exodus Rabba 42:9. See also Berakhot 32a.

Immediately afterward, Moses prays to God: וַיְחַל מֹשֶׁה אֶת פְּנֵי ה׳ אֱ־לֹהָיו וַיֹּאמֶר לָמָה ה׳ יֶחֱרֶה אַפְּךָ בְּעַמֶּךָ – "And Moses implored (*vayeḥal*) the Lord his God, saying, 'Let not Your anger, O Lord, blaze forth against Your people'" (Ex. 32:11). *Vayeḥal* is a biblical term for prayer.[5] The Hebrew comes from the word *ḥol* – profane. In other words, Moses is telling God that destroying the Jewish people is a wrongful, profane act. The Talmud makes this very point, commenting on *vayeḥal*:

רַבָּנָן אָמְרִי
מְלַמֵּד שֶׁאָמַר מֹשֶׁה לִפְנֵי הַקָּדוֹשׁ בָּרוּךְ הוּא
רִבּוֹנוֹ שֶׁל עוֹלָם חוּלִין הוּא לְךָ מֵעֲשׂוֹת כַּדָּבָר הַזֶּה.

> The rabbis say: It teaches that Moses said to the Holy One, Blessed Be He: Sovereign of the Universe, it is a profanation (*ḥullin*) for You to do this thing.[6]

In the end, God alters the decree. The prayer bears fruit; the Israelites are saved: וַיִּנָּחֶם ה׳ עַל הָרָעָה אֲשֶׁר דִּבֶּר לַעֲשׂוֹת לְעַמּוֹ – "And the Lord renounced the punishment He had planned to bring upon His people" (Ex. 32:14).

There are other examples of leaders who challenge God in private prayer. In his doctoral dissertation, my son, Dov Weiss, cites cases of "how a biblical character stood up in prayer (*amad bitefilla*) before God, and then proceeded to…confront Him with words."[7]

---

5. Note that when this event is recorded in Deuteronomy, the Torah states: וָאֶתְפַּלֵּל אֶל ה׳ וָאֹמַר אֲ־דֹנָי ה׳ אַל תַּשְׁחֵת עַמְּךָ וְנַחֲלָתְךָ אֲשֶׁר פָּדִיתָ בְּגָדְלֶךָ – "I prayed (*va'etpallel*) to the Lord and said, 'O Lord God, do not annihilate Your very own people, whom You redeemed in Your majesty'" (Deut. 9:26). Clearly, *vayeḥal* is prayer, as the Deuteronomy text uses the word *va'etpallel* instead.
6. The Talmud seems to be arguing that there were many righteous people in the wilderness not deserving of death. Why, then, should the whole people of Israel be destroyed? Moses' prayer parallels Abraham's concerning the destruction of Sodom. There, Abraham tells God: חָלִלָה לְּךָ מֵעֲשֹׂת כַּדָּבָר הַזֶּה לְהָמִית צַדִּיק עִם רָשָׁע – "It would be profane for You to do such a thing, to bring death upon the innocent as well as the guilty" (Gen. 18:25).

   The Talmud records other interpretations of *vayeḥal* that are submissive. Still, this talmudic passage indicates that one stream of thought understands *vayeḥal* as the right to engage in more demanding prayer.
7. Dov Weiss, *Confrontation with God in Late Rabbinic Literature* (Chicago: University

Joseph Heinemann lists three categories of confrontational prayer: (a) prayers of the talmudic sages, (b) prayers found in various ancient rites, and (c) fictitious prayer ascribed in the *Aggada* to biblical heroes.[8] Heinemann argues that the idea that we, as mere mortals, are empowered to confront God in prayer is a Jewish innovation. Furthermore, he maintains that this empowerment underscores an ethical worldview:

> The idea that God should allow one of His creatures to "take Him to court" and to "hurl words at heaven," which is expressed so strikingly in the confessions of Jeremiah, for example, and even more so in the book of Job, is certainly a Jewish innovation. The use of the controversy pattern (the "law court" style) indicates a certain frame of mind which involves a highly personalized approach to the problem of the individual's fate. The legal controversy of man with God presupposes the existence of an "I-Thou" relationship between the two....
>
> So, too, the use of this pattern reveals a decidedly ethical, normative conception of God and of His relationship to man, predicated on the assumption of a stable, ethical order in the universe that was established by God and is sustained by Him. "Justice" is the fundamental concept in the Jewish ethico-religious worldview.[9]

Standardized *tefilla*, too, can at times have a more challenging tone. The Jerusalem Talmud records:

---

of Chicago, 2011) p. 20 n. 56. Dr. Weiss cites the following cases of private confrontational prayer that begin with the words *amad bitefilla*: Berakhot 32b; Midrash *Tanḥuma* (Buber), *Vayishlaḥ* 10; Numbers 28; Esther Rabba 7:13; *Seder Eliya Rabba* 4, 7, 9, 28; Deuteronomy Rabba (TY) (Vilna) 11:10; and Esther Rabba II (TY) 43:1 (without the preceding word "stood").

8. Joseph Heinemann, *Prayer in the Talmud: Forms and Patterns*, trans. Richard S. Sarason (Berlin: De Gruyter Press, 1977), pp. 193–217.

9. Heinemann, *Prayer in the Talmud*, p. 208. Often, these prayers open with the phrase "Master of the Universe," or "Lord of all worlds."

זֶה שֶׁעוֹבֵר לִפְנֵי הַתֵּיבָה
אֵין אוֹמֵר לוֹ בֹּא וְהִתְפַּלֵּל
אֶלָּא בֹּא וּקְרַב
עֲשֵׂה קָרְבֵּינוּ עֲשֵׂה צְרָכֵינוּ עֲשֵׂה מִלְחֲמוֹתֵינוּ.

One who is called upon to lead services
is told not, "Come and pray,"
but "Come and *kerav* – offer our sacrifices, seek out our needs, fight our wars."[10]

The word *kerav,* here meaning "battle" or "combat," is related to the word *karov,* "close". This term perfectly captures the combative yet intimate nature of prayer – the need to draw close to God in order to challenge Him.

The *Sefat Emet* articulates how *Az Yashir* is a prayer that reflects clarity of faith, appropriately setting the tone for the larger service, which can be combative in nature. While the author of the *Sefat Emet* could be referring to the inner struggle of *tefilla* itself, he could also be relating to the struggles one may at times have with God. He writes:

אָז יָשִׁיר אֵין אָז אֶלָּא בִּטָּחוֹן כמ״ש אָז תֵּלֵךְ לָבֶטַח דַּרְכֶּךָ. דְּהִנֵּה בנ״י יָצְאוּ מִמִּצְרַיִם לִהְיוֹת צִבְאוֹת ה׳ לְהִלָּחֵם עִם מַלְכֵי כְּנַעַן... וְזֹאת הַשִּׁירָה הָיָה לָהֶם הֲכָנָה לְמִלְחָמוֹת אֵלּוּ....

וְכֵן בְּכָל יוֹם הִקְדִּימוּ חז״ל קְרִיעַת יַם סוּף וְהַשִּׁירָה קוֹדֶם הַתְּפִלָּה שֶׁהוּא בְּחִי׳ מִלְחָמָה כמ״ש שְׁעַת צְלוֹתָא שְׁעַת קְרָבָא.

"Then he [Moses (and the Israelites)] sang" [Ex. 15:1] – Wherever it says "then" (*az*), it means trust, as it says, "Then you will walk on your way securely" [Prov. 3:23]. For behold, the Children of Israel left Egypt to be the soldiers of God, to go out to battle with the kings of Canaan.... And this song was preparatory for these battles....

So too, every day, the rabbis asked us to recount the Splitting of the Sea and to sing the Song of the Sea (*Az Yashir*) prior

10. Jerusalem Talmud, Berakhot 4:4 (8b). See *Sefer Ḥaredim,* s.v. *ein omer*: "The language [*bo u'kerav*] does not have one meaning, but many."

> to our prayers, because it [prayer] is like battle. As it is said, the time of prayer is a time of combat.[11]

The language of the service itself underscores the inherent assertiveness of Jewish prayer. In the petitional passages of the *Amida*, we ask for discernment (*haskel*),[12] understanding (*bina*), and knowledge (*de'ah*) – ambitious requests by any standard. We ask that we be repeatedly forgiven (*hamarbeh lisloaḥ*) – not just marginally excused. We ask that the arrogant among us be uprooted (*te'aker*), crushed (*teshaber*), cast down (*temager*), and humbled (*takhniya*) – not just defeated.[13] We ask that Jerusalem be established for eternity (*binyan olam*) – not just built.[14]

Assertive prayer need not be an expression of anger toward God – it can express love. While it may be stern, such prayer can and should reflect a relationship so close that one feels comfortable enough to open up and cry and express upset, certain that God's concern and love will continue unconditionally. On a human level, too, if love is real, one should be able to express deep, intimate feelings, unafraid of being judged, ridiculed, or mocked; one is able to take off masks and be who he or she is. The Midrash articulates this idea when it declares:

> כָּל אַהֲבָה שֶׁאֵין עִמָּהּ תּוֹכֵחָה אֵינָהּ אַהֲבָה.
>
> Any love that does not include reprimand is not [true] love.[15]

---

11. *Sefat Emet, Pesaḥ* 5660, s.v. *Itta bamidrash az yashir.*
12. In the Sephardic rite, the term *ḥokhma* (wisdom) is used.
13. These words are part of the blessing of *VeLaMalshinim*. The blessing was composed by Shemuel HaKatan and ordained by Rabban Gamliel (see Berakhot 28b). It was directed against the early Christians who jeopardized the Jewish community by informing against it to the Roman authorities. The blessing reads:
    For the slanderers let there be no hope,
    and may all wickedness perish in an instant.
    May all Your people's enemies swiftly be cut down.
    May You swiftly uproot, crush, cast down,
    and humble the arrogant swiftly in our days.
    Blessed are You, Lord, who destroys enemies and humbles the arrogant.
14. See Rabbi Norman Lamm, *The Royal Reach: Discourses on the Jewish Tradition and the World Today* (New York: Feldheim Publishers, 1970), pp. 212–213.
15. Genesis Rabba 54.

There exists folklore of great Jewish spiritual leaders who lovingly but assertively dialogued with God. The eighteenth-century hasidic Rabbi Levi Yitzḥak of Berditchev was renowned for making demands of God. It is told that he once saw a Jew drop his *tefillin* (phylacteries). The Jew picked them up and gently kissed them. Seeing the Jew kiss his *tefillin*, the Berditchever turned to God and said, "Lord, O God, look how this holy Jew kisses his *tefillin* as an expression of his love for You. And when You, O God, drop Your *tefillin*, do You kiss it as gently, do You kiss it as emotionally? In other words, do You love us as much as we love You?"[16]

In the twentieth century, the Klausenberger Rebbe, who lost his entire family – his wife and eleven children – in the Holocaust, was known to speak to God in loving but strong terms. After the war, he came to America. One Shabbat morning, when the Torah portion of the *tokhaḥa* (curse) was read, the reader chanted it quickly and softly, as is the custom. Suddenly the Rebbe began to scream, "*Pamelekher*! Slower! – *Hekher*! Louder!" His disciples were stunned. The *tokhaḥa* was always read fast and in a hushed tone, as a way of declaring that we want no part of the curse. But the Rebbe insisted, so the *tokhaḥa* was read aloud.

After Shabbat, the students sought an explanation from the Rebbe. He replied, "I lost my entire family in Europe. I know this curse well – not only as prediction, but also as that which has already happened. I therefore insist that it be read aloud as my way of telling God: 'Listen closely, Almighty God, the curse has already come true. Now it is time for all of us to experience Your blessing of redemption!'"[17]

THE DIFFERENCE BETWEEN PRAYER AND *TEFILLA*

There is a fundamental difference between prayer and *tefilla*. While the English word "prayer" means to ask or implore, *tefilla* is associated with the Hebrew word נָפַל – *nafal,* which means "fall." Thus, unlike

16. The Talmud in Berakhot 6a declares that even God wears *tefillin*. But whereas our *tefillin* include the *Shema*, in which we express our love for God, God's *tefillin* include the words וּמִי כְעַמְּךָ כְּיִשְׂרָאֵל גּוֹי אֶחָד בָּאָרֶץ – "Who is like Your people Israel, a unique nation on earth?" (II Sam. 7:23), reflecting God's love for us.
17. I first heard this story from Rabbi Shlomo Riskin. The Klausenberger Rebbe remained in America briefly before moving to Israel.

prayer, *tefilla* entails falling before God and feeling His presence on an intimate level.

This concept of *tefilla* is captured in an early interaction between Abraham and God. When God changes Abram's name to Abraham and spells out his mission as the Patriarch of Israel who will be "a father of a multitude of nations," the Torah states: וַיִּפֹּל אַבְרָם עַל פָּנָיו, "Abram fell (*vayipol*) on his face" (Gen. 17:3–5). Here, *vayipol* is a form of *tefilla*. Even as Abraham assumes his new responsibility, he recognizes the awesomeness of the task before him and his need for God's help.[18] On a deeper level, this verse can be read as "Abram fell on His face," fully feeling God's presence.[19]

In *tefilla*, we converse directly with God. The word that appears perhaps most frequently in *tefilla* is אַתָּה (*You*). It is an "I-Thou" encounter, a close and intimate relationship.[20] Consider the *tefilla* of *Modim*, the

---

18. The verb *vayipol* is understood as the source for falling on our faces in the *Taḥanun* prayer. See *Teshuvat HaGeonim, Sha'arei Teshuva* 337, Leipzig ed.

In response to Koraḥ's rebellion against Moses and Aaron, God declares His readiness to annihilate the people. Moses and Aaron fall on their faces, demanding that only the guilty be punished:

> וַיִּפְּלוּ עַל פְּנֵיהֶם וַיֹּאמְרוּ אֵל אֱ־לֹהֵי הָרוּחֹת לְכָל בָּשָׂר הָאִישׁ אֶחָד יֶחֱטָא וְעַל כָּל הָעֵדָה תִּקְצֹף.
>
> But they fell on their faces and said, "O God of the spirits of all flesh! When one man sins, will You be wrathful with the whole community?" (Num. 16:22)

In their quest to settle the land of Canaan, the Jews are led by Joshua to victory in Jericho, but are then defeated in the city of Ai. Devastated, Joshua falls on his face, contrite and in deep mourning:

> וַיִּקְרַע יְהוֹשֻׁעַ שִׂמְלֹתָיו וַיִּפֹּל עַל פָּנָיו אַרְצָה לִפְנֵי אֲרוֹן ה׳ עַד הָעֶרֶב הוּא וְזִקְנֵי יִשְׂרָאֵל/וַיַּעֲלוּ עָפָר עַל רֹאשָׁם.
>
> Joshua thereupon rent his clothes. He and the elders of Israel lay until evening with their faces to the ground in front of the Ark of the Lord; and they strewed earth upon their heads. (Josh. 7:6)

Note that in the Korah example, Moses and Aaron assume responsibility by assertively insisting that only the guilty be punished. In the Ai example, Joshua submissively expresses reliance upon God, as he fears for the future of his people. Although the motifs of these prayers seem different – assertion and submission – they share a point of commonality: falling before God, feeling His presence.

19. Note the phrase from the *Taḥanun* prayer: אֲנַחְנוּ מַפִּילִים תַּחֲנוּנֵינוּ לְפָנֶיךָ – "We lay our pleas before You" (Dan. 9:18). Laying one's plea before God is a form of falling before Him in prayer. Here again, לְפָנֶיךָ (*lefanekha*) means "before Your face."

20. Martin Buber distinguishes between the "I-It" and "I-Thou" encounters. In the

offering of thanksgiving, with its repeated reference to "You," emphasizing our direct communication with God:

> מוֹדִים אֲנַחְנוּ לָךְ שָׁאַתָּה הוּא ה׳ אֱלֹהֵינוּ וֵאלֹהֵי אֲבוֹתֵינוּ לְעוֹלָם וָעֶד. צוּר חַיֵּינוּ, מָגֵן יִשְׁעֵנוּ אַתָּה הוּא לְדוֹר וָדוֹר. נוֹדֶה לְּךָ וּנְסַפֵּר תְּהִלָּתֶךָ עַל חַיֵּינוּ הַמְּסוּרִים בְּיָדֶךָ וְעַל נִשְׁמוֹתֵינוּ הַפְּקוּדוֹת לָךְ וְעַל נִסֶּיךָ שֶׁבְּכָל יוֹם עִמָּנוּ וְעַל נִפְלְאוֹתֶיךָ וְטוֹבוֹתֶיךָ שֶׁבְּכָל עֵת, עֶרֶב וָבֹקֶר וְצָהֳרָיִם. הַטּוֹב, כִּי לֹא כָלוּ רַחֲמֶיךָ, וְהַמְרַחֵם, כִּי לֹא תַמּוּ חֲסָדֶיךָ מֵעוֹלָם קִוִּינוּ לָךְ.
>
> We give thanks to You, for You are the Lord our God and God of our ancestors for ever and all time. You are the Rock of our lives, Shield of our salvation from generation to generation. We will thank You and declare Your praise for our lives, which are entrusted into Your hand; for our souls, which are placed in Your charge; for Your miracles, which are with us every day; and for Your wonders and favors at all times, evening, morning, and midday. You are good – for Your compassion never fails. You are compassionate – for Your loving-kindnesses never cease. We have always placed our hope in You.
>
> וְעַל כֻּלָּם יִתְבָּרַךְ וְיִתְרוֹמַם שִׁמְךָ מַלְכֵּנוּ תָּמִיד לְעוֹלָם וָעֶד.
>
> For all these things, may Your name be blessed and exalted, O our King, continually, for ever and all time.
>
> וְכֹל הַחַיִּים יוֹדוּךָ סֶּלָה, וִיהַלְלוּ אֶת שִׁמְךָ בֶּאֱמֶת הָאֵל יְשׁוּעָתֵנוּ וְעֶזְרָתֵנוּ סֶלָה. בָּרוּךְ אַתָּה ה׳, הַטּוֹב שִׁמְךָ וּלְךָ נָאֶה לְהוֹדוֹת.
>
> Let all that lives thank You, Selah! And praise Your name in truth, O God, our Savior and Help, Selah! Blessed are You, Lord, whose name is "The Good" and to whom thanks are due.[21]

"I-It," the "I" interacts with the other in the third person. The other is an object to be used for the benefit of the "I." In the "I-Thou," the other is addressed in the second person, connoting a close and personal relationship. The "I" interacts for the sake of the other. See Martin Buber, *I and Thou,* trans. Walter Kaufmann (Touchstone, 1971).

21. This prayer is found in the *Amida*.

As Rabbi Levi Yitzḥak of Berditchev wrote:

> Where I wander – You!
> Where I ponder – You!
> Only You everywhere, You, always You.
> You, You, You.
>
> When I am gladdened – You!
> And when I am saddened – You!
> Only You, everywhere You!
> You, You, You.
>
> Sky is You!
> Earth is You!
> You above! You below!
> At every bend, at every end,
> Only You, always You![22]

Tefilla as נָפַל (*nafal*) – falling before God, feeling His love, sensing that one is never alone, that God is near and caring – raises the issue of theodicy. Why direct *tefilla* to a God who oversees a world that is often wracked with evil? Given all the suffering in the world and the often painful challenges of life, why fall before God? Either God is impotent and unable to stop suffering, or God is evil, inflicting general and personal pain. The issue of theodicy is, for many, the greatest obstacle to *tefilla*.

Bracketing

Truth be told, certain *tefillot* express human struggle with God. *Kaddish*, for example, is recited not only by the leader of the service, but by mourners. Note that God is referred to in the third person rather than the second:

22. This poetic translation from the Yiddish is by Perle Besserman.

יִתְגַּדַּל וְיִתְקַדַּשׁ שְׁמֵהּ רַבָּא
בְּעָלְמָא דִּי בְרָא כִרְעוּתֵהּ....
יְהֵא שְׁמֵהּ רַבָּא מְבָרַךְ לְעָלַם וּלְעָלְמֵי עָלְמַיָּא.

> Magnified and sanctified may His great name be,
> in the world He created by His will….
> May His great name be blessed for ever and all time.

Once speaking of the greatness and holiness of God, shouldn't the prayer declare, "Magnified and sanctified may Your great name be, in the world You created by Your will" and "May Your great name be blessed forever and all time"? Why is God referred to in the third person rather than the second? Perhaps, having just experienced a devastating loss, mourners feel distant from God.[23] As a consequence, they do not use the second person *You,* a term of closeness, and instead use the third person *He,* denoting a sense of isolation from the Divine. The mourner is still connected to God, but the relationship is not intimate. It is a third person "I-He" encounter rather than a second person "I-You" relationship.[24]

On the whole, however, the liturgy speaks of the intimate encoun-

---

23. In the morning service, קָדוֹשׁ, קָדוֹשׁ, קָדוֹשׁ ה׳ צְבָאוֹת מְלֹא כָל הָאָרֶץ כְּבוֹדוֹ, "Holy, holy, holy is the Lord of hosts; the whole earth is full of His glory" (Is. 6:3), is juxtaposed to בָּרוּךְ כְּבוֹד ה׳ מִמְּקוֹמוֹ, "Blessed is the Lord's glory from His place" (Ezek. 3:12). These verses reflect two different historical experiences. קָדוֹשׁ, קָדוֹשׁ, קָדוֹשׁ – "Holy, holy, holy" was said by Isaiah, in whose time Jerusalem survived (II Kings 19). He therefore speaks of God's omnipresent holiness. בָּרוּךְ כְּבוֹד ה׳ מִמְּקוֹמוֹ – "Blessed is the Lord's glory from His place" was said by Ezekiel the prophet of the destruction of the First Temple. Thus, Ezekiel, the prophet of the exile, senses that God is distant. Still, he talks of the challenge of receiving God's blessing from "His place," even though that place, the Temple, has been destroyed.
24. Maḥzor Vitry suggests that *Kaddish* is mostly in Aramaic as Aramaic is the language of exile, reflecting the mourners' feelings of estrangement from God. See Maḥzor Vitry, ed. S. Hurwitz (Berlin, 1896-1897), p. 8. *Tosafot,* Berakhot 3a, s.v. *ve'onin,* explains that *Kaddish* is said in Aramaic as that was the language then understood by the larger community. See Rabbi Marvin Luban, *The Kaddish: Man's Reply to the Problem of Evil* (New York: Yeshiva University Press, 1969), p. 209.

    As mentioned in chapter 1, *Kaddish* is a constant reminder of our responsibility to bring God into the world. The mission is full of pitfalls; at times it is daunting, seemingly impossible. While there is an abiding belief that one day the obstacles will be overcome, *Kaddish* is in the third person, reflecting the difficulty of this endeavor.

ter between the human being and God – where God is referred to as *Atah* (You). How can this be reconciled with the understandable feeling of upset that every human being may at times, even often, feel toward God?

The question of how to reconcile the idea of a loving God with our earthly reality has been the subject of endless study. Yet *tefilla* is not study; it is a love encounter with God.[25] In moments of love, points of tension are put aside. Love allows for the bracketing of areas of disagreement, of ignoring the clutter that blocks the channels between lover and beloved.

In the first blessing recited before *Shema* every morning, we say:

> בָּרוּךְ אַתָּה ה׳ אֱ־לֹהֵינוּ מֶלֶךְ הָעוֹלָם יוֹצֵר אוֹר וּבוֹרֵא חֹשֶׁךְ עֹשֶׂה שָׁלוֹם וּבוֹרֵא אֶת הַכֹּל.
>
> Blessed are You, Lord our God, Ruler of the Universe, Former of light, Creator of darkness, Maker of peace and Creator of all things.

These last words come from Isaiah 45:7. There, however, the text states עֹשֶׂה שָׁלוֹם וּבוֹרֵא רָע – "Maker of peace and Creator of evil." Why do our daily prayers refer to God as the "Creator of all things," while Isaiah calls Him "Creator of evil"?

The Isaiah text underscores the monotheistic tenet that one God reigns over both good and evil. Isaiah proclaims that there is only one God, and He conducts the world in a way that only He understands. But in *tefilla* we declare this in a manner that avoids any direct mention of evil. In the time of intimate conversation with God, we focus on His beneficence.

The יִגְדַּל (*Yigdal*) prayer, based on Maimonides' *Thirteen Principles of Faith*, posits absolute reward and punishment: גּוֹמֵל לְאִישׁ חֶסֶד כְּמִפְעָלוֹ נוֹתֵן לְרָשָׁע רַע כְּרִשְׁעָתוֹ – "He rewards people with loving-kindness according to their deeds; He punishes the wicked according to his wickedness."[26]

---

25. Certain paragraphs from biblical and talmudic texts are part of the *tefilla*. By and large, during *tefilla* we say these texts within the framework of spiritual striving rather than intellectual debate.
26. *Yigdal* is said during the daily morning blessings. In some congregations, it is recited at the end of the Friday night service as well. Maimonides' complete *Thirteen Principles* are said by some after the daily morning service.

In the *beit midrash* (study hall), this statement would prompt endless discussion. One might ask whether this principle is empirically true, or whether this is the optimal way to serve God. Isn't it best to serve with purity of heart, without promise of reward?[27] But in *tefilla*, this principle is not only said, it is sung. For *tefilla* is the time to love God and lift our voices in song to Him. Even if we question the idea of a benevolent God, in *tefilla* we take the time to pause from our struggles – we set them aside – leaving ourselves open to feel God's embrace.[28]

Coping

At times, however, it is impossible to bracket pain, as the suffering is so overwhelming it suffuses the very core of our being. One needs, then, to lower expectations, to seek God's help in coping with, rather than solving, problems. Sometimes there are no answers. The heart condition, the cancer, the spinal injury remains; the depression, the loneliness doesn't go away; the learning disability, the speech impediment cannot be surmounted; the struggle with a marriage, a parent, a sibling, a child continues. Often, *tefilla* is a reflective rather than redemptive experience; a process of managing problems rather than solving them.[29]

In this spirit, I stood before my congregation after my mother died more than twenty-five years ago, and apologized. I said, "I'm sorry. All these years I thought my goal as a rabbi was, in time of death, to remove the pain, stop the suffering, mend the broken heart, lift the heaviness. With the death of my mother, I have come to realize that is impossible.

---

27. See Mishna Avot 1:3.
28. Sa'adia Gaon writes about the methodological doubt that necessitates bracketing even as one's belief remains intact. See Sa'adia Gaon, *Emunot VeDeot,* introduction. See also Rabbi Norman Lamm, *Faith and Doubt: Studies in Traditional Jewish Thought* (New York: KTAV Publishing House, 1986), pp. 9–16.
29. From this perspective, the term "*tefilla*" may be associated with the word הִפִּיל, as in *hipil pur* – "to cast lots" (Est. 3:7, 9:24). Whatever one's fate, during *tefilla,* one yearns to come close to the Divine.

    Tefilla may also be connected with the word פֶּלֶא – *peleh,* which means miracle. *Tefilla* is a process through which one takes cognizance of God's role in the miracle of life itself, even if His involvement is limited to dealing with, rather than eliminating, life's challenges.

One can't remove the darkness, but should try to reach out to God, to feel His embrace as He helps us go on."

In memory of my mother, I've written these words concerning the loss of someone close:

> מָשָׁל, לְמָה הַדָּבָר דּוֹמֶה, לְאָדָם שֶׁנִּכְנַס לְתוֹךְ חֶדֶר חָשׁוּךְ וְנִתְקַל בְּכָל מִינֵי דְּבָרִים שֶׁמְּפוּזָּרִים בְּתוֹךְ הַחֶדֶר. בְּכָל פַּעַם שֶׁנִּכְנָס לַחֶדֶר, הוּא לוֹמֵד יוֹתֵר וְיוֹתֵר בְּדִיּוּק אֵיפֹה הַדְּבָרִים נִמְצָאִים. וְכָךְ נִתְקָל בָּהֶם פָּחוֹת וּפָחוֹת, עַד שֶׁאַחֲרֵי זְמַן מָה, הוּא מַכִּיר אֶת הַמָּקוֹם הֵיטֵב וְלֹא נִתְקָל בְּשׁוּם דָּבָר, לַמְרוֹת שֶׁהַחֶדֶר עֲדַיִין חָשׁוּךְ.
>
> כְּמוֹ כֵן הַמָּוֶת. יֵשׁ חוֹשֶׁךְ בַּמָּוֶת שֶׁאִי אֶפְשָׁר לְגָרְשׁוֹ. אֲבָל אֶפְשָׁר לִלְמוֹד אֵיךְ לְהַמְשִׁיךְ לִחְיוֹת לַמְרוֹת הַחוֹשֶׁךְ הַזֶּה.
>
> To what can death be compared? To a person who enters a darkened room for the first time and trips over the furniture. Each time he enters the room, he learns more and more where the furniture stands. In time, he becomes familiar with the room, and despite the darkness knows how to get around.
>
> So, too, death. There is darkness in death that cannot be chased away. But it is possible to learn how to go on living despite the darkness that forever remains.[30]

The ability to navigate the dark room and, in time, make one's way is made easier and is sometimes only possible when one is able to feel the fullness of God's presence. The psalmist makes this point when calling out, כִּי אָבִי וְאִמִּי עֲזָבוּנִי וה׳ יַאַסְפֵנִי – "For my father and mother have left

30. Many thanks to Rabbi Yonah Berman for editing the Hebrew translation.
Leonard Cohen, the famed contemporary musician, sings of finding happiness in a life that is less than perfect. In a concert he gave in Israel in September 2009, Cohen offered what he called "a response to human grief; a radical, unique, 'holy, holy, holy' response to human suffering – *barukh Hashem*." He then sang his well-known "Ring the Bells":

> Ring the bells that still can ring
> Forget your perfect offering
> There is a crack in everything
> That's how the light gets in.

me, but the Lord gathers me in" (Ps. 27:10).[31] Death is final. Once dead, father and mother can never return. And yet, King David declares, God is there not necessarily to solve problems, but to cuddle us, to hug us, to gather us in by helping us cope with the situation at hand. This mindset can help us overcome other insoluble difficulties.

TEFILLA AND THE JEWISH MISSION

It can be suggested that the Torah begins with the Genesis narrative to teach the central mission of Judaism – to bring ethical monotheism into the world. The recurring theme of the first chapters is that sin results in estrangement from God. In the words of Nahmanides, עַד שֶׁגֵּירַשׁ אוֹתוֹ חֶטְאוֹ מִשָּׁם – "until his [Adam's] sin expelled him from there."[32]

After Adam and Eve disobey God and eat from the tree, the Torah states: וַיִּתְחַבֵּא הָאָדָם וְאִשְׁתּוֹ מִפְּנֵי ה׳ אֱ-לֹהִים – "Adam and his wife hid from (*mipnei*) the Lord God" (Gen. 3:8). Note the term פְּנֵי (*penei*), which means they were hidden from the face of God; they no longer felt His presence.

So, too, after Cain murders Abel, the Torah says וַיֵּצֵא קַיִן מִלִּפְנֵי ה׳, literally, "Cain left the face (*milifnei*) of God" (Gen. 4:16).

Again, in the description of the wrongdoings of the generation of the Deluge, the Torah proclaims: וַתִּשָּׁחֵת הָאָרֶץ לִפְנֵי הָאֱ-לֹהִים – "The earth was corrupt before (*lifnei*) God" (Gen. 6:11). Or more literally, the sins of the world were manifest in humankind's turning away from the face of God.

And the story of the Tower of Babel reaches its crescendo with the words וַיָּפֶץ ה׳ אֹתָם מִשָּׁם עַל פְּנֵי כָל הָאָרֶץ – "The Lord scattered them from there over the entire face of (*penei*) the earth" (Gen. 11:8). This implies that they were no longer experiencing the face, or presence, of God.

In all these accounts, the word פְּנֵי (*penei*) is used as a metaphor to describe the exile taking place – an exile from God's presence, in which God turns His face away.

---

31. This is part of *LeDavid Hashem*, Psalm 27, said in Ashkenazic synagogues from the beginning of the Hebrew month of Elul until Simḥat Torah. In some Sephardic communities it is said year round.

32. Nahmanides, Genesis 1:1, s.v. *bereshit bara E-lohim.*

It is after Adam and Eve are banished from the Garden of Eden, after Cain has killed Abel, after the world is destroyed by flood and then rebuilt, only to have its peoples dispersed by language – only then do Abraham and Sarah enter the biblical story. Their mandate, and ultimately the mandate of the Jewish people, is to bring God and God's system of ethics back into the world.[33] This mission differentiates Abraham and Sarah from the generation of the Dispersion. That generation said, וְנַעֲשֶׂה לָּנוּ שֵׁם – "let us make a name for ourselves [by building the tower]" (Gen. 11:4). In contrast, Abram did not call out in his own name, but וַיִּקְרָא בְּשֵׁם ה׳ – "He called out in the name of the Lord" (Gen. 12:8).[34]

Two generations later, as Abraham's grandson Jacob wrestles with the angel prior to his reunion with Esau, he is given the name Yisrael (Gen. 32:29). The word "Yisrael" has many possible meanings, one of them being a compound of *shur* and *El*, meaning to see or to perceive God.[35] This becomes the name of the Jewish people, as our ultimate purpose is to be aware of the Divine and bring His presence back into the world.

The Torah records the name of the place where Jacob struggled with the angel: וַיִּקְרָא יַעֲקֹב שֵׁם הַמָּקוֹם פְּנִיאֵל כִּי רָאִיתִי אֱלֹהִים פָּנִים אֶל פָּנִים וַתִּנָּצֵל נַפְשִׁי – "Jacob called the place Peniel, for I saw the Lord face to face (*panim el panim*), and my soul was saved" (Gen. 32:31). Adam and Eve, Cain, the generation of the Deluge, and the generation of the Dispersion all turn against the face of God. Yet Jacob/Yisrael sees and embraces God face to face.

As noted at the outset of Part One, this was King David's greatest wish: שִׁבְתִּי בְּבֵית ה׳ כָּל יְמֵי חַיַּי לַחֲזוֹת בְּנֹעַם ה׳ וּלְבַקֵּר בְּהֵיכָלוֹ – "to live in the House of the Lord all the days of my life, to gaze upon the beauty of the Lord, to frequent His Temple" (Ps. 27:4). Rabbi Abba in the Midrash explains David's request as *malkhut sha'al* – "he asked like a king."[36] Not

33. Ibid.
34. Note the Bible's play on the word *shem*. In the generation of the Dispersion, it refers to themselves. In the Abraham and Sarah narrative, it refers to God, as the name of God is added. I first heard this idea from Rabbi Menachem Leibtag.
35. See Genesis 49:22 and Numbers 24:17, where *shur* means "gaze" or "see."
36. *Midrash Tehillim* (Buber), Psalm 27. This midrash was brought to my attention by Rabbi Norman Lamm in his book *The Royal Reach*, p. 211.

only does David ask like a king, he literally asks for *Malkhut* – to feel the presence of God Himself.

The mission of Judaism is to encounter God, to bring God into the world. It is beautifully expressed by Dr. Samuel Soloveitchik in his poem "I See Him":

> I see Him in a sick's recovery
> In a scientific discovery
> I see Him in creative tension,
> Realization, materialization, and invention.
>
> I see Him in the voice of our Tanoim,
> In the discussion of the Amoroim.
> I see Him in the Rishonim's debate,
> And in my ancestor's faith.
>
> I see Him in my mother's devotion,
> In a little girl's emotion.
> I see Him in Beethoven's inspiration
> And in Dr. Schweitzer's devotion…
>
> I see Him in Jewish history,
> Highly complex and full of mystery.
> I see the Great Sire
> Even in Treblinka's and Oswiecim's fire.
>
> On a rainy day I see Him on the cloud's roof,
> Cold, far, distant, aloof.
> And on a warm day, in prayer I see Him clear
> Glorious, majestic, and yet close and near…
>
> I believe that all people are of one stock,
> Yet I am aware that I am of the minority bloc,
> A lost sheep of Jacob's flock,
> And God is my fortress and rock.[37]

---

37. The poem was published in the Yeshiva University student newspaper *Hamevaser*,

In searching for a person whom I can consider *mori verabbi* (my teacher and rabbi), I always look for someone who sees God as his fortress and rock. For me, that person for many years was Rabbi Ahron Soloveichik. After his death, I sought someone whom I once again could call *mori verabbi.* I found such an individual in Rabbi Yehuda Amital. A survivor of the Holocaust, Rabbi Amital was a *talmid ḥakham* (Torah sage) who became the co-leader of Yeshivat Har Etzion in Israel and one of the country's strongest voices of Jewish moral conscience in his day. It was my custom to visit him when in Israel.

I saw Rabbi Amital a few months before his death, after he had undergone a difficult medical procedure. Sitting at his kitchen table, I could see he was weak, so I stayed for only a few moments. Normally, before leaving Rav Yehuda, I would ask him to share some thoughts of Torah. Recognizing he was frail, I turned to him and said, "*Mori verabbi,* a whole Torah teaching may be too difficult for you. But share with me a word, just one word of Torah." He paused for some long seconds. Placing his hand on mine, he looked into my eyes and with an angelic smile said, "*Veha'ikkar ha'emuna* – and the main thing is to have faith." These were the last words I ever heard from him.[38]

For Rabbi Amital, a man of extraordinary courage, salvation comes through faith. Faith is the foundation through which one can sing and pray and bring about the ultimate redemption. In his words:

כְּשֶׁזּוֹכִים לִישׁוּעוֹת, הַחוֹבָה הִיא ׳שִׁירוּ לוֹ זַמְּרוּ לוֹ שִׂיחוּ בְּכָל נִפְלְאוֹתָיו׳.
אֲבָל כְּדֵי שֶׁאָדָם יָשִׁיר וּכְדֵי שֶׁאָדָם יִרְצֶה לָשִׁיר,
תְּנַאי קוֹדֵם לְכָךְ הוּא אֱמוּנָה
שֶׁאָכֵן אוֹתָם הַמַּעֲשִׂים הֵם מַעֲשֵׂי אֱלוֹקֵינוּ.
וּכְעוֹמֶק הָאֱמוּנָה עָצְמָתָהּ שֶׁל שִׁירָה.

When one merits salvation,
It is incumbent to "sing to Him, raise your voice to Him, meditate on all His wonders."

March 9, 1967, p. 3. Dr. Samuel Soloveitchik was a chemist and the brother of rabbis Joseph B. Soloveitchik and Ahron Soloveichik. To my knowledge, this poem is one of his few works pertaining to religion.

38. Rabbi Amital died on 27 Tammuz 5770 – July 9, 2010.

> But in order for a person to sing
> and in order for a person to desire to sing,
> First he must be infused with belief
> that indeed these acts of salvation are the work of God.
> The deeper the faith, the more powerful the song [the deeper the prayer].[39]

To have faith means to live and encounter God at all times, in all places, walking in His ways. This is the mission of Judaism, and this is the *nekuda hapenimit,* the innermost core, of *tefilla.*

Thus, the overarching goal of *tefilla* is conflated with the primary goal of Judaism. This is "prayer as feeling God's presence."

39. Rabbi Yehuda Amital, *HaMa'alot MiMa'amakim* (Jerusalem: Agudat Yeshivat Har Etzion, 5734 [1974]), p. 67.

Part Two

Why Set Tefilla?

When considering the biblical sources for tefilla, *Maimonides'* וּלְעָבְדוֹ בְּכָל לְבַבְכֶם – *"to serve Him with all your heart," and Nahmanides'* בְּעֵת הַצָּרוֹת – *"in distress, turn to God," one wonders why there is structure in* tefilla. *These texts speak of* tefilla *as spontaneous, emanating from the heart, or arising in moments of distress. Why, then, are there specific times, places, or texts for* tefilla*? Why can't we pray whenever, wherever, and however we wish?*

My father would often comment that the term מַזָּל (mazal), *fate, is an acronym of* מָקוֹם־זְמַן־לַעֲשׂוֹת – מָקוֹם *(place),* זְמַן *(time),* לַעֲשׂוֹת *(to do).*[1] *In essence, my father was saying that* מַזָּל *is being in the right place at the right time and doing your part. Over the years, I have come to see great truth in this formula.*

One of the key missions of Judaism is to infuse kedusha *(holiness) into the everyday; to give spiritual meaning to all aspects of life.* Kedushat makom *is the Hebrew term for holiness of space, i.e., a synagogue, the city of Jerusalem, the* Beit HaMikdash *(Temple).* Kedushat zman *is the holiness of time, i.e., the holidays, Shabbat.* Kedushat gavra *is the holiness of the individual who does the right thing at the right time.*

1. As we pointed out at the end of chapter 1, God, in His last act of creation, commands humankind *la'asot*, to do its share to complete creation and, in partnership with God, redeem the world. Here, the God who created the world with the term *vaya'as*, "and He made" (Gen. 1:7, 16, 25), turns to the human being and, using the same root, declares *la'asot*: Now you do your share.

Part Two: Why Set Tefilla?

Tefilla *encompasses all three realms: time, as we are commanded to pray three times daily; place, as the synagogue is designated for* tefilla*; and the individual, in the text of the prayers one recites.*

Chapter Four

Time

About a hundred years ago, Rabbi Isaac Meir Alter of Ger pondered over the question of what a certain shoemaker of his acquaintance should do about his morning prayer. His customers were poor men who owned only one pair of shoes. The shoemaker used to pick up their shoes at a late evening hour, work on them all night and part of the morning, in order to deliver them before their owners had to go to work. When should the shoemaker say his morning prayer? Should he pray quickly, first thing in the morning, and then go back to work? Or should he let the appointed hour of prayer go by and, every once in a while, raising his hammer from the shoes, utter a sigh: "Woe unto me, I haven't prayed yet!?" Perhaps that sigh is worth more than prayer itself.[1]

---

1. Heschel, *Quest for God*, pp. 3–4.

ACTIONS SHAPE CHARACTER

Tefilla is a love encounter between the human being and God. In love, one receives and gives. Receiving is no simple matter, as it often involves recognition of need and dependence upon others. In turn, this could lead one to feel vulnerable, as one could be rejected. The challenge of receiving is to be open and trusting that the giver will not take advantage of the receiver's limitations. Additionally, it involves being thankful and gracious. As part of the relationship, the recipient assumes a certain level of responsibility to the giver.

In *tefilla,* as we stand before God – often in need – we open up, expressing our vulnerability and trust in Him. We also must acknowledge what we've already received. When asking for life, we thank God for the gift of life we've already been given. When asking for health, we thank God for whatever our level of well-being. When asking that Israel be secure, we thank God for the miracle of the Jewish state. We show gratitude by taking responsibility for our role as receivers, by acknowledging our accountability to God for His benevolence, and our responsibility for what has been given.

The importance of receiving is stressed by Rabbi Ben-Tziyon Meir Ḥai Uziel. He writes:

> In the opening to *Pirkei Avot* it says, "Moses received Torah from Sinai." The language of this line emphasizes and highlights the act of Moses' receiving [of Torah, and not God's giving of the Torah].
>
> In general, when transmissions focus on the action of giving, the [text] is highlighting that the giver is the most important and central element in the transition and its essence. And when the focus of the transmission is on the receiving end, it shows that the act of giving was contingent on the recipient, and without him there would not have been any transmission at all.
>
> Since the essence of giving the Torah, *Matan Torah,* was in the merit of Moses, who had the ability to receive, *Pirkei Avot* begins with the words: "Moses received the Torah from Sinai." This reception of the Torah became the personal acquisition of Moses. And this ability to receive Torah must be done in the

> spirit and manner of Moses. In this way, all who follow Moses and seek to receive Torah must be prepared and fitting to receive and to guard this precious gift.[2]

As important as the act of receiving may be, the cornerstone of the love encounter is giving. The very word *ahava* (love) is commonly associated with *hav*, which means "give."[3] The renowned psychologist and humanistic philosopher Erich Fromm explains the importance of giving in a love relationship:

> Love is an activity, not a passive affect; it is a "standing in," not a "falling for." In the most general way, the active character of love can be described by stating that love is primarily giving, not receiving.[4]

Yet Rabbi E. E. Dessler teaches that love does not always precede giving. The reverse is equally true. Feelings of love often arise from giving. And the more one gives, the more one loves. In his words:

> הוּרְגַּלְנוּ לַחֲשׁוֹב אֶת הַנְּתִינָה לְתוֹלֶדֶת הָאַהֲבָה, כִּי לַאֲשֶׁר יֹאהַב הָאָדָם, יֵיטִיב לוֹ. אֲבָל הַסְּבָרָה הַשְּׁנִיָּה הִיא, כִּי יֹאהַב הָאָדָם אֶת פְּרִי מַעֲשָׂיו, בְּהַרְגִּישׁוֹ אֲשֶׁר חֵלֶק מִן עַצְמִיּוּתוֹ בָּהֶם הוּא.
>
> We have become accustomed to thinking that giving is a derivative of love, that one gives to the person he or she loves. But the opposite is also true. [Love can come from giving], as one naturally loves the fruits of his labor, feeling that part of his very essence is in what he has created.[5]

---

2. Rabbi Ben-Tziyon Meir Ḥai Uziel, *Derashot Uziel al Masekhet Avot* (Jerusalem: HaVa'ad LeHotza'at Kitvei HaRav, 5751 [1991]), p. 4. Many thanks to Rabbi Andy Kastner for this translation.
3. This is an often used association in *derash* but not likely the etymology of *ahava*.
4. Erich Fromm, *The Art of Loving* (London: Harper & Row, 1956), cited in John Powell, *The Secret of Staying in Love* (Texas: RCL, 1974), p. 37.
5. Dessler, *Mikhtav MeEliyahu*, "*Kuntres HaḤesed*." Rabbi Dessler believes that in giving to another, the other becomes an extension of the self. There is another possibility:

John Powell, in *The Secret of Staying in Love,* maintains that love is not only a feeling – it's a decision:

> Everyone knows that feelings are like yo-yos – up and down, depending on such fickle things as the barometer, amounts of sunshine, digestion, the time of the month, and the side of the bed out of which we crawl on a given morning. Feelings are fickle and people who identify love with feelings become fickle lovers….
>
> It is obvious that feelings are related to love. The first attraction of love is usually experienced in terms of very strong feelings…however, in the course of a love relationship, we will have to go through an occasional winter of emotional discontent to find a newness of our love in the springtime. As the tinsel of young love is burnished by time into the more valuable gold of mature love, there will be times when emotional satisfaction will be absent. There will be other times when negative feelings will cloud the skies of our world.[6]

It is here, Powell argues, that the idea of love as a decision comes into play. Feelings alone cannot form the foundation of a solid relationship. Rather, the relationship must be continuously nurtured. In other words, the real test of love is not only what I feel about you, but what I am prepared to do for you.

My mother, of blessed memory, and father made *aliya* in the late 1970s. Whenever my parents flew to New York, it was my responsibility, as their only child living there, to meet them at the airport. One time, my father called to inform me that at the last moment their arrival was moved up by twenty-four hours. Professing my deep love for my parents, I insisted that I couldn't change my schedule on such short notice. "You became a hotshot rabbi," my father responded, "and don't have time for your parents?" "I love you deeply," I protested, "but it's difficult to alter

---

Giving is the foundation of love, precisely because in this process I wish to help the other achieve his or her full, unique potential, even if it is distinct and apart from my own.

6. Powell, *Staying in Love*, pp. 36–37.

plans at the last minute." I'll never forget my father's response: "Don't love me so much, just pick me up at the airport!"

The idea that love is predicated on action is crucial to understanding *tefilla* and, more broadly, all of Jewish ritual. If *tefilla* is an expression of love, why should we be mandated to pray? Why not pray only when we feel like praying? In truth, however, we may not feel like praying for long periods of time. But if we're obliged to pray, we make a decision to pray. By placing ourselves in the prayerful mode, feelings of prayer may surface. As Rabbi Abraham Joshua Heschel comments:

> Many of us regretfully refrain from habitual prayer, waiting for an urge that is complete, sudden, and unexampled. But the unexampled is scarce, and perpetual refraining can easily grow into a habit. We may even come to forget what we regret, what to miss.[7]

This is the basic idea of ritual. Ritual is an expression of our love for God. Its goal is by and large to do an action from which feelings may come. Hence, Jews at Sinai first proclaimed, "We will do." Only then did they say, "We will listen" – *na'aseh venishma* (Ex. 24:7).

From this perspective, Jewish ritual is a form of behavioral psychology. As *Sefer HaḤinukh* states,

> דַּע כִּי הָאָדָם נִפְעָל כְּפִי פְּעֻלּוֹתָיו, וְלִבּוֹ וְכָל מַחְשְׁבוֹתָיו תָּמִיד אַחַר מַעֲשָׂיו שֶׁהוּא עוֹסֵק בָּהֶם אִם טוֹב וְאִם רַע. וַאֲפִילוּ רָשָׁע גָּמוּר בִּלִיבּוֹ וְכָל יֵצֶר מַחְשְׁבוֹת לִבּוֹ רַק רַע כָּל הַיּוֹם, אִם יְעָרֶה רוּחוֹ וְיָשִׂים הִשְׁתַּדְּלוּתוֹ וְעִסְקוֹ בְּהַתְמָדָה בַּתּוֹרָה וּבַמִּצְוֹת, וַאֲפִילוּ שֶׁלֹּא לְשֵׁם שָׁמַיִם, מִיָּד יִנְטֶה אֶל הַטּוֹב. וּבְכֹחַ מַעֲשָׂיו יָמִית הַיֵּצֶר הָרַע, כִּי אַחֲרֵי הַפְּעֻלּוֹת נִמְשָׁכִים הַלְּבָבוֹת.
>
> Know that a person is influenced by his actions, and his intellectual and emotional life is conditioned by the things he does, good or bad. Even if he is thoroughly wicked and his mind is dominated by evil thoughts the whole day long, if he bestirs himself and endeavors to be constantly occupied with the Torah and its precepts, though not with godly intent, he will inevitably

7. Heschel, *Quest for God*, pp. 3–4.

> veer towards the good. From the wrong motive he will be led to the right one and by the force of his actions he will kill the evil inclination, since it is actions that shape character.[8]

Action involves identifying a need. But there are several levels of needs. There is an active need; for example, a person feels hungry and eats. And then there is a latent need. Even if a person doesn't feel hungry, he or she knows that eating regularly is important. Hence, one eats even if the need is hidden. Finally, there is the unknown need. That is, a person is unaware of the existence of the need.

For some, *tefilla* is an active need. For others it is latent. And for others still, it is unknown. The goal of mandatory *tefilla* is to inspire feelings that may be latent or unknown, feelings that can surface if stirred. Every human being has a divine spark. Formal *tefilla* is the igniting of that spark, a spark that awakens our connection with God.

THREE TIMES DAILY

So we are mandated to pray. But why three times daily? Why morning, afternoon, and evening? The Jerusalem Talmud explains that there is a rhythm to the natural world, which finds a parallel in the human experience. As the sun rises, peaks, and sets, so too does the human being experience different emotions during the course of the day, as reflected in the morning, afternoon, and evening services.

> וּמֵאֵיכָן לָמְדוּ ג׳ תְּפִילּוֹת? רַבִּי שְׁמוּאֵל בַּר נַחְמָנִי אָמַר כְּנֶגֶד ג׳ פְּעָמִים שֶׁהַיּוֹם מִשְׁתַּנֶּה עַל הַבְּרִיּוֹת.
>
> בְּשַׁחַר צָרִיךְ אָדָם לוֹמַר מוֹדֶה אֲנִי לְפָנֶיךָ ה׳ אֱ־לֹהַי וֵא־לֹהֵי אֲבוֹתַי שֶׁהוֹצֵאתַנִי מֵאֲפֵילָה לְאוֹרָה.
>
> בְּמִנְחָה צָרִיךְ אָדָם לוֹמַר מוֹדֶה אֲנִי לְפָנֶיךָ ה׳ אֱ־לֹהַי וֵא־לֹהֵי אֲבוֹתַי כְּשֵׁם שֶׁזִּכִּיתַנִי לִרְאוֹת הַחַמָּה בַּמִּזְרָח כָּךְ זָכִיתִי לִרְאוֹת בַּמַּעֲרָב.
>
> בָּעֶרֶב צָרִיךְ לוֹמַר יְהִי רָצוֹן מִלְּפָנֶיךָ ה׳ אֱ־לֹהַי וֵא־לֹהֵי אֲבוֹתַי כְּשֵׁם שֶׁהָיִיתִי בַּאֲפֵילָה וְהוֹצֵאתַנִי לְאוֹרָה כָּךְ תּוֹצִיאֵנִי מֵאֲפֵילָה לְאוֹרָה.

---

8. *Sefer HaḤinukh*, commandment 16, cited in Nehama Leibowitz, *New Studies in Shemot (Exodus)* (Jerusalem: World Zionist Organization, 1993), vol. 1, pp. 179–180.

> From where do we derive that we pray three times a day? R. Shemuel b. Naḥmani said it corresponds to the three times that nature changes over creation.
>
> In the morning, a person should say, "I thank You, O Lord, my God and God of my fathers, for having delivered me from darkness to light."
>
> In the afternoon service, a person should say, "I thank You, O Lord, my God and God of my fathers, for just as I merited to see the sun in the east, so too have I merited to see the sun in the west."
>
> In the evening, a person should say, "May it be Your will, O Lord, my God and God of my fathers, that just as in the past You have delivered me from darkness to light, so may You deliver me now from darkness to light."[9]

The morning service, *Shaḥarit,* is an expression of our gratitude to God – in the words of the Jerusalem Talmud, "for having delivered [us] from darkness to light."[10] The central message of the service is one of renewal (*hitḥadshut*). Judaism does not view the morning as a mere extension of the night before. Rather, every morning is a time to celebrate rebirth – it is as if we were being recreated. We say two words that we often forget to say to those who are closest – "thank you." We offer these words to God not only for the gift of life but for the gift of being "reborn."

The afternoon service, *Minḥa,* is primarily a *tefilla* of introspection as, according to the Jerusalem Talmud, one contemplates the magnificence of the world as created by God: "Just as I merited to see the sun in the east, so too have I merited to see the sun in the west."[11] As the *Minḥa* service is offered during the day, with all its pressures, the *tefilla* is brief. It is significant, however, as it encourages self-reflection precisely when it's needed most, when we are preoccupied with the day's activities.

The theme of the evening service, *Ma'ariv,* is hope, as the Jerusalem Talmud states: "Just as in the past You have delivered me from darkness

9. Jerusalem Talmud, Berakhot 4:1.
10. The term *Shaḥarit* comes from the word *shaḥar* – dawn.
11. *Minḥa* may be a play on the word *menuḥa,* rest, as it is a prayer service that allows for a respite of quiet reflection.

to light, so may You deliver me now from darkness to light." Night in Jewish tradition is the symbol of loneliness. Night is exile. Night is encountering feelings of being forlorn, bereft, lost.[12] At night, when we are ready to go to sleep, when we are ready to lie down, we express trust and faith in God's mercy that we will survive the darkness, and the morning light will soon come.

The Babylonian Talmud seems to support the Jerusalem Talmud's reason for morning and evening *tefilla*. There it states:

> Rabba b. Ḥinena the elder said in the name of Rav: If one fails to say "true and steadfast" (*emet veyatziv*) in the morning and "true and faithful" (*emet ve'emuna*) in the evening, he has not fulfilled his obligation; for it is said, "To declare Your loving-kindness in the morning and Your faithfulness in the night" [Ps. 92:3].[13]

"True and steadfast" (literally, *yatziv* means "steady"), which is recited immediately after the morning *Shema*, is related to acknowledging God's blessings that enable us to rise. "True and faithful," which is recited after the evening *Shema*, is an articulation of the faith that one will make it through the night and awake the next morning.

While the *Tosafot* relates these *tefillot* to thanksgiving and belief that each of us, as individuals, will overcome the challenges we face,[14] Rashi posits that they pertain to the collective people of Israel. In Rashi's words:

> The blessing of "true and steadfast," which we recite in the morning, is devoted to the kindness that God showed our forefathers in redeeming them from Egypt, splitting the sea, and bringing them across it....
>
> And the blessing of "true and faithful" speaks of the hope

12. Elie Wiesel called his book about his experiences during the Holocaust, and the death of his father in the camps, *Night*.
13. Berakhot 12a.
14. *Tosafot* ad loc., s.v. *lehaggid*. In the words of the *Tosafot*, שֶׁאָדָם מַאֲמִין וּמַפְקִיד רוּחוֹ בְּיָדוֹ וּמַחֲזִירָהּ בְּלֹא יְגִיעָה – "A person believes that God will return his soul in the morning refreshed."

> that God will fulfill His promise...to redeem us from ruling oppressors...and grant us life.[15]

Whether the focus of these *tefillot* is upon the individual or the community, whether our thoughts at any given moment concern ourselves or our nation, there is no end to the praise or blessings we could impart. Ideally, one should be in a constant state of expression of thanksgiving and faith toward God. In a perfect world, one would be in a continuous, perpetual state of prayer. As the Midrash proclaims:

עַל כָּל נְשִׁימָה וּנְשִׁימָה שֶׁאָדָם נוֹשֵׁם צָרִיךְ לְקַלֵּס לַבּוֹרֵא.

> For every breath a man takes, he must give praise to the Holy One, Blessed Be He."[16]

In real life, however, left to human whims, most people would rarely pray. As a middle ground, Jewish law asks that three times a day – *Shaḥarit, Minḥa,* and *Ma'ariv* – we connect to the Source of the universe, to God Himself. Much as we eat morning, afternoon, and evening, so too do we consume food for the soul. Rabbi Judah HaLevi suggests this correspondence:

וְהַסֵּדֶר הַזֶּה מֵהַנֶּפֶשׁ כְּסֵדֶר הַמָּזוֹן מֵהַגּוּף מִתְפַּלֵּל לְנַפְשׁוֹ וְנִזּוֹן לְגוּפוֹ.

> Prayer is for the soul what nourishment is for the body. [17]

Thus, *tefilla* is mandated so we will be stirred to renew, evaluate, and hope, morning, afternoon, and evening. But how do the specific prayers help inspire these emotions? The following section-by-section explication of the daily services shows the way.

---

15. Rashi ad loc., s.v. *kol mi.*
16. Genesis Rabba 14:9. The Midrash cites, as a proof, the last verse of Psalms: כֹּל הַנְּשָׁמָה תְּהַלֵּל יָ־הּ הַלְלוּ יָ־הּ – "Let all living souls praise the Lord. Hallelujah!" (Ps. 150:6).
17. Rabbi Judah HaLevi, *Book of Kuzari,* trans. Hartwig Hirschfeld (New York: Pardes Publishing House, Inc., 1946), p. 123 (3:5).

Decoding The Daily Prayer Service

Below is a summary of the three *tefillot*. Even readers entirely conversant with the text of the *tefilla* may find that this analysis offers a fresh interpretation, a new shade of meaning to the words uttered every day. The commentary is meant to be a springboard for further reflection and discussion.

SHAḤARIT – THE MORNING SERVICE

As pointed out, the central message of *Shaḥarit* is *hitḥadshut* – renewal, thanking God for the gift of rebirth as the new day begins. The service can be summarized in this manner:

Rebirth of body and soul	בִּרְכוֹת הַשַּׁחַר *Birkhot HaShaḥar*	Morning Blessings
Recreation of nature	פְּסוּקֵי דְזִמְרָה *Pesukei DeZimra*	Verses of Praise
Reenergizing Israel as a people	בִּרְכוֹת שְׁמַע *Birkhot Shema*	Blessings of the *Shema*[18]
Reaffirmation of principles of faith	שְׁמַע *Shema*	*Shema*
Recommitment to personal and covenantal relationship	עֲמִידָה *Amida*	Silent Meditation
Reinvigoration of redemptive hope	אַשְׁרֵי, וּבָא לְצִיּוֹן, עָלֵינוּ *Ashrei, Uva LeTziyon, Aleinu*	Concluding Prayers

What follows is a brief analysis of each of these sections.[19]

18. The first two blessings are said before *Shema*, the last after.
19. While this chapter covers most of the service, other prayers are discussed elsewhere in this work.

Birkhot HaShaḥar – Morning Blessings

The service begins with *Birkhot HaShaḥar,* the morning blessings, which stress the rebirth of body and soul. At the outset, we recite the blessing for washing hands:

> בָּרוּךְ אַתָּה ה׳ אֱ־לֹהֵינוּ מֶלֶךְ הָעוֹלָם אֲשֶׁר קִדְּשָׁנוּ בְּמִצְוֹתָיו וְצִוָּנוּ עַל נְטִילַת יָדָיִם.
>
> Blessed are You, Lord our God, King of the Universe, who has made us holy through His commandments, and has commanded us about washing hands (*Al Netilat Yadayim*).[20]

In the Torah, water is a symbol of creation. The world started when "the spirit of God hovered over the face of the waters" – וְרוּחַ אֱ־לֹהִים מְרַחֶפֶת עַל פְּנֵי הַמָּיִם (Gen. 1:2). We became a people when we marched through the sea (Ex. 14:29). We are born when the sac of amniotic fluid – the water – breaks. Appropriately, the ritual that marks the dawn of day is the washing of hands, symbolic of being reborn. The recitation of *Al Netilat Yadayim* ("about washing hands") hopefully inspires us to approach the day as a time of personal renaissance.

In the *Asher Yatzar* ("who fashioned") blessing that follows, one becomes more specific, offering detailed thanksgiving for physical rejuvenation:

> בָּרוּךְ אַתָּה ה׳ אֱ־לֹהֵינוּ מֶלֶךְ הָעוֹלָם
> אֲשֶׁר יָצַר אֶת הָאָדָם בְּחָכְמָה
> וּבָרָא בוֹ נְקָבִים נְקָבִים חֲלוּלִים חֲלוּלִים
> גָּלוּי וְיָדוּעַ לִפְנֵי כִסֵּא כְבוֹדֶךָ
> שֶׁאִם יִפָּתֵחַ אֶחָד מֵהֶם אוֹ יִסָּתֵם אֶחָד מֵהֶם
> אִי אֶפְשָׁר לְהִתְקַיֵּם וְלַעֲמוֹד לְפָנֶיךָ
> בָּרוּךְ אַתָּה ה׳
> רוֹפֵא כָל בָּשָׂר וּמַפְלִיא לַעֲשׂוֹת.

20. See *Shulḥan Arukh, Oraḥ Ḥayyim* 4:1.

> Blessed are You, Lord our God, King of the Universe,
> who fashioned the human being with wisdom,
> and created in him many orifices and cavities.
> It is revealed and known before the throne of Your glory
> that were one of them to be ruptured or blocked,
> it would be impossible to survive and stand before You.
> Blessed are You, Lord,
> Healer of all flesh, who does wondrous deeds.

While these words are usually associated with ingesting and expelling foods,[21] following my cardiac surgery I have come to think of them as a prayer that the vessels to my heart remain open. Whatever the association, it is a powerful reminder that God plays a major role in our physical well-being.

The last word of the blessing, *la'asot,* may be lifted from the creation story. *La'asot* is God's mandate to the human being to do his or her share to redeem the world (Gen. 2:3).[22] Similarly, the *Asher Yatzar* blessing ends with *la'asot,* recording the human responsibility to assist others medically. The seal of the blessing could therefore mean: Blessed are You, Lord, who heals all flesh and gives humankind the wondrous capacity to cure and make others well.

According to the Vilna Gaon, *Asher Yatzar* is immediately followed by *E-lohai, Neshama* ("My God, the Soul"), a blessing that speaks in precise terms about spiritual revitalization.[23] The verbs used in the blessing – *bara* (created), *yatzar* (formed), and *nafaḥ* (breathed) – are taken from the Genesis narrative dealing with the creation of the spiritual aspects of the human being:

וַיִּבְרָא אֱ־לֹהִים אֶת הָאָדָם בְּצַלְמוֹ.

> And God created Adam in His image. (Gen. 1:27)

21. This prayer is also said when leaving the lavatory.
22. See the discussion of *brit* in chapter 1.
23. See *Mishna Berura, Shulḥan Arukh, Oraḥ Ḥayyim* 6:12.

וַיִּיצֶר ה׳ אֱ־לֹהִים אֶת הָאָדָם עָפָר מִן הָאֲדָמָה וַיִּפַּח בְּאַפָּיו נִשְׁמַת חַיִּים.

And the Lord formed Adam from the dust of the ground and breathed into him the breath of life. (Gen. 2:7)

The spiritual component of the human being experiences rebirth every day, much like Adam and Eve when they were first created. The blessing proclaims:

אֱ־לֹהַי, נְשָׁמָה שֶׁנָּתַתָּ בִּי טְהוֹרָה הִיא
אַתָּה בְרָאתָהּ אַתָּה יְצַרְתָּהּ אַתָּה נְפַחְתָּהּ בִּי
וְאַתָּה מְשַׁמְּרָהּ בְּקִרְבִּי.

My God, the soul You placed within me is pure.
You created it, You formed it, You breathed it into me,
And You guard it while it is within me.

These physical and spiritual blessings of *Asher Yatzar* and *E-lohai, Neshama* are juxtaposed, as they accentuate the interfacing of body and soul. Each is dependent on the other. A soul as it exists in this world cannot function without a body. And a body without a soul is a body without direction, without meaning, without purpose.

Following these blessings are *Birkhot HaTorah*, blessings over the Torah. They are recited here as the Torah is a manual for living nobly, teaching us how to dedicate body and soul to the service of God, Israel, and humankind.

The blessings over the Torah are all-encompassing, as they deal with the full corpus of Jewish law – the Written Torah and the Oral Law.

בָּרוּךְ אַתָּה ה׳ אֱ־לֹהֵינוּ מֶלֶךְ הָעוֹלָם, אֲשֶׁר קִדְּשָׁנוּ בְּמִצְוֹתָיו, וְצִוָּנוּ לַעֲסוֹק בְּדִבְרֵי תוֹרָה. וְהַעֲרֶב נָא ה׳ אֱ־לֹהֵינוּ אֶת דִּבְרֵי תוֹרָתְךָ בְּפִינוּ וּבְפִי עַמְּךָ בֵּית יִשְׂרָאֵל. וְנִהְיֶה אֲנַחְנוּ וְצֶאֱצָאֵינוּ וְצֶאֱצָאֵי עַמְּךָ בֵּית יִשְׂרָאֵל, כֻּלָּנוּ יוֹדְעֵי שְׁמֶךָ וְלוֹמְדֵי תוֹרָתְךָ לִשְׁמָהּ. בָּרוּךְ אַתָּה ה׳, הַמְלַמֵּד תּוֹרָה לְעַמּוֹ יִשְׂרָאֵל.

בָּרוּךְ אַתָּה ה׳ אֱ־לֹהֵינוּ מֶלֶךְ הָעוֹלָם, אֲשֶׁר בָּחַר בָּנוּ מִכָּל הָעַמִּים וְנָתַן לָנוּ אֶת תּוֹרָתוֹ. בָּרוּךְ אַתָּה ה׳, נוֹתֵן הַתּוֹרָה.

Blessed are You, Lord our God, King of the Universe, who has made us holy through His commandments, and has commanded

> us to engage in study of the words of Torah. And please, Lord our God, make the words of Your Torah sweet in our mouths and in the mouths of Your people, the House of Israel, so that we, our descendants (and their descendants) and the descendants of Your people, the House of Israel, may all know Your name and study Your Torah for its own sake. Blessed are You, Lord, who teaches Torah to His people Israel.
>
> Blessed are You, Lord our God, King of the Universe, who has chosen us (*Asher Baḥar Banu*) from all the peoples and given us His Torah. Blessed are You, Lord, Giver of the Torah.

Note that the first blessing includes the word *la'asok* – "to engage" – as it deals with the Oral Law, which requires intensive intellectual pursuit. It goes on to discuss the transmission of Torah from generation to generation – a central motif of the oral tradition. This is followed by the blessing *Asher Baḥar Banu* – "who has chosen us," as this relates to the time when the Torah, the Written Law, was given. In sum, these blessings remind us that the Oral Law is based on the Torah. Both play critical roles in guiding us through the day.[24]

After the Torah blessings, the liturgy cites passages from the Torah and Oral Law, which teach basic lessons of life. The biblical passage is the Priestly Benediction, which is divided into three sentences – each including God's blessing, and a prayer to avoid the potential pitfalls of that blessing.

---

24. This is the view of the *Tosafot*, Berakhot 46a, s.v. *kol haberakhot kulan*. According to the *Tosafot*, one would add the conjunctive *vav* (*ve*) before *ha'arev* (sweeten) to indicate its link to *la'asok*.

 Maimonides (*Code*, Laws of Prayer 7:10–11) disagrees, maintaining that *ha'arev* is an independent blessing (without the conjunctive *vav*), and hence there are three blessings, probably corresponding to the major types of blessings: *birkhat hamitzva*, said when performing a commandment ("and has commanded us to... study... Torah"); *birkhat hanehenin*, said over pleasurable activities ("make the words of Your Torah sweet"); and *birkhat hoda'a, a* blessing of thanksgiving ("who has chosen us from all the peoples"). So encompassing is Torah that it requires all forms of blessings. See David Abudarham, *Sefer Abudarham HaShalem* (Jerusalem: Hotza'at Usha, 5723) p. 44. The Torah blessings as recorded in the Siddur are found in Berakhot 11b.

יְבָרֶכְךָ ה׳ וְיִשְׁמְרֶךָ
יָאֵר ה׳ פָּנָיו אֵלֶיךָ וִיחֻנֶּךָּ
יִשָּׂא ה׳ פָּנָיו אֵלֶיךָ וְיָשֵׂם לְךָ שָׁלוֹם.

> May the Lord bless you and protect you
> May the Lord make His face shine on you and be gracious to you
> May the Lord turn His face toward you and grant you peace. (Num. 6:24–26)

Blessing (*berakha*), as found in "May the Lord bless you," is associated with wealth. But money can corrupt. Therefore, we ask that we be "protect[ed]" from its dangers.[25] Light (*ohr*) as found in "May the Lord make His face shine on you" may refer to Torah knowledge or general knowledge.[26] But knowledge can lead to arrogance. So we implore that it be a knowledge of "gracious[ness]." Finally, we ask to feel God's presence (*panav*) – "May the Lord turn His face toward you." But people have done wicked things in the name of God. Thus, the blessing concludes with the hope that we be embraced by a God of *shalom* – "peace."[27]

Serving as the centerpiece of the morning blessings are the *Birkhot Hoda'a*, a series of blessings thanking God for each stage of wakefulness. As the Talmud explains:

כִּי שָׁמַע קוֹל תַּרְנְגוֹלָא, לֵימָא: בָּרוּךְ אֲשֶׁר נָתַן לַשֶּׂכְוִי בִינָה לְהַבְחִין בֵּין יוֹם וּבֵין לַיְלָה.
כִּי פָּתַח עֵינֵיהּ, לֵימָא: בָּרוּךְ פּוֹקֵחַ עִוְרִים.
כִּי תָּרֵיץ וְיָתֵיב, לֵימָא: בָּרוּךְ מַתִּיר אֲסוּרִים.
כִּי לָבֵישׁ, לֵימָא: בָּרוּךְ מַלְבִּישׁ עֲרוּמִּים.
כִּי זָקֵיף, לֵימָא: בָּרוּךְ זוֹקֵף כְּפוּפִים.
כִּי נָחֵית לְאַרְעָא, לֵימָא: בָּרוּךְ רוֹקַע הָאָרֶץ עַל הַמַּיִם.

---

25. See Sifrei, Numbers 40, s.v. *ye'varekhekha;* Rashi, Numbers 6:24, s.v. *yevarekhekha*.
26. See Proverbs 6:23, כִּי נֵר מִצְוָה וְתוֹרָה אוֹר – "For the commandment is a lamp, and the Torah is light."
27. The Oral texts cited in the Siddur deal primarily with interpersonal ethics (Pe'ah 1:1 and Shabbat 127a – *Eilu Devarim*). See the end of chapter 1 for a discussion of these texts.

כִּי מַסְגֵּי, לֵימָא: בָּרוּךְ הַמֵּכִין מִצְעֲדֵי גָבֶר.
כִּי סָיֵּים מְסָאנֵיהּ, לֵימָא: בָּרוּךְ שֶׁעָשָׂה לִי כָּל צָרְכִּי.
כִּי אָסַר הֶמְיָינֵיהּ, לֵימָא: בָּרוּךְ אוֹזֵר יִשְׂרָאֵל בִּגְבוּרָה.
כִּי פָּרֵיס סוּדָרָא עַל רֵישֵׁיהּ, לֵימָא: בָּרוּךְ עוֹטֵר יִשְׂרָאֵל בְּתִפְאָרָה.

When one hears the rooster crow, one says: Blessed are You who gives the heart understanding to distinguish between day and night.
When one opens the eyes, one says: Blessed are You who gives sight to the blind.
When one straightens and sits up, one says: Blessed are You who releases the bound.
When one dresses, one says: Blessed are You who clothes the naked.
When one stands up, one says: Blessed are You who raises those bowed down.
When one steps upon the ground, one says: Blessed are You who spreads the earth above the waters.
When one walks, one says: Blessed are You who makes firm the steps of the human being.
When one puts on shoes, one says: Blessed are You who has provided me with all I need.
When one fastens the belt, one says: Blessed are You who girds Israel with strength.
When one spreads a cloth upon the head, one says: Blessed are You who crowns Israel with glory.[28]

Today, the morning blessings are recited as a unit during the service itself.[29]

At first glance, these blessings seem unnecessary. Why thank God for the mundane? But that's precisely the point. Upon awakening, everything we do – even a simple, everyday action, like thinking, seeing, standing, walking, using our fingers – is acknowledged as a wondrous gift from God. In Jewish thought, the everyday occurrence, often taken for granted, is viewed as miraculous. In fact, the term *nes*, the Hebrew

28. Berakhot 60b.
29. *Shulḥan Arukh, Oraḥ Ḥayyim* 46:2. The order of the blessings in the Siddur is slightly different.

word for miracle, more literally means "banner" or "flag." The function of a banner is to direct the attention of an onlooker to what it symbolizes. A banner is one-dimensional; what it represents is often far deeper. Similarly, an everyday occurrence like eating or breathing may appear simple, but deeper observation reveals God's hand in its miraculous complexities.

Incorporated into the morning blessings is a series of three blessings relating to personal identity, introduced in the second century by R. Meir, thanking God for not having been made a gentile, a slave, and a woman.[30] Much has been written about why these blessings are framed in the negative,[31] and even more has been written about the blessing of gender.[32] What is important for us in this book is to recognize that these blessings were composed so that upon waking, in addition to expressing gratitude for everything God has given us, we take a moment to thank Him for our identity as men or women who are free and part of the Jewish covenantal community.

A story is told about the Volozhin Yeshiva during the latter half of the nineteenth century. Students who attended studied day and night. One student, however, began missing classes. Soon he disappeared from the *beit midrash*. He was approached by his rebbe, who reminded him of his responsibilities. The student responded, "But, Rebbe, you don't understand. Just recently I was given a gift – a new invention, a phonograph.

30. See Menahot 43b.

31. Women recite the gender blessing in the positive, thanking God for having "made me according to His will" – שֶׁעָשַׂנִי כִּרְצוֹנוֹ.

32. The recitation of the blessing thanking God "for not having created me a woman" – שֶׁלֹּא עָשַׂנִי אִשָּׁה continues to arouse great passion and controversy within the Orthodox community, as this blessing touches directly on the tension of fidelity to traditional formulations that are rooted in talmudic directives versus other Torah values, such as *kevod haberiyot* (human dignity), not causing pain to others, and affirming the *tzelem E-lohim* in every person. How this issue will ultimately play out in the Modern and Open Orthodox communities remains to be seen. At our synagogue, we have opted to avoid the public dimension of this issue by reciting all the morning blessings silently, with the leader of the service beginning from "*Rabbi Yishmael Omer*." See Dr. Joel B. Wolowelsky, "A Quiet Berakha," *Women, Jewish Law, and Modernity: New Opportunities in a Post-Feminist Age* (KTAV Publishing House, 1977), pp. 75-84.

It's a box on which you place something circular, a record – and voices miraculously come out. If the ultimate goal of Torah is to feel the miracle of God's wisdom, through the phonograph, through this box, I feel it more profoundly." The rebbe thought for a moment. With a cherubic smile, he looked into his student's eyes and softly said, "And tell me, my dear student, is the box in your throat any less miraculous?" It wasn't long before the student returned to the *beit midrash*.[33]

Pesukei DeZimra – Verses of Praise

Psalm 30, *Mizmor Shir*, מִזְמוֹר שִׁיר חֲנֻכַּת הַבַּיִת לְדָוִד – "A psalm of David, a song for the dedication of the House" – serves as the transition from the morning blessings (the blessings of rebirth of body and soul) to *Pesukei DeZimra* (the verses celebrating the recreation of nature). The psalm emphasizes the greatness of God, who has the capacity to transform even the most difficult of moments into moments of glory – to transform the night and all it symbolizes into day. It concludes with these words of hope:

הָפַכְתָּ מִסְפְּדִי לְמָחוֹל לִי
פִּתַּחְתָּ שַׂקִּי וַתְּאַזְּרֵנִי שִׂמְחָה.
לְמַעַן יְזַמֶּרְךָ כָבוֹד וְלֹא יִדֹּם
ה׳ אֱ-לֹהַי לְעוֹלָם אוֹדֶךָּ.

> You have turned my sorrow into dancing.
> You have removed my sackcloth and clothed me with joy,
> So that my soul may sing to You and not be silent.
> Lord my God, forever I will thank You. (Ps. 30:12–13)

As *Pesukei DeZimra* begins, we note the power of words. With words, God created the world:

בָּרוּךְ שֶׁאָמַר וְהָיָה הָעוֹלָם...
בָּרוּךְ אוֹמֵר וְעוֹשֶׂה.

33. I first heard this story at a Torah Leadership Seminar sponsored by Yeshiva University in the late 1960s.

Birkhot HaShaḥar
Renewal of Body and Soul

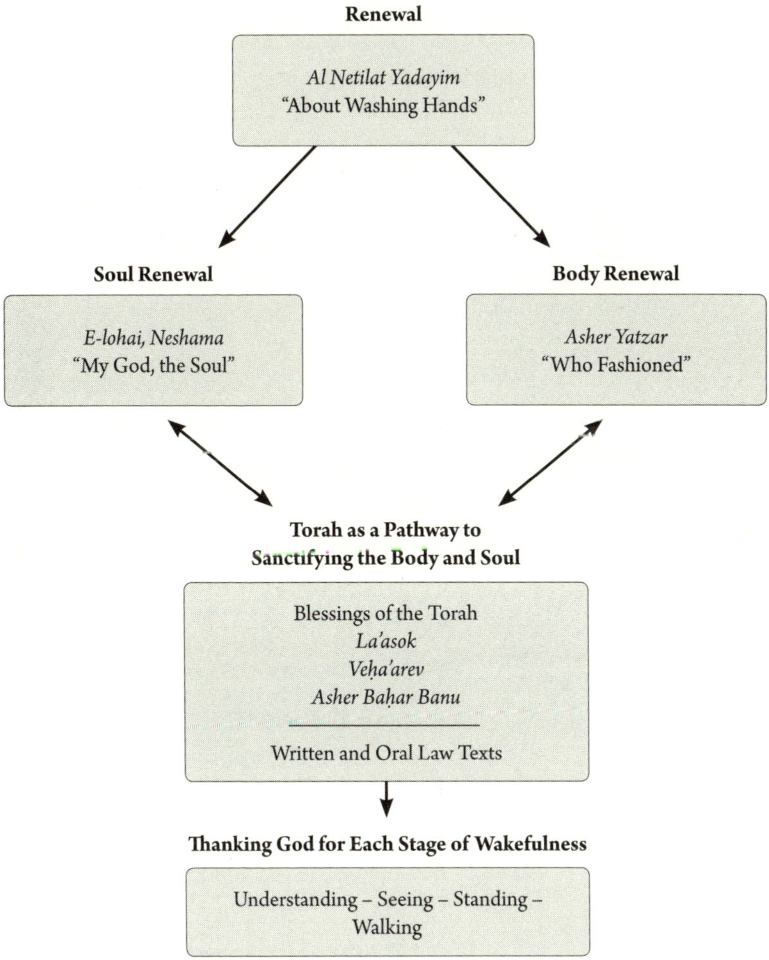

> Blessed be He who spoke (*Barukh SheAmar*) and the world came into being…
> Blessed be He who speaks and creates.

It follows that just as well-used words have the power to create, so can words misused destroy.[34]

In *Barukh SheAmar*, God is blessed as the One who not only created the world, but is constantly recreating it. As the *Sefat Emet* notes:

> מַאֲמָר אוֹמֵר וְעוֹשֶׂה פֵּירוּשׁ לְבַד הַמְּצִיאוּת שֶׁהִמְצִיא יֵשׁ מֵאַיִן רַק שֶׁנּוֹתֵן בָּהֶם כֹּחַ חָדָשׁ תָּמִיד.
>
> The meaning of "He … speaks and creates" is that aside from having created the world ex nihilo, God instills within the world the potential for constant renewal.[35]

Soon afterward, we utter the actual words "thank you" to God for His creation:

> מִזְמוֹר לְתוֹדָה, הָרִיעוּ לַה׳ כָּל הָאָרֶץ…
> כִּי טוֹב ה׳ לְעוֹלָם חַסְדּוֹ,
> וְעַד דֹּר וָדֹר אֱמוּנָתוֹ.
>
> A psalm of thanksgiving (*Mizmor LeToda*). Shout joyously to the Lord, all the earth…
> For the Lord is good, His loving-kindness is everlasting,
> and His faithfulness is for every generation. (Ps. 100:1, 5)[36]

---

34. It is interesting that the prayer service, which includes so much verbiage, is bracketed by prayers that deal with the importance of words: בָּרוּךְ שֶׁאָמַר ("Blessed be He who spoke") as we begin *Pesukei DeZimra*, and אֱ־לֹהַי נְצוֹר לְשׁוֹנִי מֵרָע ("My God, guard my tongue from evil") as we end the *Amida*. See chapter 8 for further discussion of these prayers.
35. *Sefat Emet*, Leviticus, *Behar* 5735, s.v. *BeRashi ma inyan.*
36. Today, a special blessing of thanksgiving – *HaGomel* – is recited after surviving a dangerous situation (i.e., illness, captivity, a hazardous journey). See *Shulḥan Arukh, Oraḥ Ḥayyim* 219:1–3.

    In the Torah, human beings never say "thank you" to one another. People bow to or kiss each other in gratitude, but "thank you" is never said. So focused were Jews

This is not the first time we thank God in the morning. When we rise we declare:

מוֹדֶה אֲנִי לְפָנֶיךָ
מֶלֶךְ חַי וְקַיָּם
שֶׁהֶחֱזַרְתָּ בִּי נִשְׁמָתִי בְּחֶמְלָה
רַבָּה אֱמוּנָתֶךָ.

> I thank You,
> living and eternal King,
> for giving me back my soul in mercy.
> Great is Your faithfulness.

The precise Hebrew for "I thank You" is אֲנִי מוֹדֶה (*ani modeh*). It has been noted that the order in this prayer is reversed – מוֹדֶה אֲנִי (*modeh ani*) – as the first word we utter when waking should be not "I," but "thank."[37]

The central paragraph of *Pesukei DeZimra* is *Ashrei* (Psalm 145).[38] The Talmud states, "Whoever says *Tehilla LeDavid* [*Ashrei*] three times daily is sure to inherit the World to Come."[39] The passage goes on to record the reasons *Ashrei* is of special importance. First, it follows the order of the *Aleph-Beit,* and second, it includes the sentence פּוֹתֵחַ אֶת יָדֶךָ וּמַשְׂבִּיעַ לְכָל חַי רָצוֹן – "You open Your hand and satisfy the desire of every living being" (Ps. 145:16). For Rabbi Meir Simḥa HaKohen of Dvinsk, these reasons conflate. The alphabetical order of the prayer symbolizes the natural order of creation, which has the resources to provide for all creatures. Thus, every morning when reciting this *tefilla,* we thank God for the everyday wonder of nature, which has the capacity

on recognizing God, and no other, that only He was thanked. Indeed, the Hebrew term for Jews, יְהוּדִים – *Yehudim,* comes from the name Judah (יְהוּדָה – *Yehuda*), the fourth son of Jacob. The word is associated with הוֹדָאָה – *hoda'a* (thanksgiving). When Judah is born, his mother, Leah, declares הַפַּעַם אוֹדֶה אֶת ה׳ – "This time, let me offer thanksgiving to the Lord" (Gen. 30:35).

As we thank God for the continuous gift of creation, we may also consider how to acknowledge others for all they do for us – including those who join in partnership with God in keeping the world and our communities vibrant and strong.

37. I recently heard this thought from Rabbi Shai Held.
38. *Ashrei* includes two introductory verses, Psalms 84:5 and 144:15.
39. Berakhot 4b.

to support and sustain the whole world. In his words, "Everything is [constantly] arranged [by God]...according to the natural order."[40]

Ashrei is followed by several psalms, as inspired by the talmudic passage that declares, "R. Yose said: May my portion be among those who recite *Hallel* every day...this refers to the Verses of Praise."[41] These include Psalm 148, which evokes the imagery of the Genesis story, listing God's creation in sequence.

הַלְלוּ יָ־הּ הַלְלוּ אֶת ה׳ מִן הַשָּׁמַיִם הַלְלוּהוּ בַּמְּרוֹמִים....
הַלְלוּהוּ שֶׁמֶשׁ וְיָרֵחַ הַלְלוּהוּ כָּל כּוֹכְבֵי אוֹר
הַלְלוּהוּ שְׁמֵי הַשָּׁמָיִם וְהַמַּיִם אֲשֶׁר מֵעַל הַשָּׁמָיִם....
הַלְלוּ אֶת ה׳ מִן הָאָרֶץ תַּנִּינִים וְכָל תְּהֹמוֹת
אֵשׁ וּבָרָד שֶׁלֶג וְקִיטוֹר רוּחַ סְעָרָה עֹשָׂה דְבָרוֹ
הֶהָרִים וְכָל גְּבָעוֹת עֵץ פְּרִי וְכָל אֲרָזִים
הַחַיָּה וְכָל בְּהֵמָה רֶמֶשׂ וְצִפּוֹר כָּנָף
מַלְכֵי אֶרֶץ וְכָל לְאֻמִּים שָׂרִים וְכָל שֹׁפְטֵי אָרֶץ
בַּחוּרִים וְגַם בְּתוּלוֹת זְקֵנִים עִם נְעָרִים
יְהַלְלוּ אֶת שֵׁם ה׳.

Hallelujah! Praise the Lord from the heavens, praise Him in the heights....
Praise Him, sun and moon; praise Him, all shining stars.
Praise Him, highest heavens, and the waters above the heavens....
Praise the Lord from the earth: sea monsters and all the deep seas;
fire and hail, snow and mist, storm winds that obey His word;
mountains and all hills, fruit trees and all cedars;
wild animals and all cattle, creeping things and winged birds;
kings of the earth and all nations, princes and all judges on earth;
youths and maidens, old and young.
Let them praise the name of the Lord. (Ps. 148:1–14)

---

40. See Rabbi Meir Simḥa HaKohen, *Meshekh Ḥokhma* (Jerusalem, 5751 [1991]), Leviticus 26:4, s.v. *venatati*. This teaching suggests that God created the world with enough food for everyone, if only human beings learn to "distribute" food properly.
41. Shabbat 118b. Psalms 145–150 are called *Hallel* as the term "praise" (הַלֵּל) is repeatedly found in them.

Like the climax of a symphony orchestra, these psalms conclude with the recitation of the last chapter of the book of Psalms. Here God is praised in the Temple and in all places. Instruments of every kind – wind, string, percussion – join in song. All of creation exalts God, proclaiming as one: *Hallelujah!*

הַלְלוּ יָהּ הַלְלוּ אֵל בְּקָדְשׁוֹ הַלְלוּהוּ בִּרְקִיעַ עֻזּוֹ...
הַלְלוּהוּ בְּתֵקַע שׁוֹפָר הַלְלוּהוּ בְּנֵבֶל וְכִנּוֹר.
הַלְלוּהוּ בְתֹף וּמָחוֹל הַלְלוּהוּ בְּמִנִּים וְעוּגָב...
כֹּל הַנְּשָׁמָה תְּהַלֵּל יָהּ הַלְלוּ יָהּ.

> *Hallelujah*! Praise God in His holy place; Praise Him in the heavens of His power...
> Praise Him with blasts of the shofar; praise Him with the harp and lyre.
> Praise Him with timbrel and dance; praise Him with strings and flute...
> Let all living souls praise the Lord. Hallelujah! (Ps. 150:1–6)

These paragraphs of *Pesukei DeZimra,* which opened with בָּרוּךְ שֶׁאָמַר וְהָיָה הָעוֹלָם – "Blessed be He who spoke and the world came into being" – now close:

בָּרוּךְ ה׳ לְעוֹלָם, אָמֵן וְאָמֵן.
וּבָרוּךְ שֵׁם כְּבוֹדוֹ לְעוֹלָם
וְיִמָּלֵא כְבוֹדוֹ אֶת כָּל הָאָרֶץ
אָמֵן וְאָמֵן.

> Blessed be the Lord forever. Amen and amen. (Ps. 89:53)
> Blessed be His glorious name forever,
> and may all the earth be filled with His glory.
> Amen and amen. (Ps. 72:19)

This section can therefore be viewed as one long blessing (beginning and ending with "blessed") praising God for His daily recreation of nature.

Pesukei DeZimra concludes with a second blessing, which begins:

וַיְבָרֶךְ דָּוִיד אֶת ה׳...
בָּרוּךְ אַתָּה ה׳
אֱלֹהֵי יִשְׂרָאֵל אָבִינוּ,
מֵעוֹלָם וְעַד עוֹלָם.

David blessed the Lord...
Blessed are you, Lord,
God of our father Israel,
for ever and ever. (1 Chr. 29:10)

This blessing ends with the paragraph of *Yishtabaḥ* (May [Your name] be praised), which itself ends:

בָּרוּךְ אַתָּה ה׳...
מֶלֶךְ אֵל, חֵי הָעוֹלָמִים.

Blessed are You, Lord...
King, God, Giver of life to the world.[42]

The second blessing's central paragraph is אָז יָשִׁיר (*Az Yashir*), the song that Moses, Miriam, and the Israelites sang after the Exodus from Egypt when crossing the sea (Ex. 15:1–21).

While the first blessing of *Pesukei DeZimra* praises God for His role in creating and sustaining the natural world, the second blessing recognizes that sometimes God operates outside of the natural order. The Splitting of the Sea was a paradigmatic moment. It was then that God saved the Israelites, reversing the laws of nature by performing this miracle.

In a very real sense, *Pesukei DeZimra* is multi-directional. On its surface, it moves from recognizing the hand of God in the natural order to recognizing it in the supernatural realm. The reverse is also true. By experiencing God in a supernatural way, one may be inspired to a greater awareness of God's presence in the more natural occurrences of life. Thus, when contemplating the Splitting of the Sea, one may gain a greater appreciation of its everyday miracles – of its water being contained

42. I first heard the idea that *Pesukei DeZimra* can be broken into two long blessings from Rabbi Saul Berman.

within its banks, of the wondrous marine life it sustains, of the water it supplies, and the passageway it provides. In the words of Nahmanides:

> וּמִן הַנִּסִּים הַגְּדוֹלִים הַמְפוּרְסָמִים אָדָם מוֹדֶה בְּנִסִּים הַנִּסְתָּרִים שֶׁהֵם יְסוֹד הַתּוֹרָה כֻּלָּהּ.
>
> And from the great, well-known miracles, one is able to acknowledge the hidden miracles, which are the foundation of the entire Torah.[43]

From this perspective, the supernatural miracles highlighted at the end of *Pesukei DeZimra* not only reflect God's ultimate power, but serve as a means to better appreciate the miraculous hand of God in the natural order, as stressed in the earlier part of *Pesukei DeZimra.*

Having extolled God for His creative powers in both the natural and supernatural realms, *Pesukei DeZimra* reaches its crescendo with the paragraph of יִשְׁתַּבַּח שִׁמְךָ לָעַד מַלְכֵּנוּ – "May Your name be praised forever, our King."[44] It is not God who needs these praises. Rather, it is the human being who, in *tefilla,* hopefully feels a passionate desire to say, "thank You." It's much like love. If I love you, truly love you, I am driven to reach out and express my love to you.[45]

I remember giving Rabbi Joseph B. Soloveitchik a note soon after his mother, brother, and wife died within a short span of time. In the note, I expressed my deepest appreciation for "the Rav" and offered the blessing that he be spared more pain.[46] I signed it, "*BeAhava,* your student, Avraham." Years later, in private conversation, I brought up the note. He generously thanked me for having written it, but went on to say that there was no need for me to go out of my way to express my appreciation. I responded that my admiration, respect, and love for him

43. Nahmanides, Exodus 13:15, s.v. *uletotafot.*
44. For an understanding of *Pesukei DeZimra* as introductory to *Birkhot Shema,* see chapter 8.
45. The Half Kaddish concluding the morning blessings and *Pesukei DeZimra* is now said. For an analysis of *Kaddish* as the model of "prayer as responsibility," see the end of chapter 1.
46. Rabbi Joseph B. Soloveitchik was affectionately called "the Rav" (the Rabbi).

Pesukei DeZimra

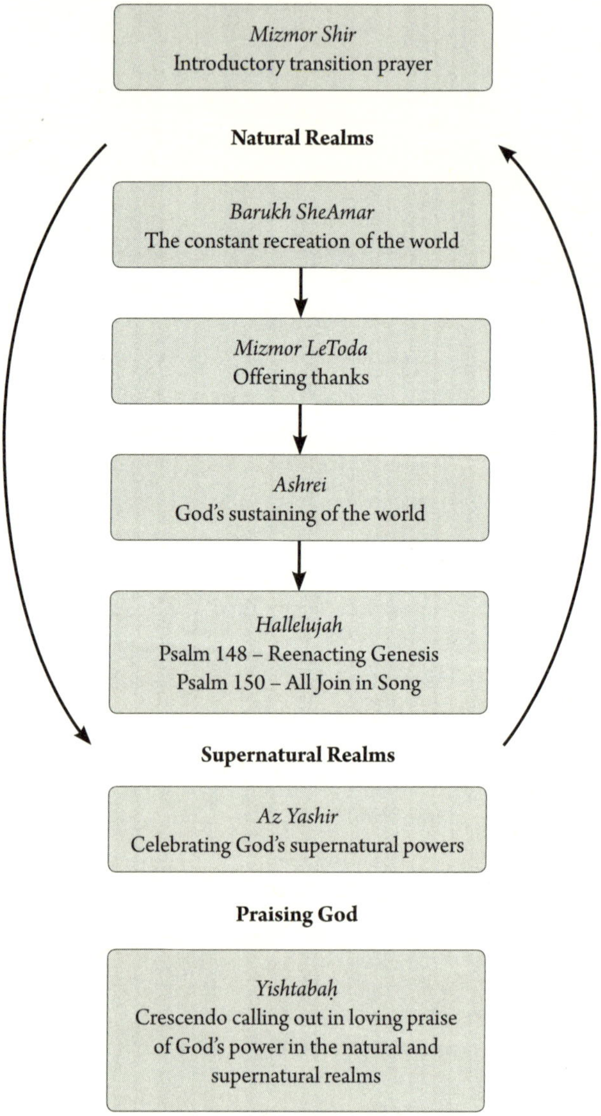

impelled me to write – not only for him, but for myself. I needed to thank him, to say, "*BeAhava*." The Rav gently nodded – he understood.

Birkhot Shema – The *Shema* Blessings

Pesukei DeZimra is followed by the blessings of *Shema* (*Birkhot Shema*), focusing on the renewal of Israel as a people. There are, as the Mishna states, three blessings: "In the morning one recites two blessings before [the *Shema*] and one blessing after [the *Shema*]."[47] As a composite, the three blessings relate to the way the nation of Israel constantly reenergizes its relationship with God.

The first blessing focuses on God as the universal Creator. Hence, throughout this blessing, God is referred to as *Melekh*, King, Ruler. Here we affirm our place in God's larger world.

הַמֵּאִיר לָאָרֶץ וְלַדָּרִים עָלֶיהָ...
הַמֶּלֶךְ הַמְרוֹמָם לְבַדּוֹ מֵאָז...
בָּרוּךְ אַתָּה ה׳ יוֹצֵר הַמְּאוֹרוֹת.

> He illuminates the earth [and provides light] for those who dwell on it…
> He is the King exalted alone from the beginning of time…
> Blessed are You, Lord, who forms the radiant lights (*Yotzer HaMe'orot*).

The second blessing is more particularistic. Every day we recall that moment when God invited us to become His treasured people, giving us the Torah and the Land of Israel:

אַהֲבָה רַבָּה אֲהַבְתָּנוּ ה׳ אֱ־לֹהֵינוּ...
אָבִינוּ הָאָב הָרַחֲמָן, הַמְרַחֵם רַחֵם עָלֵינוּ...
וְהָאֵר עֵינֵינוּ בְּתוֹרָתֶךָ...
וַהֲבִיאֵנוּ לְשָׁלוֹם מֵאַרְבַּע כַּנְפוֹת הָאָרֶץ
וְתוֹלִיכֵנוּ קוֹמְמִיּוּת לְאַרְצֵנוּ

47. Mishna Berakhot 1:4 (Berakhot 11a).

כִּי אֵל פּוֹעֵל יְשׁוּעוֹת אָתָּה
וּבָנוּ בָחַרְתָּ מִכָּל עַם וְלָשׁוֹן
וְקֵרַבְתָּנוּ לְשִׁמְךָ הַגָּדוֹל סֶלָה בֶּאֱמֶת
לְהוֹדוֹת לְךָ וּלְיַחֶדְךָ בְּאַהֲבָה
בָּרוּךְ אַתָּה ה׳ הַבּוֹחֵר בְּעַמּוֹ יִשְׂרָאֵל בְּאַהֲבָה.

> You have loved us with great love, Lord our God...
> Our Father, Compassionate Father (*Av HaRaḥaman*), ever compassionate...
> Enlighten our eyes with Your Torah...
> Bring us back in peace from the four quarters of the earth,
> and lead us upright to our land.
> For You are a God who performs acts of salvation,
> and You chose us from all peoples and tongues,
> bringing us close to Your great name forever in truth,
> that we may thank You and proclaim your Oneness in love.
> Blessed are You, Lord, who chooses His people Israel with love (*HaBoḥer BeAmo Yisrael BeAhava*).

In this particularistic blessing, God is referred to no longer as *Melekh*, but as *Av HaRaḥaman* – "Compassionate Father."[48] In fact, the term *Raḥaman* is feminine, as its root is ר.ח.ם (R-Ḥ-M), which literally means "womb," reflecting the infinite and endless love of a mother. God is a God who is close, intimate, and loving. This is the only blessing that begins and ends with the word *ahava* (love).

Shema

The *Shema* is the fulcrum of the service. Recited after the first two blessings of the *Shema* – the blessings descriptive of God's universal and particularistic reach – the opening sentence of *Shema* powerfully reaffirms our faith in God. Thus we proclaim: שְׁמַע יִשְׂרָאֵל – "Listen, O Israel," ה׳ –

48. Note also the blessing's particularistic stress on the ingathering of the exiles to Israel. Alternatively, after speaking of God's endless power in the first blessing, the second stresses God's concern for the minutiae of life. The Creator of the cosmos is also the loving *Av HaRaḥaman*.

"the Lord [God of mercy and love]," אֱ־לֹהֵינוּ – "our God [God of power and titanic strength]," ה׳ אֶחָד – "the Lord [God of both characteristics] is One" (Deut. 6:4). There is only one perfect God, the absolute Unity who possesses the traits of immanence and transcendence, who is particularistic and universalistic.[49]

The more appropriate translation of the word *Shema* is "listen" rather than "hear." There is a great difference between the two. "Hear" is superficial; the words do not penetrate. "Listen" means to integrate; to take in, to ingest the words being said. A husband and wife, for example, often hear each other but do not listen to each other. In the *Shema* we pray that Israel "listen," not just "hear," as the Oneness of God is declared.

For the *Sefat Emet*, that declaration is a continuation of God's pronouncement made at Sinai that He is the Lord. *Shema Yisrael* is, therefore, nothing less than God's call to all of Israel to listen clearly to these words. As the *Sefat Emet* states:

וְאוֹמְרִים בְּכָל יוֹם
שְׁמַע יִשְׂרָאֵל ה׳ אֱ־לֹהֵינוּ ה׳ אֶחָד
וְהוּא הַמַּאֲמָר
אָנֹכִי ה׳ אֱ־לֹהֶיךָ
אֲשֶׁר לֹא פָּסַק.

Every day we say,
"Listen, O Israel, the Lord our God, the Lord is One" (Deut. 6:4).
This is the Voice [of God] saying,
"I am the Lord your God" (Ex. 20:2),
which has never stopped.[50]

---

49. Note that before the *Shema,* the blessings move from the universal to the particularistic (from יוֹצֵר הַמְּאוֹרוֹת, "who forms the radiant lights," to הַבּוֹחֵר בְּעַמּוֹ יִשְׂרָאֵל בְּאַהֲבָה, "who chooses His people Israel with love"). Whatever one's involvement in the broader world of social justice, one should never forget his or her national responsibility. The progression is reversed in the *Shema,* teaching that involvement with one's people should not obviate one's sacred commitment to the outside world.

50. *Sefat Emet,* Genesis, *Va'era* 5659, s.v. *Bapasuk hein Benei Yisrael.* See chapter 8 for further explication.

A fascinating passage from the Talmud understands *Shema Yisrael* as the words recited by Jacob's sons to their father, who was also called *Yisrael* (Israel):

> Jacob wished to reveal to his sons the end of days [the final universal redemption], whereupon the *Shekhina* departed from him. Jacob said, "Perhaps, Heaven forbid, there is one unfit among my children."... But his sons answered him, "Listen, O Israel, the Lord our God, the Lord is One" [Deut. 6:4]. [In plain words, addressing Jacob by his other name, Israel, the sons said:] "Just as there is only One in your heart, so there is only One in our heart." In that moment our father Jacob opened [his mouth] and exclaimed, "Blessed be the name of His glorious kingdom for ever and ever (בָּרוּךְ שֵׁם כְּבוֹד מַלְכוּתוֹ לְעוֹלָם וָעֶד)."[51]

Like Jacob's sons of old, the Children of Israel reaffirm their belief in the One and Only God when reciting *Shema*. Thus, *Shema* is a chorus of God speaking to Israel, declaring the first of the Sinaitic revelations, and Israel speaking to God, reaffirming its commitment to the One, the only One.

The *Shema* continues with an expression of Israel's love for God. This may be a response to the seal of the blessing immediately prior to the *Shema*, which speaks of God's love for Israel (*HaBoḥer Be'amo Yisrael Be'ahava*). In this unit of liturgy, God initiates the love relationship; with the *Shema*, Israel responds.

By definition, love involves full commitment. This too is spelled out in the *Shema* as we dedicate heart (*levavekha*),[52] soul (*nafshekha*), and body (*me'odekha*)[53] to God. The sentence reads:

> וְאָהַבְתָּ אֵת ה׳ אֱלוֹהֶיךָ בְּכָל לְבָבְךָ וּבְכָל נַפְשְׁךָ וּבְכָל מְאֹדֶךָ.
>
> Love the Lord your God with all your heart, with all your soul, and with all your might. (Deut. 6:5)

---

51. Pesaḥim 56a. See also Maimonides, *Code*, Laws of Recitation of the *Shema* 1:4.
52. *Lev*, literally the heart, is interchangeable with the mind in biblical and rabbinic literature.
53. *Uvekhol me'odekha*, literally "with all your might," relates to the body, to physically doing all we can to serve God.

This is followed by the paragraph beginning *VeHaya,* which renews our commitment to the mitzvot (commandments). Note that the word *vehaya* (וְהָיָה) is an anagram of God's holiest name – the Tetragrammaton, the Y-H-V-H – as there is recognition that the mitzvot come from God.

> וְהָיָה אִם שָׁמֹעַ תִּשְׁמְעוּ אֶל מִצְוֹתַי אֲשֶׁר אָנֹכִי מְצַוֶּה אֶתְכֶם הַיּוֹם לְאַהֲבָה אֶת ה׳ אֱ־לֹהֵיכֶם וּלְעָבְדוֹ בְּכָל לְבַבְכֶם וּבְכָל נַפְשְׁכֶם.
>
> If you indeed heed My commandments with which I charge you today, to love the Lord your God and worship Him with all your heart and with all your soul. (Deut. 11:13)

The third paragraph, that of the *tzitzit,* offers tools through which one may reinforce belief in God and observance of His commandments:

> וַיֹּאמֶר ה׳ אֶל מֹשֶׁה לֵּאמֹר דַּבֵּר אֶל בְּנֵי יִשְׂרָאֵל וְאָמַרְתָּ אֲלֵהֶם וְעָשׂוּ לָהֶם צִיצִת עַל כַּנְפֵי בִגְדֵיהֶם לְדֹרֹתָם וְנָתְנוּ עַל צִיצִת הַכָּנָף פְּתִיל תְּכֵלֶת וְהָיָה לָכֶם לְצִיצִת וּרְאִיתֶם אֹתוֹ וּזְכַרְתֶּם אֶת כָּל מִצְוֹת ה׳ וַעֲשִׂיתֶם אֹתָם.
>
> The Lord spoke to Moses, saying: Speak to the Israelites and tell them to make a tassel (*tzitzit*) on the corners of their garments for all generations. They shall attach to the tassel at each corner a thread of blue (*tekhelet*). This shall be your tassel, and you shall see it and remember all the Lord's commandments and observe them. (Num. 15:37–39)

Tekhelet is the biblical term for the blue string wrapped around the white ones. The Talmud suggests that it is colored blue to remind us of the heavens, the seat of God: "*Tekhelet* can be likened to the sea, the sea to the heavens, and the heavens to the glorious throne of God."[54] Moreover, the numerical value of *tzitzit* (600 = צִיצִית) plus the number of threads (8) and knots (5) in the fringes add up to 613, the number of mitzvot.[55]

The passage ends:

---

54. Menaḥot 43a. *Tekhelet* (תְּכֵלֶת) too, as indicated in the introduction to this work, may be a play on the word *takhlit* (תַּכְלִית), the Ultimate Purpose – God Himself.
55. See Rashi, Numbers 15:39, s.v. *uzekhartem*.

וּרְאִיתֶם אֹתוֹ וּזְכַרְתֶּם אֶת כָּל מִצְוֹת ה׳ וַעֲשִׂיתֶם אֹתָם.

> And you shall see it [the *tzitzit*] and remember all the Lord's commandments and observe them. (Num. 15:39)

The progression in *Shema* from belief in God to adherence to mitzvot is noted in the Talmud:

> R. Yehoshua b. Korḥa said, Why was the section of "Listen" (*Shema*) placed before that of "If you… heed My commandments" (*VeHaya*)? So that one should first accept the yoke of the Kingdom of Heaven and then take upon himself the yoke of the commandments.[56]

Yet another way to understand the relationship between these three paragraphs is by recalling that the best reward for a good deed is the deed itself. Belief in God and loving Him with all our heart and soul – *Shema* – leads us to be happy with our lot in life. Whatever occurs, we feel inwardly blessed – *VeHaya*. In turn, it yields feelings of protection and redemption, the hallmark of the portion of *tzitzit*.[57]

Indeed, the third paragraph of the *Shema* deals with deliverance: אֲנִי ה׳ אֱ־לֹהֵיכֶם, אֲשֶׁר הוֹצֵאתִי אֶתְכֶם מֵאֶרֶץ מִצְרַיִם – "I am the Lord Your God, who brought you out of the land of Egypt" (Num. 15:41). Appropriately, it is followed by the third and final blessing of *Shema*, which recalls the moment in history when God delivered us from Egypt:

מִמִּצְרַיִם גְּאַלְתָּנוּ ה׳ אֱ־לֹהֵינוּ
וּמִבֵּית עֲבָדִים פְּדִיתָנוּ.

> From Egypt You liberated us, Lord our God,
> And from the slave house You delivered us.

---

56. Berakhot 13a. For some, rather than being the result of belief, the mitzvot may be a means of coming to believe. See Jerusalem Talmud, Ḥagiga 1:7, paraphrasing God: Better the Jews forsake Me and observe My Torah, for through observance they will come to believe.

57. This approach is not meant to take away from the literal meaning of these paragraphs with all their inherent problems, as the good are not necessarily rewarded and the bad punished. Rather, it is meant as an additional spiritual insight.

Birkhot Shema
Reenergizing Israel as a People

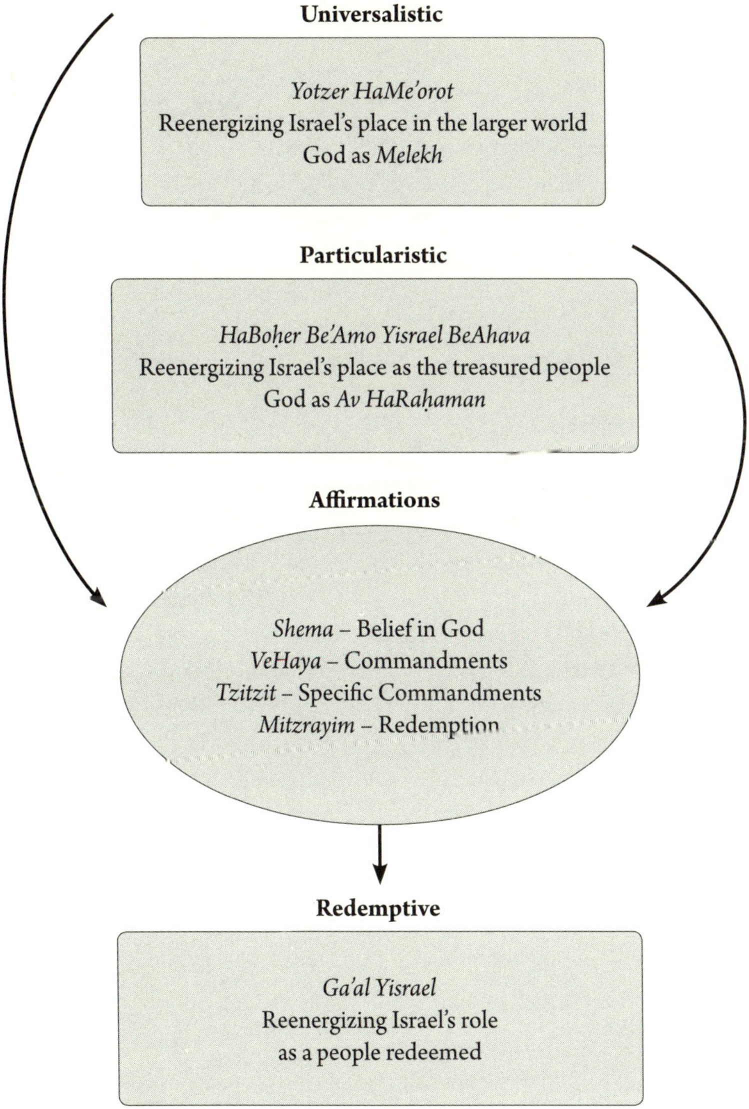

Recited every morning, the blessing shifts from the past tense to the present, expressing the belief that God will forever be with us. No matter the challenges, we will prevail:

צוּר יִשְׂרָאֵל קוּמָה בְּעֶזְרַת יִשְׂרָאֵל
וּפְדֵה כִנְאֻמֶךָ יְהוּדָה וְיִשְׂרָאֵל
גֹּאֲלֵנוּ ה׳ צְבָ־אוֹת שְׁמוֹ קְדוֹשׁ יִשְׂרָאֵל
בָּרוּךְ אַתָּה ה׳ גָּאַל יִשְׂרָאֵל.

Rock of Israel! Arise to the help of Israel.
Deliver, as You promised, Judah and Israel.
Our Redeemer, the Lord of hosts is His name,
The Holy One of Israel.
Blessed are You, Lord, who redeemed Israel (*Ga'al Yisrael*).[58]

Amida – The Silent Meditation

While the *Shema*'s central theme is *ahavat Hashem*, loving God, וְאָהַבְתָּ אֵת ה׳ אֱ־לֹהֶיךָ – "Love the Lord your God," the *Amida* stresses *yirat Hashem*, being in awe of God: הָאֵ־ל הַגָּדוֹל הַגִּבּוֹר וְהַנּוֹרָא אֵ־ל עֶלְיוֹן – "The great, mighty, and awesome God Most High."[59] Love draws one near; awe elicits instinctive retreat. Together, *ahavat Hashem* and *yirat Hashem* forge a delicate balance of closeness and distance, intimacy with boundaries. Like the major organs of the body, the *Shema* and the *Amida* are the heart and brain of the morning service, with other prayers serving as connecting vessels to and from these central *tefillot*.

In rabbinic literature, the term "*tefilla*" refers to the *Amida*,[60] as the *Amida* marks the high point of the service. In it, one supplicates God regarding personal and communal concerns. Not surprisingly, the blessing of deliverance precedes the *Amida*, as this blessing reaffirms one's belief in a God who has the power to deliver and help His people. At this point, one is properly prepared to begin the *Amida*, in which one petitions God for private and public needs. The Talmud makes this point:

58. For further analysis of the blessings of the *Shema*, see chapter 8.
59. See Maimonides, *Code*, Laws of the Foundations of the Torah 2:1, 2.
60. See, for example, Berakhot 4:1.

> R. Yoḥanan said: Who is worthy of the World to Come? One who juxtaposes the blessing of redemption to the *tefilla* [*Amida*].[61]

The opening of the *Amida* contains three *Birkhot Shevaḥ*, blessings of praise. They begin with a blessing describing God's presence in the past:

בָּרוּךְ אַתָּה ה׳ אֱ־לֹהֵינוּ וֵא־לֹהֵי אֲבוֹתֵינוּ
אֱ־לֹהֵי אַבְרָהָם אֱ־לֹהֵי יִצְחָק וֵא־לֹהֵי יַעֲקֹב...
בָּרוּךְ אַתָּה ה׳ מָגֵן אַבְרָהָם.

> *Avoteinu*: Blessed are You,
> Lord our God and God of our fathers,
> God of Abraham, God of Isaac, and God of Jacob....
> Blessed are You, Lord, Shield of Abraham.

It continues with a blessing describing God's power in the present:

אַתָּה גִּבּוֹר לְעוֹלָם, אֲ־דֹנָי...
סוֹמֵךְ נוֹפְלִים וְרוֹפֵא חוֹלִים, וּמַתִּיר אֲסוּרִים...
בָּרוּךְ אַתָּה ה׳ מְחַיֵּה הַמֵּתִים.

> *Ata Gibbor*: You are eternally mighty, Lord....
> He supports the fallen, heals the sick, sets captives free....
> Blessed are You, Lord, who revives the dead.

The contemplation of God's involvement from the beginning of time to the present evokes mounting awe of His exaltedness. Thus, the blessings of praise peak with a declaration of God's holiness:

אַתָּה קָדוֹשׁ וְשִׁמְךָ קָדוֹשׁ
וּקְדוֹשִׁים בְּכָל יוֹם יְהַלְלוּךָ סֶּלָה.
בָּרוּךְ אַתָּה ה׳ הָאֵ־ל הַקָּדוֹשׁ.

> *Ata Kadosh*: You are holy and Your name is holy,
> and holy ones praise You daily, Selah!
> Blessed are You, Lord, the holy God.

61. Ibid. 4b.

Yet, as exalted as God may be, He still allows people to come close and pour forth their needs. So the *Amida* now ventures into the terrain of *bakashot* – requests.[62]

In no small measure, what we ask for defines who we are, as requests spell out what is important to us. Indeed, the prayer service can be seen not only as a forum to express one's needs but as an educational tool to learn what we should be asking for. Hence, when beginning the *Birkhot Bakasha,* blessings of request, we go through a process of self-evaluation, as such reflection should be important to us. We begin with the blessing of understanding, the foundation of self-assessment:

אַתָּה חוֹנֵן לְאָדָם דַּעַת,
וּמְלַמֵּד לֶאֱנוֹשׁ בִּינָה.
חָנֵּנוּ מֵאִתְּךָ דֵּעָה בִּינָה וְהַשְׂכֵּל.
בָּרוּךְ אַתָּה ה׳, חוֹנֵן הַדָּעַת.

> *Ata Ḥonen*: You grace humanity with knowledge
> and teach mortals understanding.
> Grace us with the knowledge, understanding
> and discernment that come from You.
> Blessed are You, Lord, who graciously grants knowledge.

Once we are blessed with the capacity to understand our strengths and weaknesses, we can move forward on the path toward self-improvement:

הֲשִׁיבֵנוּ אָבִינוּ לְתוֹרָתֶךָ
וְקָרְבֵנוּ מַלְכֵּנוּ לַעֲבוֹדָתֶךָ
וְהַחֲזִירֵנוּ בִּתְשׁוּבָה שְׁלֵמָה לְפָנֶיךָ
בָּרוּךְ אַתָּה ה׳ הָרוֹצֶה בִּתְשׁוּבָה.

> *Hashiveinu Avinu*: Bring us back, our Father, to Your Torah.
> Draw us near, our King, to Your service.
> Lead us back to You in perfect repentance.
> Blessed are You, Lord, who desires repentance.

62. In chapter 2, we pointed out that one hopes for an affirmative response to a request. But at their core, requests in *tefilla* are expressions of fellowship with God. The petitioner no longer feels alone.

This process of self-evaluation concludes with a blessing that we be forgiven:

סְלַח לָנוּ אָבִינוּ כִּי חָטָאנוּ
מְחַל לָנוּ מַלְכֵּנוּ כִּי פָשָׁעְנוּ
כִּי מוֹחֵל וְסוֹלֵחַ אָתָּה.
בָּרוּךְ אַתָּה ה׳, חַנּוּן הַמַּרְבֶּה לִסְלוֹחַ.

Selaḥ Lanu: Forgive us, our Father, for we have sinned;
pardon us, our King, for we have transgressed;
for You pardon and forgive.
Blessed are You, Lord, the gracious One who repeatedly forgives.

In general terms, these three blessings parallel the formula for self-renewal as outlined by Maimonides – recognition of wrong (*hakarat haḥet*), repentance (*teshuva*), and forgiveness (*seliḥa*).[63]

The blessings that follow form a distinct unit dealing with personal well-being. They open with a request for inner peace – that we be free of personal crisis and turmoil:[64]

רְאֵה בְעָנְיֵנוּ, וְרִיבָה רִיבֵנוּ
וּגְאָלֵנוּ מְהֵרָה לְמַעַן שְׁמֶךָ
כִּי גּוֹאֵל חָזָק אָתָּה.
בָּרוּךְ אַתָּה ה׳, גּוֹאֵל יִשְׂרָאֵל.

Re'eh VeOnyeinu: Look on our affliction, plead our cause,
and redeem us soon for Your name's sake,
for You are a powerful Redeemer.
Blessed are You, Lord, the Redeemer of Israel.

There is a powerful connection between emotional and physical well-being. Hence, *Re'eh Ve'Onyeinu* is followed by the blessing for healing:

63. See Maimonides, *Code*, Laws of Repentance 1:1.
64. Later blessings of request deal with national redemption.

רְפָאֵנוּ ה׳ וְנֵרָפֵא
הוֹשִׁיעֵנוּ וְנִוָּשֵׁעָה, כִּי תְהִלָּתֵנוּ אָתָּה
וְהַעֲלֵה רְפוּאָה שְׁלֵמָה לְכָל מַכּוֹתֵינוּ
כִּי אֵל מֶלֶךְ רוֹפֵא נֶאֱמָן וְרַחֲמָן אָתָּה.
בָּרוּךְ אַתָּה ה׳, רוֹפֵא חוֹלֵי עַמּוֹ יִשְׂרָאֵל.

Refa'einu: Heal us, Lord, and we shall be healed;
save us and we shall be saved;
for You are our praise.
Bring about a complete recovery from all our ailments,
for You, God, King, are a faithful and compassionate Healer.
Blessed are You, Lord, Healer of the sick of His people Israel.

Once feeling emotionally and physically strengthened, we are in a better position to ask God for help in providing for ourselves. Thus, the blessing for prosperity follows:

בָּרֵךְ עָלֵינוּ ה׳ אֱ־לֹהֵינוּ אֶת הַשָּׁנָה הַזֹּאת
וְאֶת כָּל מִינֵי תְבוּאָתָהּ, לְטוֹבָה
וְתֵן בְּרָכָה/וְתֵן טַל וּמָטָר לִבְרָכָה
עַל פְּנֵי הָאֲדָמָה, וְשַׂבְּעֵנוּ מִטּוּבָהּ
וּבָרֵךְ שְׁנָתֵנוּ כַּשָּׁנִים הַטּוֹבוֹת.
בָּרוּךְ אַתָּה ה׳, מְבָרֵךְ הַשָּׁנִים.

Barekh Aleinu: Bless this year for us, Lord our God,
and all its types of produce for good.
[*In winter:*] Grant dew and rain as a blessing
[*In other seasons:*] Grant blessing
on the face of the earth, and from its goodness satisfy us,
blessing our year as the best of years.
Blessed are You, Lord, who blesses the years.

In the *Amida*'s communal requests, we reaffirm our commitment to covenant. Covenant involves three elements: mission, people, and land. In the *Amida*, we articulate what our goals are, who merits to carry them out, and how in particular they will be achieved. Our mission is outlined in the blessing for justice. Note that the last two words of the blessing are lifted from the Torah, where God shares the mission of Judaism: **וְשָׁמְרוּ דֶּרֶךְ ה׳ לַעֲשׂוֹת צְדָקָה וּמִשְׁפָּט** – "to safeguard the way of the Lord, to do righteousness and justice" (Gen. 18:19).

הָשִׁיבָה שׁוֹפְטֵינוּ כְּבָרִאשׁוֹנָה, וְיוֹעֲצֵינוּ כְּבַתְּחִלָּה,
וְהָסֵר מִמֶּנּוּ יָגוֹן וַאֲנָחָה
וּמְלוֹךְ עָלֵינוּ אַתָּה ה׳ לְבַדְּךָ בְּחֶסֶד וּבְרַחֲמִים
וְצַדְּקֵנוּ בַּמִּשְׁפָּט.
בָּרוּךְ אַתָּה ה׳ מֶלֶךְ אוֹהֵב צְדָקָה וּמִשְׁפָּט.

Hashiva Shofteinu: Restore our judges as at first
and our counselors as at the beginning,
and remove from us sorrow and sighing.
May You alone, Lord,
reign over us with loving-kindness and compassion,
and vindicate us in justice.
Blessed are You, Lord,
the King who loves righteousness and justice.

In the blessing for individuals who carry out the mission, we refer to an array of people, from lofty leaders to the common folk – with special mention of converts, who too often are shunned and pushed aside. All take part in the dream of Israel and the world redeemed:

עַל הַצַּדִּיקִים וְעַל הַחֲסִידִים
וְעַל זִקְנֵי עַמְּךָ בֵּית יִשְׂרָאֵל
וְעַל פְּלֵיטַת סוֹפְרֵיהֶם
וְעַל גֵּרֵי הַצֶּדֶק,
וְעָלֵינוּ
יֶהֱמוּ רַחֲמֶיךָ ה׳ אֱ־לֹהֵינוּ
וְתֵן שָׂכָר טוֹב לְכָל הַבּוֹטְחִים בְּשִׁמְךָ בֶּאֱמֶת
וְשִׂים חֶלְקֵנוּ עִמָּהֶם, וּלְעוֹלָם וְלֹא נֵבוֹשׁ כִּי בְךָ בָּטָחְנוּ.
בָּרוּךְ אַתָּה ה׳, מִשְׁעָן וּמִבְטָח לַצַּדִּיקִים.

Al HaTzaddikim: To the righteous, the pious,
the elders of Your people the House of Israel,
the remnant of their scholars,
the righteous converts,
and to us,
may Your compassion be aroused,
Lord our God.
Grant a good reward to all who sincerely trust in Your name.
Set our lot with them,
so that we may never be ashamed, for in You we trust.
Blessed are You, Lord,
who is the support and trust of the righteous.[65]

We focus on Israel in the blessing for Jerusalem. It is there that the destiny of the Jewish people is forged.

וְלִירוּשָׁלַיִם עִירְךָ בְּרַחֲמִים תָּשׁוּב
וְתִשְׁכֹּן בְּתוֹכָהּ כַּאֲשֶׁר דִּבַּרְתָּ
וּבְנֵה אוֹתָהּ בְּקָרוֹב בְּיָמֵינוּ בִּנְיַן עוֹלָם
וְכִסֵּא דָוִד מְהֵרָה לְתוֹכָהּ תָּכִין.
בָּרוּךְ אַתָּה ה׳, בּוֹנֵה יְרוּשָׁלָיִם.

VeLiYerushalayim: To Jerusalem, Your city,
may You return in compassion,
and may You dwell in it as You promised.
May You rebuild it rapidly in our days
as an everlasting structure,
and install within it soon the throne of David.
Blessed are You, Lord, who builds Jerusalem.[66]

---

65. This blessing is preceded by that of *VeLaMalshinim*, וְלַמַּלְשִׁינִים אַל תְּהִי תִקְוָה וְכָל הָרִשְׁעָה כְּרֶגַע תֹּאבֵד – "And for slanderers let there be no hope, and may all wickedness perish in an instant." Before listing those who are part of the mission, we list those who are not.
66. The unit of blessings dealing with the covenantal mission is introduced by תְּקַע בְּשׁוֹפָר גָּדוֹל לְחֵרוּתֵנוּ – "Sound the great shofar for our freedom," which calls for the redemptive period to begin. It is followed by a closing blessing, אֶת צֶמַח דָּוִד עַבְדְּךָ

The request blessings end with a generic request that God listen to our voices:

שְׁמַע קוֹלֵנוּ ה׳ אֱ־לֹהֵינוּ,
חוּס וְרַחֵם עָלֵינוּ,
וְקַבֵּל בְּרַחֲמִים וּבְרָצוֹן אֶת תְּפִלָּתֵנוּ,
כִּי אֵל שׁוֹמֵעַ תְּפִלּוֹת וְתַחֲנוּנִים אָתָּה.
וּמִלְּפָנֶיךָ מַלְכֵּנוּ רֵיקָם אַל תְּשִׁיבֵנוּ,
כִּי אַתָּה שׁוֹמֵעַ תְּפִלַּת עַמְּךָ יִשְׂרָאֵל בְּרַחֲמִים.
בָּרוּךְ אַתָּה ה׳
שׁוֹמֵעַ תְּפִלָּה.

Shema Koleinu: Listen to our voice, Lord our God.
Spare us and have compassion on us,
and in compassion and favor accept our prayer,
for You, God, listen to prayers and pleas.
Do not turn us away, O our King,
empty-handed from Your presence,
for You listen with compassion
to the prayer of Your people Israel.
Blessed are You, Lord, who listens to prayer.

The first time the phrase "listen to a voice" is found in the Torah is when Adam and Eve "listened to the voice of the Lord God walking in the garden" – וַיִּשְׁמְעוּ אֶת קוֹל ה׳ אֱ־לֹהִים מִתְהַלֵּךְ בַּגָּן (Gen. 3:8). The blessing in the *Amida* complements this biblical passage, as it deals with God's listening to the voices of human beings. The human-God relationship thrives when each listens to the voice of the other.[67]

מְהֵרָה תַצְמִיחַ – "May You speedily cause the offspring of Your servant David to flourish," which offers the hope that our covenantal mission will soon be fulfilled in the Messianic Era.

67. For a discussion of the request blessings as reverberating and assertive prayers, see chapters 1 and 3.

Birkhot Bakasha of the *Amida*

Individual blessings

Self Evaluation

Ata Ḥonen – Recognition
Hashiveinu Avinu – Repentance
Selaḥ Lanu – Forgiveness

Personal Well-Being

Re'eh Ve'Onyeinu – Emotional Stability
Refa'einu – Health
Barekh Aleinu – Prosperity

Communal Blessings

Covenant

Teka BeShofar – Introductory Call
Hashiva Shofteinu – Mission
VeLaMalshinim – People
Al HaTzaddikim – People
VeLiYerushalayim – Place
Et Tzemaḥ – Realization of Redemption

Closing Blessing

Culmination

Shema Koleinu – All-Inclusive

The final blessings of the *Amida* begin with:

רְצֵה ה׳ אֱ-לֹהֵינוּ
בְּעַמְּךָ יִשְׂרָאֵל
וּבִתְפִלָּתָם....

Retzeh: Find favor, Lord our God,
in Your people Israel
and their prayer....

Here we ask that God willingly accept our prayers. But the word *retzeh* echoes the hope that we make God's will our will, that the prayers heretofore recited were said with personal depth and meaning.[68] The phrase וְכֵן יְהִי רָצוֹן, which on its surface means "and so may it be God's will," reverberates with the flip side, "and so may it be our will."[69]

The *Amida* continues its concluding section with *Birkhot Hoda'a*, blessings of thanksgiving:

מוֹדִים אֲנַחְנוּ לָךְ....
בָּרוּךְ אַתָּה ה׳,
הַטּוֹב שִׁמְךָ
וּלְךָ נָאֶה לְהוֹדוֹת.

Modim: We give thanks to You....
Blessed are You, Lord,
whose name is "The Good,"
and to You it is pleasant to give thanks.

Lehodot is commonly translated "to give thanks." But *lehodot* is also associated with recognition of finitude – in modern Hebrew, it means both "to thank" and "to admit" – and of our natural human limitations, which should impel us to declare: *ani modeh* or *ani moda* – "I admit to my failings."

68. See Seforno, Leviticus 22:29, s.v. *lirtzonkhem*, who interprets *ratzon* as human will and intention instead of the simple meaning of God's favoring the human offerer.
69. I am grateful to Rabbi Steven Exler for inspiring this thought on *Retzeh*. For an analysis of *Retzeh* as a farewell prayer, see chapter 8.

How do we reconcile these two ideas? How can *lehodot* mean "thank you" on the one hand and "limitation" on the other? The answer lies in understanding that there are two kinds of "thank yous."

There is the "thank you" that is perfunctory – the kind we say when someone opens the door for us or serves us as we sit down to eat.

And then there is what can be called a substantive "thank you," the kind that is deep and real. Such thanks come from recognition of limits; the recognition that I can't do it all; that I truly need you to help me in my moment of distress.

In this way, the idea of thanks has been turned on its head. In place of the one receiving the thanks being the important one, it can be suggested that the focus should be on the thanker, who is acknowledging his or her natural human shortcomings and deficiencies. This might be why many people have difficulty saying thank you, as it involves recognition of finitude, that one is limited – that one cannot do it alone.

No wonder, then, that in the daily liturgy, after reciting the *Amida*'s blessings of request – in which we overflow with need – we immediately recite the blessings of thanksgiving. It is not God who needs the thanks, but we who feel impelled to reveal our inadequacies, as we display our deep need for Him. Even if God does not intervene, we thank Him for His fellowship and unconditional love.[70]

The *Amida* draws to a close with שִׂים שָׁלוֹם (*Sim Shalom*), the prayer for peace. Other prayers end with a similar hope (*Kaddish*, Grace After Meals), but here, in the context of peace, we are told that we have been given a תּוֹרַת חַיִּים (*Torat ḥayyim*), a Torah of life. Torah is not foisted upon us by God without reason. It is given lovingly by God as a blueprint of how to live life properly. Torah teaches life lessons, offering a pathway to living a life of "kindness, righteousness … compassion … and peace" – outer peace and inner peace.[71]

70. For a further discussion of *Modim*, see chapter 3.

71. For further analysis of *Sim Shalom*, see chapter 1. The silent *Amida* concludes with *E-lohai Netzor* – see chapter 8; regarding the repetition of the *Amida*, see chapter 6. *Taḥanun* is said at the conclusion of the *Amida*. For a brief analysis of this prayer, see the end of chapter 2. *Taḥanun* is followed by the Half Kaddish concluding the central part of the service – see chapter 1.

Concluding Prayers

The morning service concludes with prayers emphasizing the hope for ultimate redemption. In *Ashrei*, for example, we long for the time when all people will be provided for:

פּוֹתֵחַ אֶת יָדֶךָ וּמַשְׂבִּיעַ לְכָל חַי רָצוֹן.

> You open Your hand and satisfy the desire of every living being. (Ps. 145:16)

In *LaMenatze'aḥ*, we express our desire for universal peace:

אֵלֶּה בָרֶכֶב וְאֵלֶּה בַסּוּסִים וַאֲנַחְנוּ בְּשֵׁם ה׳ אֱ־לֹהֵינוּ נַזְכִּיר.

> Some [rely] upon chariots and some upon horses, but as for us, upon the name of the Lord our God we call. (Ps. 20:8)

In *Uva LeTziyon* we yearn for the coming of the redeemer:

וּבָא לְצִיּוֹן גּוֹאֵל...
וְנִירַשׁ טוֹבָה וּבְרָכָה לִשְׁנֵי יְמוֹת הַמָּשִׁיחַ.

> The redeemer shall come to Zion...
> and we will inherit the goodness and blessing of the messianic days.

The verse קָדוֹשׁ, קָדוֹשׁ, קָדוֹשׁ ה׳ צְבָ־אוֹת מְלֹא כָל הָאָרֶץ כְּבוֹדוֹ. "Holy, holy, holy (*kadosh, kadosh, kadosh*) is the Lord of hosts: the whole world is filled with His glory" (Is. 6:3), as found in *Uva LeTziyon* is most telling. This is the third time it appears in the morning service. The first time, in the first blessing before the *Shema*, it is the angels who proclaim the holiness of God, thus reinforcing the Unity of God, i.e., there is only One God to whom everyone – including angels – is beholden.

On Monday and Thursday mornings, and other occasions, e.g., *Rosh Ḥodesh*, the Torah is read. At the conclusion of the reading, *Ḥatzi Kaddish* is recited.

The second time, recited in the *Kedusha* during the repetition of the *Amida,* has the human being hoping to sanctify God in this world, in sync with the angels sanctifying Him from above.

The third mention, in *Uva LeTziyon,* carries one to the redemptive period, to an era of peace, tranquility, and holiness, when human beings will recite *kadosh, kadosh, kadosh* spontaneously, of their own accord. In the original context in Isaiah 6:3, the complete verse is וְקָרָא זֶה אֶל זֶה וְאָמַר: קָדוֹשׁ, קָדוֹשׁ, קָדוֹשׁ ה' צְבָ־אוֹת – "And one [angel] called to another, saying: 'Holy, holy, holy is the Lord of hosts.'" However, in *Uva LeTziyon,* this phrase, I believe, refers to human beings – in the time of redemption, people will call to one another and say *kadosh, kadosh, kadosh.*[72]

Next comes *Aleinu,* which consists of two paragraphs. The first sets Israel apart, as we declare: שֶׁלֹּא שָׂם חֶלְקֵנוּ כָּהֶם וְגוֹרָלֵנוּ כְּכָל הֲמוֹנָם – "for He has not made our portion like theirs, or our destiny like all their multitudes." The second embraces all of humankind: עַל כֵּן נְקַוֶּה – "We therefore hope." In it, we hope for a time when "the world will be perfected under the reign of the Almighty" – לְתַקֵּן עוֹלָם בְּמַלְכוּת שַׁ־דַּי. This movement teaches that an enlightened sense of national identity, rather than contradicting universal consciousness, is, in fact, a prerequisite to it.[73] *Aleinu* therefore concludes the process of *tefilla* that gradually expands our consciousness from within ourselves as individuals to

72. We recite *kadosh, kadosh, kadosh* on three different occasions in the morning service, representing three different periods, or worlds:

In the blessings of the *Shema, kadosh, kadosh, kadosh* brings us back to the primordial, angelic world, where celestial beings alone proclaimed God's holiness. This is the world of Eden where Adam and Eve lived. (See Dessler, *Mikhtav MeEliyahu, vol.* 2, pp. 137–154, who argues that Adam and Eve in Eden were angelic beings.)

The *Kedusha* of the *Amida* represents the post-Eden world, the world as we know it – the "real world." Here, human beings hopefully follow the path of angels and sanctify God's name in word and deed. *Kadosh, kadosh, kadosh* is said for the last time in *Uva LeTziyon.* This *Kedusha* describes the ideal world – the world as it will one day be, the world redeemed. There, human beings will have achieved the noble state of being enabling them call to one another with voices raised in holiness, living a life of *kedusha.*

See the end of chapter 1 for a discussion of the Whole Kaddish, which follows *Uva LeTziyon.*

73. For further understanding of *Aleinu,* see the end of chapter 1.

Shaḥarit

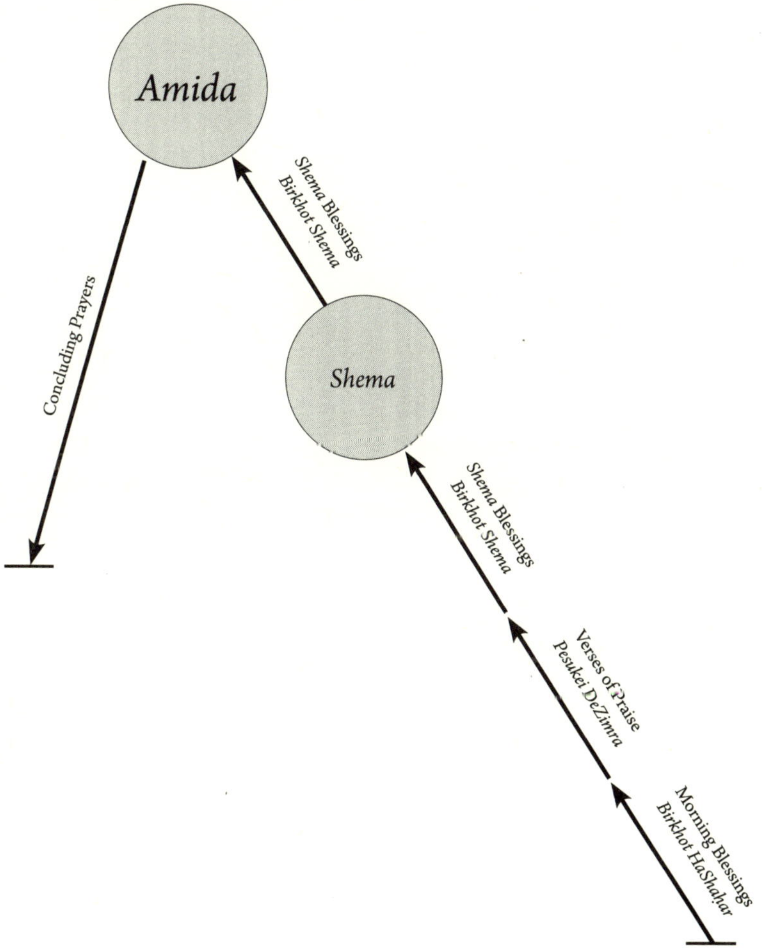
Amida
Shema Blessings
Birkhot Shema
Concluding Prayers
Shema
Shema Blessings
Birkhot Shema
Verses of Praise
Pesukei DeZimra
Morning Blessings
Birkhot HaShaḥar

those around us, our nation, and ultimately, to the entire world. Awakening and connecting us to our role within the universe, its immediate relevance accompanies us as we leave the haven of the synagogue and rejoin the outside world.

In the Daily Psalm (*Shir Shel Yom*) that follows, we recall the song chanted by the Levites in the Temple. By reciting this prayer, we express our longing for the time when the Temple will be rebuilt.[74]

The morning service can be viewed as a symphony of preparatory prayers, elevating us to the *Shema* and higher still to the *Amida*. After this pinnacle, the prayer service gently accompanies us down as we dream of redemption.[75] Coming to rest, we hopefully have impacted our psyche and inner nature, leaving the morning service and beginning our day on a higher spiritual plane.

MINḤA – THE AFTERNOON SERVICE

As noted, the *Minḥa* service is primarily a *tefilla* of introspection. It begins with *Ashrei*, whose key phrase in the afternoon service is רְצוֹן יְרֵאָיו יַעֲשֶׂה – "He fulfills the wishes of those who fear Him" (Ps. 145:19). During *Shaḥarit*, emphasis is placed on the verse פּוֹתֵחַ אֶת יָדֶךָ וּמַשְׂבִּיעַ לְכָל חַי רָצוֹן – "You open Your hand and satisfy the desire of every living being," as part of the morning process of acknowledging the daily renewal of creation. However, in the middle of the day, *Ashrei* serves as a reminder of the importance of following in God's ways.[76]

Ashrei is followed by the meditative *Amida*, a welcome, quiet relief from the humdrum of the busy day. As always, the service concludes with *Aleinu*, wherein we offer the hope that all our endeavors will contribute to repairing the world and reminding us of our roles within the world moments before we rejoin it.

---

74. The Mourner's Kaddish (*Kaddish Yatom*) and the Rabbis' Kaddish (*Kaddish DeRabbanan*) are said toward the beginning and at the end of the service. See chapters 1 and 9 for a discussion of these prayers.
75. See chapter 8 for a discussion of the end blessings of the *Amida*, which serve as farewell blessings.
76. *Tur Shulḥan Arukh, Oraḥ Ḥayyim* 93:1; *Arukh HaShulḥan, Oraḥ Ḥayyim* 93:6.

MA'ARIV – THE EVENING SERVICE

Ma'ariv is about hope. Hence, we begin the service by entreating God as the merciful One:

וְהוּא רַחוּם
יְכַפֵּר עָוֹן וְלֹא יַשְׁחִית.

> He is compassionate.
> He forgives iniquity and does not destroy.

Unlike the morning service, wherein we recite two blessings before *Shema* and one after, in the evening, we recite two before and two after. As the Mishna states, "In the evening two [blessings] are said before [*Shema*] and two after it."[77]

The two preceding blessings parallel the morning blessings of the *Shema*, which deal with God's universal and particularistic reach. The first blessing after *Shema* also corresponds to the morning's hope for redemption. The added blessing *Hashkiveinu*, "Help us lie down," spells out in more detail how redemption is achieved. Called *geula arikhta* – the long blessing of redemption[78] – it focuses on the hope that we be physically and spiritually sheltered by God.

הַשְׁכִּיבֵנוּ ה׳ אֱ־לֹהֵינוּ לְשָׁלוֹם,
וְהַעֲמִידֵנוּ מַלְכֵּנוּ לְחַיִּים,
וּפְרוֹשׂ עָלֵינוּ סֻכַּת שְׁלוֹמֶךָ,
וְתַקְּנֵנוּ בְּעֵצָה טוֹבָה מִלְּפָנֶיךָ,
וְהוֹשִׁיעֵנוּ לְמַעַן שְׁמֶךָ.
וְהָגֵן בַּעֲדֵנוּ, וְהָסֵר מֵעָלֵינוּ אוֹיֵב דֶּבֶר וְחֶרֶב וְרָעָב וְיָגוֹן,
וְהָסֵר שָׂטָן מִלְּפָנֵינוּ וּמֵאַחֲרֵינוּ וּבְצֵל כְּנָפֶיךָ תַּסְתִּירֵנוּ.
כִּי אֵל שׁוֹמְרֵנוּ וּמַצִּילֵנוּ אָתָּה,
כִּי אֵל מֶלֶךְ חַנּוּן וְרַחוּם אָתָּה.
וּשְׁמוֹר צֵאתֵנוּ וּבוֹאֵנוּ, לְחַיִּים וּלְשָׁלוֹם מֵעַתָּה וְעַד עוֹלָם.
בָּרוּךְ אַתָּה ה׳, שׁוֹמֵר עַמּוֹ יִשְׂרָאֵל לָעַד.

---

77. Mishna Berakhot 1:4 (Berakhot 11a).
78. See ibid. 4b.

Help us lie down, O Lord our God, in peace,
and rise up, O our King, to life.
Spread over us Your canopy of peace.
Direct us with Your good counsel,
and save us for the sake of Your name.
Shield us and remove from us every enemy,
plague, sword, famine, and sorrow.
Remove the adversary from before and behind us.
Shelter us in the shadow of Your wings,
for You, God, are our Guardian and Deliverer;
You, God, are a gracious and compassionate King.
Guard our going out and our coming in,
for life and peace, from now and forever.
Blessed are You, Lord, who guards His people Israel forever.

While *Hashkiveinu* stresses God's protection of Israel, the *Ḥatzi Kaddish* that follows speaks of the human contribution to this effort.[79] Together, *Hashkiveinu* and the *Ḥatzi Kaddish* reflect the covenantal partnership between God and humans to redeem Israel and the world. The evening service concludes with the *Amida* and the *Aleinu* prayers.

Permeating this chapter – and, indeed, this entire study – is the motif of prayer as a love encounter with God. In love, it is important to feel the beauty of the other, both from a distance and up close.

On the one hand, it is prudent to step back, to watch from afar and gain perspective. Coming too close might reveal the conflicts that are an inevitable part of every relationship. So it is important to love from a distance.

On the other hand, love is in the details. The test of love is how

79. See the end of chapter 1 for an analysis of this approach to *Kaddish*.

one deals with smaller issues, the seemingly insignificant ones that measure the quality of a relationship. It is therefore important to love up close.

It is the same with *tefilla*. In its broad conceptual sweeps, as well as its specific meaning, prayer has intersecting dimensions, textures, and motifs. Much like love, prayer has many faces. On both its macro and micro levels, prayer ranges from morning "rebirth" to afternoon "reflection" to evening "hope." This majestic tapestry is reflected in these poetic words:

> Love has no other desire but to fulfill itself…
> To wake at dawn with a wingèd heart and give thanks for another day of loving;
> To rest at the noon hour and meditate love's ecstasy;
> To return home at eventide with gratitude;
> And then to sleep with a prayer for the beloved in your heart and a song of praise upon your lips.[80]

80. Khalil Gibran, "Love," *The Prophet*, 1923. Many thanks to Rabbi Avi Orlow for bringing this poem to my attention.

Chapter Five

Place

Rabbi Shlomo Carlebach tells the story of a Munkatcher Hasid who needed a passport to travel from Munkatch to Berlin. He went to his rebbe and pleaded for help. The rebbe went to his room and came out many hours later, giving the Hasid a blank piece of paper drenched with his tears and with what seemed to be the tears of the Jewish people exiled for over two thousand years. "This will serve as your passport," the rebbe said.

When the Hasid came to the border, the German guard demanded to see his passport. He showed him the blank piece of paper. The guard reviewed it carefully. Suddenly he snapped to attention, saluted, and said, "Sir, I don't think Germany has ever had such an honored guest. You will be protected and given VIP treatment wherever you go."

Just before the war broke out in 1939, the Hasid died. On his deathbed, he asked that the Munkatcher passport be placed in his coffin. "If it could get me from Munkatch to Berlin in 1935, perhaps it will open the Gates of Heaven when I leave this world for the next."

The truth, Reb Shlomo explained, is that barriers exist not only between nations. There are "walls" between people – husband and wife, parents and children, human beings and God. What we need most is the Munkatcher passport. What is this passport?

When a child is born and cries, and is comforted by its mother – that's the Munkatcher passport. When a bride circles her groom under the *ḥuppa,* and in silence they look at each other – no words, just deep, emotional love – that's the Munkatcher passport. When we study the

Talmud, one notes that the Gemara begins with daf beit – page two. Page one, daf aleph, is empty, absolutely empty. What is daf aleph? That's the Munkatcher passport. And when we enter a holy place like a synagogue and gather to pray, and the synagogue helps touch our souls, and our prayers ascend – that's the Munkatcher passport.[1]

"A WALKING SINAI"

Having discussed specific times of prayer, it is important to understand why there are specific places for prayer, as theoretically the encounter could occur anywhere. A good starting point is an analysis of the intersection of time and place on a religious/spiritual level.

When considering the realms of holiness, it seems that the Torah places more emphasis on time than on place. In the sacred literature of many religions, God's creation of the world is followed by a description of where God can be worshipped, i.e., in the form of a statue, on a mountain, or at a temple. In contrast, Rabbi Abraham Joshua Heschel, in his seminal book *The Sabbath,* demonstrates that after describing God's creation of the world, the Torah introduces us not to the *kedusha* (holiness) of place, but to the *kedusha* of time: וַיְבָרֶךְ אֱ־לֹהִים אֶת יוֹם הַשְּׁבִיעִי וַיְקַדֵּשׁ אוֹתוֹ – "And God blessed the seventh day and sanctified it" (Gen. 2:3).

Similarly, when the Children of Israel stand at Sinai and become a people, God introduces Himself from the nexus of time and not place, אָנֹכִי ה׳ אֱ־לֹהֶיךָ אֲשֶׁר הוֹצֵאתִיךָ מֵאֶרֶץ מִצְרַיִם – "I am the Lord your God, who brought you out of the land of Egypt" (Ex. 20:2). Here, God refers to Himself not as the God of Creation, but rather as the God who intervened in history; who, at a particular moment in time, redeemed the Israelites from Egypt.[2]

1. While this story is Reb Shlomo's, some of its interpretations – including how it relates to a synagogue – are not.
2. Rabbi Abraham Joshua Heschel, *The Sabbath* (New York: Farrar, Straus and Giroux, 1991), p. 9.

After the destruction of the Second Commonwealth, the Jewish people, bereft of land, sustained itself by venerating time through the observance of Shabbat, *tefilla*, and other rituals. Rabbi Ahron Soloveichik has commented that the Jewish people survived because it carved out an empire not only in space, but in time.[3]

Rabbi Saul Berman takes this a step further, noting that there is no Hebrew equivalent for the English word "ownership," suggesting a de-emphasis of the value of "space." *Ba'al*, a term used for "husband," cannot mean ownership, as one's wife cannot be owned. *Adon* is the word normally associated with being a "master" of an *eved* (servant). Here too, it cannot fully mean ownership, as an *eved* has inherent human rights.[4] *Yesh li* means "I have," but to have does not mean to own – and there is not even an infinitive for the word *yesh*, no proper verb root that means "have." *Kinyan* means "to acquire," relating to acquisition – not ownership.

This does not mean that the Torah attaches no importance to the physical world. After all, God created the world and declared it very good: וַיַּרְא אֱ־לֹהִים אֶת כָּל אֲשֶׁר עָשָׂה וְהִנֵּה טוֹב מְאֹד – "And God saw every thing that He had made, and, behold, it was very good" (Gen. 1:31). Moreover, God promised Abraham and Sarah the Land of Israel, telling them to go "to the land I will show you" – אֶל הָאָרֶץ אֲשֶׁר אַרְאֶךָּ (Gen. 12:1). *Ra'a* (ראה) is a covenantal term; the Land of Israel is inextricably bound with covenant.

But prayer is not confined to any place. When God heard prayer on behalf of Ishmael – the son of Abraham and Hagar – an angel declared that the child would be called Ishmael, כִּי שָׁמַע אֱ־לֹהִים אֶל קוֹל הַנַּעַר בַּאֲשֶׁר הוּא שָׁם – "because God has heeded the cry of the boy where he is" (Gen. 21:17). Nahmanides interprets this to mean "in the place where he was."[5] Even there, in the desert, as Ishmael struggled for life, God heard his prayer. Sincere *tefilla* is accepted no matter where it is offered. Why, then, are there designated places – like synagogues – for prayer?

---

3. I heard this idea in a class given by Rabbi Soloveichik.
4. For an analysis of the Torah concept of *eved*, see Rabbi Samson Raphael Hirsch's commentary on Exodus 21:1–6.
5. Nahmanides, Genesis 21:17, s.v. *ba'asher hu sham*.

To answer this question, let us consider the first time the Israelites entered a holy place – when God revealed the Torah at Sinai. One might ask, why was it necessary for God to reveal the Torah in a specific location? Couldn't He have transmitted the Torah into the hearts and minds of the Jewish people without addressing them at Mount Sinai? Here, it is important to recognize the challenge for the finite, limited human being of dialogue with the infinite, unlimited God. The chasm is just too great. As a consequence, God revealed the Torah at Sinai. Sinai was necessary as a medium through which the people could experience Revelation.

When leaving Sinai, *Am Yisrael* felt forlorn, bereft of the physical place that had inspired it to feel God's presence. As a consequence, God commanded the nation to construct the *Mishkan*, a portable Sanctuary. The *Mishkan* became, as Umberto Cassuto points out, a "walking Sinai":

> עַד שֶׁהָיוּ חוֹנִים בְּמָקוֹם, מַרְגִּישִׁים הָיוּ אֶת קִרְבַת אֱ־לוֹקִים. נָסְעוּ, נִדְמֶה הָיָה בְּעֵינֵיהֶם כְּאִילוּ נִתְפָּרְדָה הַחֲבִילָה. אִלְמָלֵא שֶׁיִּהְיֶה בְּתוֹכָם מֵעֵין סֵמֶל מוּחָשִׁי לְנוֹכְחוּת ה׳ בְּתוֹכָם. לְשַׁמֵּשׁ סֵמֶל כָּזֶה נוֹעַד הַמִּשְׁכָּן.
>
> As long as they were encamped at Sinai, they [*Am Yisrael*] felt God's presence. Once they left Sinai, it seemed to them as though they were separated from their Source, unless a tangible symbol of God could be established in their midst. The Tabernacle was established to be this symbol.[6]

Similarly, Nahmanides argues, the command to build the *Mishkan* is given immediately after the Revelation chapter[7]:

> וְסוֹד הַמִּשְׁכָּן הוּא שֶׁיִּהְיֶה הַכָּבוֹד אֲשֶׁר שָׁכַן עַל הַר סִינַי שׁוֹכֵן עָלָיו בְּנִסְתָּר... וְהָיָה בַּמִּשְׁכָּן תָּמִיד עִם יִשְׂרָאֵל הַכָּבוֹד שֶׁנִּרְאָה לָהֶם בְּהַר סִינַי.
>
> The secret of the Tabernacle is that the Glory which abode upon Mount Sinai [openly] should abide upon it in a concealed

6. Umberto Cassuto, A *Commentary on the Book of Exodus,* trans. Israel Abrahams *(Jerusalem: Magnes Press, Hebrew University, 1967),* beginning of *Parashat Teruma.*
7. The Revelation and the command to build the *Mishkan* are described in Exodus 24 and 25, respectively.

> manner.... Thus, Israel always had with them in the Tabernacle the Glory which appeared to them on Mount Sinai.[8]

In Nahmanides' view, the *Mishkan*, like Sinai, provided a way through which Israel could experience the Divine.[9]

Sefer HaḤinukh extends the reasoning for building the *Mishkan* to later places of worship:

> בִּנְיַן בַּיִת... וַעֲשׂוֹתֵינוּ בָּהּ תְּפִלּוֹת... הַכֹּל לְהָכִין הַלְּבָבוֹת לַעֲבוֹדָתוֹ יִתְעַלֶּה... וְהַשֵּׁם חָפֵץ בְּטוֹבָתָן שֶׁל בְּרִיּוֹת... וְעַל כֵּן צִיוָּנוּ לִקְבּוֹעַ מָקוֹם שֶׁיִּהְיֶה טָהוֹר... לְטַהֵר שָׁם מַחְשְׁבוֹת בְּנֵי אִישׁ וּלְתַקֵּן לְבָבָם אֵלָיו.
>
> [The reason God commanded us] to build a Sanctuary... wherein we could pray... was to prepare our hearts to worship Him.... God wishes what is best for humankind.... Therefore He mandated that we establish a place which is pure... to purify the thoughts of people and to direct their hearts to Him.[10]

So conducive is the synagogue to *tefilla* that one is encouraged to pray there even when praying alone. This is referred to as *tefilla bemakom tzibbur* (*tefilla* in the place where the community normally prays, i.e., the synagogue). As Rabbi Aharon Lichtenstein writes:

> *Beit haknesset* (the synagogue) is a *mikdash me'at* (miniature Temple) and there is a particular *kiyyum* (fulfillment) of *tefilla* in relation to *mikdash*. There is a certain presence of *Shekhina* (the Omnipresence) in there. In some sense, we do feel that *Shekhina* is more of an indwelling presence in certain times and in certain places than in others, and *mikdash* has this element.[11]

---

8. Nahmanides, introduction to *Parashat Teruma*.
9. Rashi, unlike Nahmanides, posits that God commands the construction of the *Mishkan* after the Israelites worshipped the Golden Calf. See Rashi, Exodus 35:1, s.v. *vayak'hel Moshe*, and 35:2, s.v. *sheshet yamim*. For Rashi, the *Mishkan* was a response to Israel's worshipping the Golden Calf, as the *Mishkan* showed the people the right path for worshipping God.
10. *Sefer HaḤinukh*, commandment 95.
11. Rabbi Aharon Lichtenstein, "Imperatives and Advantages of Communal Prayer

AS HOLY AS WE MAKE THEM

This leads us to another question. While it is necessary for people to have a place in which to feel God's presence, is it possible for God to be contained in any particular space? King Solomon makes this point when he dedicates the Holy Temple. He declares: הִנֵּה הַשָּׁמַיִם וּשְׁמֵי הַשָּׁמַיִם לֹא יְכַלְכְּלוּךָ אַף כִּי הַבַּיִת הַזֶּה אֲשֶׁר בָּנִיתִי – "Behold, heaven and the heaven of heavens cannot contain You; nor can this House that I have built" (1 Kings 8:27). Isaiah echoes these sentiments: כֹּה אָמַר ה׳ הַשָּׁמַיִם כִּסְאִי וְהָאָרֶץ הֲדֹם רַגְלָי אֵיזֶה בַיִת אֲשֶׁר תִּבְנוּ לִי וְאֵי זֶה מָקוֹם מְנוּחָתִי – "So says the Lord: The heaven is My throne, and the earth is My footstool; what house could you build for Me? And what place could be My resting place?" (Is. 66:1).[12]

Abarbanel succinctly expresses the tension between the infinity of God and His command that we build Him a Sanctuary to dwell in: "Why did God command… [the] *Mishkan* to be built… as if the Blessed One were physically limited to a place? This is contrary to the truth."[13]

To answer this question, it is important to distinguish between a sign and a symbol. A sign is an entity unto itself; it is self-contained. Outside its parameters, it has no meaning. In contrast, a symbol represents something beyond itself. It is an object or place that points in a direction beyond its own limits. The symbol catapults us to experience a message that transcends its immediacy.[14]

Sinai, the *Mishkan*, and contemporary synagogues are all symbols of God, not God Himself. While God cannot be contained in a

---

Studied in Depth," *Hamevaser* 6, no. 5 (28 Adar 5728/March 28, 1968), p. 5.

12. In the morning liturgy, we recite the verse קָדוֹשׁ, קָדוֹשׁ, קָדוֹשׁ ה׳ צְבָאוֹת מְלֹא כָל הָאָרֶץ כְּבוֹדוֹ – "Holy, holy, holy is the Lord of hosts; the whole earth is full of His glory" (Is. 6:3). Holy (*kadosh*) can mean separate, apart, transcendent; "the whole earth is full of His glory" speaks of God being close, of His immanence. This suggests the following formula, which I have heard over the years: G – W = G, God minus the world equals God; W – G = 0, the world minus God equals nothing. Here, the simultaneous transcendence and immanence of God suggests that He cannot be contained in any place.
13. Abarbanel, beginning of *Parashat Teruma*.
14. See Paul Tillich, *The Courage to Be* (New Haven and London: Yale University Press, 1952), pp. 179–180, 189–190.

space, a space can become a symbol of God. Whether or not the symbol inspires us to integrate its teaching into our lives depends upon us. It's not automatic. While the symbol can help catapult us to a higher plane, the journey requires intense human effort.

The verse that offers the rationale for the *Mishkan* reads: וְעָשׂוּ לִי מִקְדָּשׁ וְשָׁכַנְתִּי בְּתוֹכָם – "And let them make Me a Sanctuary, that I may dwell among them" (Ex. 25:8). One wonders, why *betokham,* "among them," and not *betokho,* "within it"? The answer is that *betokho* would imply that God could be contained by the *Mishkan,* whereas *betokham* emphasizes that through the *Mishkan,* God has the potential to dwell among the people – if only we receive Him.

This concept applies not only to places (i.e., Sinai, the *Mishkan*) but to objects as well. Consider one of the holiest objects – the Tablets (*Luḥot*). Rabbi Meir Simḥa of Dvinsk explains why Moses shattered them after witnessing Israel worshipping the Golden Calf. After the Exodus from Egypt, the Israelites perceived Moses as a demigod, bridging the gap between themselves and the Divine. When Moses was late descending Mount Sinai, they lost faith in him and transferred their understanding of Moses as the intermediary to the Golden Calf.[15] They did so because they were accustomed to the Egyptian model of worshipping calves; this form of worship had become synonymous with their understanding of God. Once told that *Am Yisrael* built the Golden Calf, Moses feared that even if it were destroyed, the people would replace it with the Tablets – and they would become their new sub-god. Moses therefore shattered the Tablets to show that even they were not intrinsically holy. In the words of Rabbi Meir Simḥa:

> Had Moses left the Tablets intact, he feared they [the people] would substitute them for the calf and not reform their ways. But now that he had broken the Tablets, they realized how far they had fallen short of true faith....
>
> For this reason God approved of Moses' action.... By this he had demonstrated that the Tablets themselves possessed

15. See Shabbat 89a, which records that the people had miscalculated. In reality, Moses returned on time. See also Rashi, Exodus 32:1, s.v. *ki voshesh Moshe.*

> no intrinsic holiness other than that invested in them by Israel's observance of the Torah in accordance with the will of the Creator and His holy name.[16]

Here, Rabbi Meir Simḥa posits that holy objects are only as holy as people make them. The Tablets made by God were broken, teaching that even a God-made object is not automatically holy. In contrast, the second Tablets, hewn by Moses, remained whole, as the people had invested them with *kedusha*.[17]

> It was the first Tablets, which were the work of God, [that were broken].... But the [second] Tablets, hewn by Moses, remained whole. This demonstrates that no holiness resides in any created thing other than that invested in it by Israel's observance of the Torah in accordance with the will of the Blessed Name.[18]

16. Rabbi Meir Simḥa HaKohen, *Meshekh Ḥokhma*, Exodus 32:19, s.v. *vayehi ka'asher karav el hamaḥaneh*.
17. See Exodus 34:1, where Moses is told by God: פְּסָל לְךָ שְׁנֵי לֻחֹת אֲבָנִים כָּרִאשֹׁנִים – "Hew for yourself two Tablets of stone like the first ones." Whereas the second *Luḥot* were hewn by Moses, the first ones were hewn by God.
18. Rabbi Meir Simḥa HaKohen, *Meshekh Ḥokhma*, Exodus 34:1. For a complete analysis of the *Meshekh Ḥokhma* on the breaking of the Tablets, see Leibowitz, *New Studies in Shemot*, vol. 2, pp. 612–618.

   From a certain perspective, the second *Luḥot* were much "humbler" than the first. The first were given amidst "thunder and lightning and a thick cloud upon the mountain, and the sound of the shofar exceedingly loud" (Ex. 19:16). The second, hewn by Moses, were given with no fanfare (Ex. 34:1–5). This accentuates the importance of symbols remaining modest. When symbolism is cluttered, ornate, or expensive, it can serve as a barrier rather than a pathway to God.

   For this reason, Jewish ritual symbols are, by and large, simple. Consider, for example, the basic rituals of the Passover and Sukkot festivals – matza and sukka. Matza is flat bread, and the sukka, a flimsy temporary dwelling. Neither is ostentatious. They are both plain. This teaches that the symbol should not be confused with what it represents. In this spirit, holy objects, even holy spaces like synagogues, should be humble. Perhaps for this reason, Sinai – the place of Revelation – was a low mountain.

Vessels like the Ark, which contained the Tablets, also function as symbols. An important narrative recounting Israel's defeat at the hands of the Philistines in the book of Samuel illustrates this point:

> וַיַּעַרְכוּ פְלִשְׁתִּים לִקְרַאת יִשְׂרָאֵל וַתִּטֹּשׁ הַמִּלְחָמָה וַיִּנָּגֶף יִשְׂרָאֵל לִפְנֵי פְלִשְׁתִּים וַיַּכּוּ בַמַּעֲרָכָה בַּשָּׂדֶה כְּאַרְבַּעַת אֲלָפִים אִישׁ.
>
> The Philistines arrayed themselves against Israel; and when the battle was fought, Israel was routed by the Philistines, who slew about four thousand men on the field of battle. (I Sam. 4:2)

The Israelites concluded that they'd lost the battle because the Ark had not been with them. They believed the Ark *was* God. They therefore decided to bring the Ark into the camp so that God, in their minds, had no choice but to grant them victory.

> וַיָּבֹא הָעָם אֶל הַמַּחֲנֶה וַיֹּאמְרוּ זִקְנֵי יִשְׂרָאֵל לָמָּה נְגָפָנוּ ה׳ הַיּוֹם לִפְנֵי פְלִשְׁתִּים נִקְחָה אֵלֵינוּ מִשִּׁלֹה אֶת אֲרוֹן בְּרִית ה׳ וְיָבֹא בְקִרְבֵּנוּ וְיֹשִׁעֵנוּ מִכַּף אֹיְבֵינוּ.
>
> When the [Israelite] troops returned to the camp, the elders of Israel asked, "Why did the Lord put us to rout today before the Philistines? Let us fetch the Ark of the Covenant of the Lord from Shilo; thus He will be present among us and will deliver us from the hands of our enemies." (I Sam. 4:3)

The Ark is then described with the *keruvim* (cherubs) on top. In addition, Ḥofni and Pinḥas, the two sons of Eli previously described as wicked,[19] are mentioned as tending to the Ark.

> וַיִּשְׁלַח הָעָם שִׁלֹה וַיִּשְׂאוּ מִשָּׁם אֵת אֲרוֹן בְּרִית ה׳ צְבָ־אוֹת יֹשֵׁב הַכְּרֻבִים וְשָׁם שְׁנֵי בְנֵי עֵלִי עִם אֲרוֹן בְּרִית הָאֱ־לֹהִים חָפְנִי וּפִינְחָס.
>
> So the troops sent men to Shilo; there Eli's two sons, Ḥofni and Pinḥas, were in charge of the Ark of the Covenant of the Lord,

19. See I Samuel 2:12.

> and they brought down from there the Ark of the Covenant of the Lord of hosts enthroned on the *keruvim*. (1 Sam. 4:4)

The narrative goes on to recount that although the Ark was brought into the camp, Israel was again defeated. The Ark was captured, and Ḥofni and Pinḥas were killed:

> וַיִּלָּחֲמוּ פְלִשְׁתִּים וַיִּנָּגֶף יִשְׂרָאֵל וַיָּנֻסוּ אִישׁ לְאֹהָלָיו וַתְּהִי הַמַּכָּה גְּדוֹלָה מְאֹד וַיִּפֹּל מִיִּשְׂרָאֵל שְׁלֹשִׁים אֶלֶף רַגְלִי. וַאֲרוֹן אֱ־לֹהִים נִלְקָח וּשְׁנֵי בְנֵי עֵלִי מֵתוּ חָפְנִי וּפִינְחָס.
>
> The Philistines fought; Israel was routed, and they all fled to their homes. The defeat was very great, thirty thousand foot soldiers of Israel fell there. The Ark of God was captured, and Eli's two sons, Ḥofni and Pinḥas, were slain. (1 Sam. 4:10–11)

Here we see how deeply the people had misunderstood how God is manifest. They thought the Ark was God, when in fact it was a *symbol* of God. Furthermore, with the wicked Ḥofni and Pinḥas tending to the Ark, it was of little value. It was, in a sense, "*kedusha*-less." Hence, Israel was defeated. Malbim makes this point:

> חָשְׁבוּ בַּאֲשֶׁר בְּהֶכְרֵחַ יַצִּיל אֶת אֲרוֹן עוּזוֹ וְיִשְׁמְרֵהוּ מִיַּד פְּלִשְׁתִּים וְעַל יְדֵי זֶה יִנָּצְלוּ וְיִשָּׁמְרוּ גַּם הֵם. וְזֶה מַחְשֶׁבֶת דוֹפִי, כִּי בְּרִית הָאָרוֹן אֵינוֹ תַּכְלִית לְעַצְמוֹ רַק בַּעֲבוּר יִשְׁמְרוּ אֶת הַכָּתוּב בּוֹ.
>
> They thought God would necessarily save His mighty Ark and protect it from the Philistines, and through this they [the Jewish people] would be saved and protected. This is foolishness, as the covenantal Ark is not an end unto itself, but has holiness only if the Jewish people observes what is written in it.[20]

Thus, we learn that vessels are not intrinsically holy. This message is underscored in the epilogue of Pinḥas' wife giving birth:

---

20. Malbim, 1 Samuel 4:3, s.v. *nikḥa eleinu.*

וְכַלָּתוֹ אֵשֶׁת פִּינְחָס הָרָה לָלַת וַתִּשְׁמַע אֶת הַשְּׁמֻעָה אֶל הִלָּקַח אֲרוֹן הָאֱ-לֹהִים וּמֵת חָמִיהָ וְאִישָׁהּ וַתִּכְרַע וַתֵּלֶד כִּי נֶהֶפְכוּ עָלֶיהָ צִרֶיהָ...
וַתִּקְרָא לַנַּעַר אִיכָבוֹד לֵאמֹר גָּלָה כָבוֹד מִיִּשְׂרָאֵל אֶל הִלָּקַח אֲרוֹן הָאֱ-לֹהִים וְאֶל חָמִיהָ וְאִישָׁהּ.
וַתֹּאמֶר גָּלָה כָבוֹד מִיִּשְׂרָאֵל כִּי נִלְקַח אֲרוֹן הָאֱ-לֹהִים.

His daughter-in-law, the wife of Pinḥas, was with child, about to give birth. When she heard the report that the Ark of God had been captured and that her father-in-law and her husband were dead, she was seized with labor pains, and she crouched down and gave birth….

She named the boy Ikhavod, meaning, "The glory has departed from Israel" – referring to the capture of the Ark of God and to [the death of] her father-in-law and her husband.

"The glory had departed from Israel," she said, "for the Ark of God has been captured." (I Sam. 4:19, 21, 22)

Here, the wife of Pinḥas is notified of Israel's losing the battle, of the taking of the Ark, and the death of her husband and father-in-law. She gives birth and calls the child אִיכָבוֹד (Ikhavod) – "Un-glory," proclaiming: גָּלָה כָבוֹד מִיִּשְׂרָאֵל – "glory has departed from Israel." Note that when God's glory rests in the *Mishkan*, the Torah states, וּכְבוֹד ה׳ מָלֵא אֶת הַמִּשְׁכָּן – "and the glory of God filled the *Mishkan*" (Ex. 40:34). This echoes the Torah's description of "the glory of the Lord resting on Mount Sinai" – וַיִּשְׁכֹּן כְּבוֹד ה׳ עַל הַר סִינַי (Ex. 24:16).

There, at Sinai, the honor of God's glory suffused the *Mishkan*, whose centerpiece was the Ark, as the people infused the place with *kedusha*. Here, in I Samuel, the people were void of holiness; therefore the Ark's physical presence had little impact. The child born is Ikhavod, a name that literally means "there is no *kavod*," no honor, no glory.

In sum, *kedusha*, holiness, can be initiated only by the human being. While objects, vessels, and places have the potential to become holy, their holiness is proportional to the degree that we infuse them with *kedusha*. Rabbi Moshe Soloveitchik expands this concept to include all of the Land of Israel:

> There are two conceptual frameworks relative to the Land of Israel. The first is the concept of the holiness of the land, *kedushat ha'aretz,* that it was sanctified through its conquest by Israel, resulting in our obligation to fulfill the commandments linked to the land.
>
> Besides this is the concept of the name of the Land of Israel, *shem Eretz Yisrael,* which is not dependent on its sanctity. Rather, it applies to all the places God chose to give us, and this is the chosen land....
>
> And it appears...that the holiness of the land can be nullified, as in the idea that the first sanctification was not eternal (קְדוּשָּׁה רִאשׁוֹנָה לֹא קִידְּשָׁה לֶעָתִיד לָבֹא). But the name of the Land of Israel that applies from the fact that God chose it to be given to us, eternally applies.[21]

Rabbi Soloveitchik is suggesting that Israel's status as the chosen land does not necessarily entail its status as the Holy Land – rather, its level of holiness depends on us.[22] Similarly, a synagogue or temple's designation as a place of prayer does not automatically render it a holy place. The level of *kedusha* of any synagogue building is directly proportional to the holiness with which we infuse it.

This idea is articulated at the dedication of the First Temple. There, God tells King Solomon that His presence in the Temple is dependent upon Israel's adherence to His dictates:

> וַיְהִי דְּבַר ה׳ אֶל שְׁלֹמֹה לֵאמֹר. הַבַּיִת הַזֶּה אֲשֶׁר אַתָּה בֹנֶה אִם תֵּלֵךְ בְּחֻקֹּתַי וְאֶת מִשְׁפָּטַי תַּעֲשֶׂה וְשָׁמַרְתָּ אֶת כָּל מִצְוֹתַי לָלֶכֶת בָּהֶם וַהֲקִמֹתִי אֶת דְּבָרִי אִתָּךְ אֲשֶׁר דִּבַּרְתִּי אֶל דָּוִד אָבִיךָ. וְשָׁכַנְתִּי בְּתוֹךְ בְּנֵי יִשְׂרָאֵל וְלֹא אֶעֱזֹב אֶת עַמִּי יִשְׂרָאֵל.
>
> Then the word of the Lord came to Solomon: "With regard to this House you are building – if you follow My laws and observe

21. Rabbi Ḥayyim Avraham Shiyovitz, ed., *Shiurei HaRav Yosef Dov HaLevi Soloveitchik, Zatzal, al Mesekhet Ḥalla* (Jerusalem: Mesora, 2003), pp. 127, 128.
22. It can also be suggested that our being the chosen people doesn't necessarily mean we're a holy people. That holiness must be earned.

> My rules and faithfully keep My commandments, I will fulfill for you the promise that I made to your father, David: I will abide among the Children of Israel, and I will never forsake My people Israel." (I Kings 6:11–13)[23]

Thus, the encounter with *kedushat makom* presents us with three basic tenets. First, finite human beings need a space in which to bridge the chasm with God. Second, that space is not God Himself, but a symbol of the Divine. Third, the holiness of that symbol depends on the meaning we give it.

This is the way one should view even the holiest of places, Jerusalem itself.[24] Natan Sharansky articulated this idea at the wedding of his daughter, Rachel, to Micha Danziger. Beneath the *ḥuppa* in Jerusalem, overlooking the hills of Judea as the sun broke through that cold, cloudy January morning, Natan said:

> This moment takes me back to our *ḥuppa*, Avital's and mine, thirty-four years ago. It was in a small, one-room Moscow apartment where four friends held a sheet above our heads. The number of guests hardly reached a *minyan* (quorum).
>
> It was the first *ḥuppa* in our lives that we ever saw, and all that we could do was simply repeat after the rabbi every move and every word – while hardly understanding many of them.
>
> But when it came to breaking the glass, the rabbi spoke about Jerusalem, and we became instantly reconnected to our reality. It was so obvious to us that we were in the very last stages of the thousands of years of struggle to return to Jerusalem. And

23. These words reverberate with the language of the biblical mandate וְעָשׂוּ לִי מִקְדָּשׁ וְשָׁכַנְתִּי בְּתוֹכָם – "And let them make Me a Sanctuary, that I may dwell among them" (Ex. 25:8).

24. Maimonides understands the holiness of Jerusalem to fall into the category of *kedushat Shekhina*, a holiness that emanates from God. He argues that "the holiness of the Temple in Jerusalem is caused by the *Shekhina*. And, just as the *Shekhina* is eternal, [so, too, is Jerusalem]." In his words, לְפִי שֶׁקְּדוּשַּׁת הַמִּקְדָּשׁ וִירוּשָׁלַיִם מִפְּנֵי הַשְּׁכִינָה וּשְׁכִינָה אֵינָהּ בְּטֵלָה. Still, Jerusalem first had to be liberated by *Am Yisrael* in order for the *Shekhina* to be present there. See Maimonides, *Code*, Laws of the Temple 6:16.

> this *ḥuppa*, ours, invigorated our determination to win this battle and made us feel powerful.
>
> Today, we are standing here: We are in Jerusalem! The dream has come true.
>
> But if we are here already, in the unified capital of the reborn Jewish state, what is the meaning today of breaking the glass? What is the dream we still yearn for? What is our – your – challenge?
>
> When I compare your *ḥuppa* and our *ḥuppa*, I think that the challenge you face is much more difficult. Our aim was so simple and so clear. We had to win the battle, and nothing could deter us.
>
> Today, on the one hand, you have to be builders and guardians of Jerusalem, and at the same time guardians of the idea of Jerusalem. You have to physically build the earthly Jerusalem, and keep alive the power, energy, and uniqueness of the heavenly Jerusalem.
>
> The power of unity and connection to the generations of our people is in heavenly Jerusalem, in *Yerushalayim shel ma'ala*.[25]

Synagogues are as holy as the spiritual meaning we give them. The purpose of places of prayer is to intensify our inner spiritual quest. These places are mediums through which we can come to feel the presence of God. Within the larger sanctuary of the synagogue, we may come to create inner sanctuaries within our souls. In the words of Rabbi Elazar Azikri:

בִּלְבָבִי מִשְׁכָּן אֶבְנֶה לַהֲדַר כְּבוֹדוֹ
וּבַמִּשְׁכָּן מִזְבֵּחַ אָשִׂים לְקַרְנֵי הוֹדוֹ,
וּלְנֵר תָּמִיד אֶקַּח לִי אֶת אֵשׁ הָעֲקֵדָה,
וּלְקָרְבָּן אַקְרִיב לוֹ אֶת נַפְשִׁי הַיְּחִידָה.

25. The wedding took place on January 4, 2008. Natan's comments under the *ḥuppa* were widely disseminated. See, for example, the op-ed page of *The Jerusalem Post*, January 10, 2008.

In my heart a Sanctuary I shall build, for the splendor of His honor;
and in the Sanctuary an altar I shall place, for the rays of His glory.
And for an eternal flame I shall take for myself the fire of the *Akeda* [Isaac's would-be sacrifice];
and for a sacrifice I shall offer Him my soul, my one and only soul.[26]

26. Rabbi Elazar Azikri, *Sefer Ḥaredim.*

Chapter Six

Text

A couple had faithfully attended services on a weekly basis. As cold as it was, Berel and Golda would make their way to the synagogue. In time, however, they began to miss services – first for one Shabbat, and then for more. The rabbi became concerned. He asked their friends if they had any idea why the loyal couple had stopped coming. The answer was unequivocal: Berel and Golda found it more meaningful to pray by themselves. Alone, they could reach higher levels, unencumbered by folks who sometimes distracted them from offering what they felt was purer prayer.

One cold Friday morning, the rabbi made his way to Berel and Golda's home. Answering the knock on the door, they were astounded to see their rabbi. They invited him in, and the rabbi took a seat near the fireplace. "To what do we owe this honor?" Golda asked. The rabbi said nothing. "Why are you here?" Berel chimed in. And still, the rabbi remained silent. He sat for many moments and then took the stoker lying near the fireplace and gently lifted one of the coals that, amidst the others, was white-hot. The rabbi placed the solitary piece on the side of the fire. He stared at it as it turned from white-hot to red-hot, and then the color completely faded. Finally, the "lonely" lump of coal had lost its heat. Only then did the rabbi leave.

The next Shabbat, Golda and Berel returned to the synagogue.[1]

1. This is a contemporary formulation of a story I heard years ago.

PRAYER AS EQUALIZER AND UNIFIER

Ideally, *tefilla* should be an expression of what we feel in those moments when our souls are inspired, or when we feel the pressures of life. This, in fact, is the way *tefilla* was offered before the destruction of the First Temple. In the words of Maimonides:

> אִם הָיָה רָגִיל מַרְבֶּה בִּתְחִנָּה וּבַקָּשָׁה, וְאִם הָיָה עֲרַל שְׂפָתַיִם מְדַבֵּר כְּפִי יָכְלוֹ וּבְכָל עֵת שֶׁיִּרְצֶה. וְכֵן מִנְיַן הַתְּפִלּוֹת כָּל אֶחָד כְּפִי יְכָלְתּוֹ. יֵשׁ שֶׁמִּתְפַּלֵּל פַּעַם אַחַת בַּיּוֹם, וְיֵשׁ שֶׁמִּתְפַּלֵּל פְּעָמִים הַרְבֵּה. וְהַכֹּל הָיוּ מִתְפַּלְּלִין נֹכַח הַמִּקְדָּשׁ בְּכָל מָקוֹם שֶׁיִּהְיֶה. וְכֵן הָיָה הַדָּבָר תָּמִיד מִמֹּשֶׁה רַבֵּנוּ וְעַד עֶזְרָא.
>
> If one were accustomed, one could extend supplications and requests. If unaccustomed to speech, one could speak according to one's ability at any desired time. And so, too, the number of *tefillot*: everyone according to his ability. There were those who would pray once a day, and those who would pray many times. And everyone would pray facing the Temple from wherever each happened to be. This is the way it was from Moses our teacher until Ezra.[2]

Here, Maimonides paints a picture of a community in which prayer was fundamentally spontaneous, with no prescribed set of texts or specially designated times, as long as one prayed daily. Among the members of the Jewish community in Jerusalem until the time of Ezra, *tefilla* was an individualized form of personal expression. One could pray with or without words, as often as one felt the need.

So why today are we bound to a set formula of prayer? If there is a historical precedent for unscripted *tefilla*, why do we have a structured text? Maimonides explains the historical and political factors that led to the standardization of the prayer service:

---

2. Maimonides, *Code*, Laws of Prayer 1:3.

כֵּיוָן שֶׁגָּלוּ יִשְׂרָאֵל בִּימֵי נְבוּכַדְנֶצַּר הָרָשָׁע, נִתְעָרְבוּ בְּפָרַס וְיָוָן וּשְׁאָר הָאֻמּוֹת וְנוֹלְדוּ לָהֶם בָּנִים בְּאַרְצוֹת הַגּוֹיִם, וְאוֹתָן הַבָּנִים נִתְבַּלְבְּלָה שְׂפָתָם וְהָיְתָה שְׂפַת כָּל אֶחָד וְאֶחָד מְעֹרֶבֶת מִלְּשׁוֹנוֹת הַרְבֵּה, וְכֵיוָן שֶׁהָיָה מְדַבֵּר אֵינוֹ יָכוֹל לְדַבֵּר כָּל צְרָכוֹ בְּלָשׁוֹן אַחַת אֶלָּא בְּשִׁבּוּשׁ... וּמִפְּנֵי זֶה כְּשֶׁהָיָה אֶחָד מֵהֶם מִתְפַּלֵּל תִּקְצַר לְשׁוֹנוֹ לִשְׁאוֹל חֲפָצָיו אוֹ לְהַגִּיד שֶׁבַח הַקָּדוֹשׁ בָּרוּךְ הוּא בִּלְשׁוֹן הַקֹּדֶשׁ עַד שֶׁיְּעָרֵב עִמָּהּ לְשׁוֹנוֹת אֲחֵרוֹת.

וְכֵיוָן שֶׁרָאָה עֶזְרָא וּבֵית דִּינוֹ כָּךְ, עָמְדוּ וְתִקְּנוּ לָהֶם שְׁמוֹנֶה עֶשְׂרֵה בְּרָכוֹת עַל הַסֵּדֶר: שָׁלֹשׁ רִאשׁוֹנוֹת שֶׁבַח לַה׳, וְשָׁלֹשׁ אַחֲרוֹנוֹת הוֹדָיָה, וְאֶמְצָעִיּוֹת יֵשׁ בָּהֶן שְׁאֵלַת כָּל הַדְּבָרִים, שֶׁהֵן כְּמוֹ אָבוֹת לְכָל חֶפְצֵי אִישׁ וָאִישׁ וּלְצָרְכֵי הַצִּבּוּר כֻּלָּן;

כְּדֵי שֶׁיִּהְיוּ עֲרוּכוֹת בְּפִי הַכֹּל וְיִלְמְדוּ אוֹתָן בִּמְהֵרָה וְתִהְיֶה תְּפִלַּת אֵלּוּ הָעִלְּגִים תְּפִלָּה שְׁלֵמָה כִּתְפִלַּת בַּעֲלֵי הַלָּשׁוֹן הַצָּחָה.

וּמִפְּנֵי עִנְיָן זֶה תִּקְּנוּ כָּל הַבְּרָכוֹת וְהַתְּפִלּוֹת הַסְּדוּרוֹת בְּפִי כָּל יִשְׂרָאֵל כְּדֵי שֶׁיְּהֵא כָּל עִנְיַן בְּרָכָה עָרוּךְ בְּפִי הָעִלֵּג.

When the people of Israel went into exile in the days of the wicked Nebuchadnezzar, they mingled with the Persians, Greeks, and other nations. In those foreign countries, children were born to them whose language was confused. Everyone's speech was a mixture of many tongues. No one was able, when he spoke, to express his thoughts adequately in any one language.... Consequently, when any one of them prayed in Hebrew, he was unable adequately to express his needs or recount the praises of God without mixing Hebrew with other languages.

When Ezra and his council realized this condition, they ordained the Eighteen Benedictions (*Shemoneh Esreh*) in their present order. The first three are praises of God and the last three are thanksgiving. The intermediate contain requests for all those things that serve as general categories for the desires of each and every person and the needs of the whole community.

The objective was that these prayers should be in an orderly form in everyone's mouth; that all should learn them, and thus the prayer of those whose speech was inarticulate would be as perfect as that of those who had command of a pure [Hebrew] style.

> For the same reason, they arranged [in a fixed form] all the blessings and prayers of all Jews, so that the form of every blessing would be familiar and relevant to those whose speech was inarticulate.[3]

After the destruction of the First Temple and the exile to Babylon, the Jewish people lost its ability to speak articulately in Hebrew, and for that matter, in any language. Living in Babylon (*Bavel,* which literally means "mixture"), Jews began to speak in a combination of many tongues. In that setting, some individuals lost their ability to fully express themselves. A hierarchal model emerged in which Jews found themselves on different levels – some prayed eloquently, others with difficulty, and some perhaps not at all. Thus, a standard text was introduced to equalize the entire populace; it was a way to declare that all Jews are equal in the eyes of God.

The theme of our equality before God is highlighted in a talmudic passage that describes how the rabbis of Yavne understood individual roles within a community:

> מַרְגְּלָא בְּפוּמַיְיהוּ דְּרַבָּנַן דְּיַבְנֶה אֲנִי בְּרִיָּה וַחֲבֵרִי בְּרִיָּה אֲנִי מְלַאכְתִּי בָּעִיר וְהוּא מְלַאכְתּוֹ בַּשָּׂדֶה אֲנִי מַשְׁכִּים לִמְלַאכְתִּי וְהוּא מַשְׁכִּים לִמְלַאכְתּוֹ כְּשֵׁם שֶׁהוּא אֵינוֹ מִתְגַּדֵּר בִּמְלַאכְתִּי כָּךְ אֲנִי אֵינִי מִתְגַּדֵּר בִּמְלַאכְתּוֹ וְשֶׁמָּא תֹּאמַר אֲנִי מַרְבֶּה וְהוּא מַמְעִיט שָׁנִינוּ אֶחָד הַמַּרְבֶּה וְאֶחָד הַמַּמְעִיט וּבִלְבַד שֶׁיְּכַוֵּין לִבּוֹ לַשָּׁמַיִם.
>
> A favorite saying of the rabbis of Yavne was: I am God's creature and my fellow is God's creature. My work is in the town and his work is in the country. I rise early for my work and he rises early for his work. Just as he does not presume to do my work, so I do not presume to do his work. Will you say, I do much and he does little? We have learned: One may do much or one may do little; it is all one, provided he directs his heart to heaven.[4]

---

3. Ibid. 1:4. Translation by Moses Hyamson (New York: Feldheim Publishers, 1981), p. 98b.
4. Berakhot 17a.

Here, the rabbis of Yavne stress that, regardless of one's profession or economic status, one's *tefilla* is received with only one proviso: וּבִלְבַד שֶׁיְּכַוֵּין לִבּוֹ לַשָּׁמַיִם – that "he directs his heart to heaven."

A story is told about a pious Jew who *davened* (prayed) in the *shteibel* (small synagogue) of the Karliner Rebbe. The Rebbe was impressed by the way this individual immersed himself in *tefilla*, and inquired as to what his secret was. The man responded, "I am a water carrier, hardly noticed by anyone. Once, feeling lonely, I stood in the central marketplace, trying to get the attention of passersby. No one would stop. Even you, dear Rebbe, passed me by without giving me the time of day. So when I stand in *tefilla*, and recite the same prayers as you do, and realize that even if it takes me longer, God patiently listens – of course, I *daven* with great fervor."

Just as fixed *tefilla* had the power to level the playing field between the humble water carrier and the great Karliner Rebbe, structured prayer reminds us that we are all equal in God's eyes. In the simple but beautiful words of Rabbi Yehuda Amital:

> כְּאוֹתָהּ אֵם, שֶׁפִּטְפּוּטֵי תִּינוֹקָהּ עֲרֵבִים עָלֶיהָ, כָּךְ, כִּבְיָכוֹל, עֲרֵבָה תְּפִילָּתוֹ שֶׁל אָדָם מִיִּשְׂרָאֵל עַל הקב"ה. הֲיֵשׁ שִׂמְחָה גְּדוֹלָה מִזּוֹ? מִישֶׁהוּ שׁוֹמֵעַ, מוּכָן לְהַקְשִׁיב.
>
> לְעִתִּים עוֹבְרִים אָנוּ לְיַד קַבְּצָן בָּרְחוֹב, נוֹתְנִים לוֹ מַטְבֵּעַ, וְהוּא מְבָרֵךְ אוֹתָנוּ בַּאֲרִיכוּת. וְכִי אָנוּ עוֹצְרִים לְרֶגַע כְּדֵי לִשְׁמוֹעַ? אֲבָל הוּא בְּשֶׁלּוֹ, מַרְגִּישׁ צוֹרֶךְ לְהוֹדוֹת... אֲבָל אֵצֶל הקב"ה... אַדְּרַבָּה, הקב"ה פּוֹנֶה, כִּבְיָכוֹל, אֶל הָאָדָם וְאוֹמֵר לוֹ: הִנְנִי מְבַקֵּשׁ לִשְׁמוֹעַ אוֹתְךָ.[5]
>
> Like a mother who enjoys listening to the babbling of her infant, so, as it were, God enjoys listening to our prayers. Can there be any greater joy than this? Someone is hearing us; someone is ready to listen.
>
> Sometimes, we pass a beggar in the street and give him a few coins, and he thanks us over and over again. We do not stop to listen to him, but he continues nevertheless, feeling a need to

5. Rabbi Yehuda Amital, *VeHaAretz Natan Livnei Adam* (Alon Shvut, Israel: Mikhlelet Ya'akov Hertzog, 5765 [2005]), p. 90.

> thank us.... But in the case of our prayers to God.... God turns to man, as it were, and says, "I am waiting and eager to hear you."[6]

Moreover, set text has the ability to unite Jews regardless of geographical location or level of Jewish observance. One can enter a synagogue in France, India, or Russia and feel a powerful sense of connection in reciting the same *Shema*, the same *Amida*. I felt this most powerfully in the spring of 1989, when I was present at a conference in Riga, which was probably the first gathering of Jews from the former Soviet Union since the Communist revolution.

On the Shabbat before the conference, I prayed in the central Riga synagogue. Atop the Ark was a quote from Psalms, בָּרוּךְ ה׳ שֶׁלֹּא נְתָנָנוּ טֶרֶף לְשִׁנֵּיהֶם – "Blessed be the Lord, who has not delivered us to be preyed upon by our enemies" (Ps. 124:6). An older man explained to me that lots of people associated the text with the Soviets' liberation of many Jews from the Nazi death camps. His voice dropped, and he went on in Yiddish. In truth, he said, the enemy was the Soviets, who had, in effect, incarcerated the Jewish community, preventing its members from practicing Judaism or emigrating. Pointing to the words on the Ark, the elderly Jew said, "With God's help, the Soviet tyrants will not succeed."

Asked to share some words of Torah with those gathered at the synagogue, I wondered what I could say to a congregation that had suffered so terribly; a congregation whose native tongue was not my own. And then it hit me. I began by singing out the first verse of the *Shema*, שְׁמַע יִשְׂרָאֵל ה׳ אֱ־לֹהֵינוּ ה׳ אֶחָד – "Listen, O Israel, the Lord our God, the Lord is One." Suddenly, I could see tears in the eyes of many people. Some were tears of sadness. Others were tears of joy. What happened next was extraordinary: the congregation spontaneously echoed the words. *Shema Yisrael A-donai E-loheinu A-donai Eḥad* reverberated throughout the sanctuary. At that moment, I felt the power of the *Shema* to unite Jews with no common language or background.

The next day, the Riga conference opened with a klezmer rendition of the Shabbat songs *Shalom Aleikhem* and *Yah Ribbon*. The tunes

6. Rabbi Yehuda Amital, *Jewish Values in a Changing World* (Alon Shevut, Israel: Yeshivat Har Etzion; New Jersey: KTAV Publishing House, 2005), p. 119.

being sung were the old ones, melodies so ancient that I generally refused to sing them. For years they had seemed out of touch with contemporary music. On that day in Riga, however, something spiritually ecstatic occurred. As I heard those *niggunim* (tunes), I felt transported to the past. I felt a deep connection to my roots, going back to my grandparents and great-grandparents and even further. Listening to these songs, I felt at one with what came before me, even as I imagined a oneness with the future.

That is the power of standardized *tefilla*. Not only does set prayer connect us to our fellow Jews in what can be called horizontal unification, it also fosters a sense of connection to past generations of Jews who recited these same *tefillot*.[7] And not only does this unification reach backward in time, it projects a link into the future, when our children and our children's children will recite the same *tefillot*. Its sameness connects past to future, forging a glorious present.

In fact, when standardized *tefilla* was introduced after the First Temple was destroyed, it served as a substitute for the sacrificial service, forever connecting us to our past. The Talmud makes this point when it declares: תְּפִלּוֹת כְּנֶגֶד תְּמִידִין תִּקְּנוּם – "The prayer service was established to parallel the daily sacrifices."[8]

THE COVENANT OF FAMILY

While there is unanimity among Jewish religious thinkers that the primary covenant with God took place at Sinai (*Brit Sinai*), there is disagreement as to what constitutes its precursor.[9] In my understanding, the

7. For a further elaboration of horizontal unification, see the discussion of *beit knesset* in chapter 9.
8. Berakhot 26b.
9. For Rabbi Joseph B. Soloveitchik, the foundational covenant is *Brit Mitzrayim,* forged in Egypt. This is the Covenant of Fate, in particular, shared suffering. See Soloveitchik, *Kol Dodi Dofek,* as found in *BeSod HaYaḥid VeHaYaḥad* (Jerusalem: Orot, 1976), p. 369.

   Rabbi Abraham Isaac HaKohen Kook sees the foundational covenant as emerging from an inner soulful superiority that Jews intrinsically possess – what he calls *Brit Avot,* Covenant of the Patriarchs. See his *Iggrot HaRe'iyah* (Jerusalem: Mossad Harav Kook, 5722–5725 [1961–1965]), 2:555.

foundational covenant is that of family. The book of Genesis provides the basis for this view, as it tells the story of a family, beginning with Abraham and Sarah, and continuing through Isaac and Rebecca, Jacob, Rachel, and Leah. The covenant that binds this family together also generates its shared values and aspirations. In the words of the Torah: כִּי יְדַעְתִּיו לְמַעַן אֲשֶׁר יְצַוֶּה אֶת בָּנָיו וְאֶת בֵּיתוֹ אַחֲרָיו וְשָׁמְרוּ דֶּרֶךְ ה׳ לַעֲשׂוֹת צְדָקָה וּמִשְׁפָּט – "For I love him [Abraham], as he will instruct his children and family after him to safeguard the way of the Lord, by doing what is just and right" (Gen. 18:19). What sets the Jewish people apart is our mission to bring ethical monotheism into the world. And it is this mission that emerges from and remains forever linked to what can be called *Brit Mishpaḥa*, Covenant of Family.

Covenant of Family begins when God tells Abram to go to Canaan, have children, inherit the land, and be a blessing to the world (Gen. 12:1–3, 7). The formula "and be a blessing to the world, and all the families on earth shall be blessed through you" – וְנִבְרְכוּ בְךָ כֹּל מִשְׁפְּחֹת הָאֲדָמָה is the covenantal mission to disseminate the values of ethical monotheism. This mission is repeated to Isaac and Jacob and their families.[10] It courses through the whole of Genesis, when we were not yet a nation – we were family.

---

10. Covenant, as already mentioned, is a contract with God. It involves a mission, people who will carry out this mission, and the place where it will unfold. In biblical terms, the mission is the spreading of ethical monotheism to the world, the people are the Children of Israel, and the place is the Land of Israel. These three elements are found in the narrative of each of the patriarchs:

To Abraham, God proclaims, וְנִבְרְכוּ בְךָ כֹּל מִשְׁפְּחֹת הָאֲדָמָה – "and all the families on earth shall be blessed through you" (Gen. 12:3). The covenantal formula continues as God says to Abraham, לְזַרְעֲךָ אֶתֵּן אֶת הָאָרֶץ הַזֹּאת – "to your seed I will give this land" (Gen. 12:7). The covenantal promise is repeated in Genesis 13:15; 15:18; and 17:3–9.

To Isaac, God similarly says, וְהִרְבֵּיתִי אֶת זַרְעֲךָ כְּכוֹכְבֵי הַשָּׁמַיִם וְנָתַתִּי לְזַרְעֲךָ אֵת כָּל הָאֲרָצֹת הָאֵל וְהִתְבָּרֲכוּ בְזַרְעֲךָ כֹּל גּוֹיֵי הָאָרֶץ – "I will make your descendants as numerous as the stars of heaven, and give to your descendants all these lands, so that all the nations of the earth shall be blessed through your offspring" (Gen. 26:4). The entire covenantal promise is laid out in Genesis 26:2–5.

And to Jacob, God says, אֲנִי ה׳ אֱ־לֹהֵי אַבְרָהָם אָבִיךָ וֵאלֹהֵי יִצְחָק הָאָרֶץ אֲשֶׁר אַתָּה שֹׁכֵב עָלֶיהָ לְךָ אֶתְּנֶנָּה וּלְזַרְעֶךָ. וְהָיָה זַרְעֲךָ כַּעֲפַר הָאָרֶץ...וְנִבְרֲכוּ בְךָ כָּל מִשְׁפְּחֹת הָאֲדָמָה וּבְזַרְעֶךָ – "I am the Lord, the God of your father, Abraham, and the God of Isaac. The ground on which you are lying I will assign to you and to your offspring. Your descendants

At first glance, the book of Genesis seems unnecessary.[11] After all, the Bible deals with the nation of Israel and its mission in the book of Exodus. The mission given to the Patriarchs and their families is given to the people of Israel at Sinai. There, the Israelites are told they will become an עַם סְגֻלָּה, "a treasured nation" (Ex. 19:5), and a מַמְלֶכֶת כֹּהֲנִים וְגוֹי קָדוֹשׁ – "a kingdom of priests and a holy nation" (Ex. 19:6). Priests are teachers responsible for bringing holiness, that is, ethical monotheism, into the world.[12]

But Genesis precedes Exodus not only because the Patriarchs and Matriarchs and their families generated the Jewish nation, but also to teach that the best model of nation is family. If one wishes to understand one's obligation to the Jewish nation, a good idea would be to substitute the word "nation" with "family." As family members are united by common history and goals, so are the people of Israel. It is this underlying sense of commonality that is reflected in the standardized *tefilla*, whose ultimate purpose is to bring the family together.

---

shall be as [numerous as] the dust of the earth… and all the families of the earth shall be blessed through you and your descendants" (Gen. 28:13–14). After Jacob receives an additional name, Yisrael (Israel), God repeats the covenantal promise. See Genesis 35:11–12.

Note the repetition of the formula "and all the families on earth shall be blessed through you," which, as mentioned in our text, is the mission. Note also the repetition of the promise of land and children.

11. Rashi, in his first comment on the Torah, asks this very question. See Rashi, Genesis 1:1, s.v. *bereshit*.

12. See Seforno, Exodus 19:6, s.v. *ve'atem tiheyu li mamlekhet kohanim*:

> For you have the responsibility to be a "kingdom of priests," to understand and teach the entire human race that all shall call in the name of God and serve Him in one accord.

Seforno succinctly summarizes God's special relationship with Israel while underscoring His love for all of humankind. In his words on Exodus 19:5, s.v. *viheyitem li segula mikol ha'amim*:

> Although the entire human race is more precious to Me than all other inferior creatures, for he [man] alone represents My intention, as our sages say, "Precious is man, who was created in the image [of God]" (חָבִיב אָדָם שֶׁנִּבְרָא בְּצֶלֶם) [Mishna Avot 3:14], still, you shall be to Me a treasure beyond all of them.

Translation of Seforno from his *Commentary on the Torah,* trans. Raphael Pelcovitz (New York: Mesorah Publications, 1987).

The Jewish concept of community – perhaps drawn from this understanding of its familial nature – is not merely a collection of individuals, but a whole that is greater than the sum of its parts. This idea is conveyed by the term *Knesset Yisrael*. In the words of Rabbi Joseph B. Soloveitchik:

> The community [in Judaism] is not just an assembly of people who work together for their mutual benefit, but a metaphysical entity, an individuality; I might say, a living whole. In particular, Judaism has stressed the wholeness and the unity of *Knesset Yisrael*, the Jewish community. The latter is not a conglomerate. It is an autonomous entity, endowed with a life of its own. We, for instance, lay claim to *Eretz Yisrael*. God granted the land to us as a gift. To whom did He pledge the land? Neither to an individual, nor to a partnership consisting of millions of people. He gave it to the *Knesset Yisrael*, to the community as an independent unity, as a distinct juridic metaphysical person. He did not promise the land to me, to you, to them; nor did He promise the land to all of us together. Abraham did not receive the land as an individual, but as the father of a future nation. The owner of the Promised Land is the *Knesset Yisrael*, which is a community persona. However strange such a concept may appear to the empirical sociologist, it is not at all a strange experience for the halakhist and the mystic, to whom *Knesset Yisrael* is a living, loving, and suffering mother.[13]

It follows that if a person is missing from an "assembly of people," it is hardly noticeable. The group is fundamentally the same – a conglomerate minus an individual. But if the community is a "metaphysical entity," a missing person significantly alters the very essence of the group. As an "individuality," each person plays an essential role in the makeup of the whole. As a family, every person plays a vital, irreplaceable part – no one is dispensable.

This idea lends itself to the theory of Rabbi Judah HaLevi, who

13. Rabbi Joseph B. Soloveitchik, "The Community," *Tradition* 17, no. 2 (Spring 1978), pp. 12–13.

writes that the advantage of communal prayer is that, individually, our weaknesses are glaring. Together, however, we make up for each other's deficiencies; my strength is your weakness, your strength is my weakness. Only in a *tzibbur* – a community with common prayer – can *tefilla* be whole again. In his words:

> Common prayer has many advantages.... An individual rarely accomplishes his prayer without slips and errors. Therefore it has been established that the individual should pray with a community, and if possible with a community of not less than ten persons, so that one makes up for the forgetfulness or error of the other.... In this way, a complete prayer is gained, read with wholly pure devotion. Its blessing rests on everyone, each receiving his portion.[14]

PERSONAL EXPRESSION IN *TEFILLA*

Notwithstanding the influences that join our people and fashion a nation, it is crucial to remember that the nation is made up of individuals, each of whom is unique. While Judaism stresses the importance of community, on both a national and universal level, one must never lose one's sense of individuality. According to Rabbi Soloveitchik, the lone creation of Adam was meant to teach the importance of each individual. The value of our individuality can never been underestimated. In the words of Rabbi Soloveitchik:

> Why was it necessary to create lonely man? Why was social man not created at the very outset?
>
> 1. The originality and creativity in man are rooted in his loneliness – experience, not in his social awareness.... Social man is superficial: he imitates, he emulates. Lonely man is profound: he creates, he is original.
> 2. Lonely man is free: social man is bound by many rules and ordinances. God willed man to be free. Man is required, from

14. HaLevi, *Kuzari*, pp. 137–138 (3:19).

> time to time, to defy the world, to replace the old and obsolete with the new and relevant. Only lonely man is capable of casting off the harness of bondage to society.[15]

The tension between the subjective experience of the "lonely man" and the structured experience of communal obligation is reflected in the following talmudic discussion about the source of *tefilla*. This passage discusses two possible precedents for prayer: the Patriarchs' prayer and the sacrificial offerings brought during the Temple period. How we understand the origins of prayer is important, as these two views present us with two different models of approaching prayer today.

> אִיתְּמַר, רַבִּי יוֹסֵי בְּרַבִּי חֲנִינָא אָמַר תְּפִלּוֹת אָבוֹת תִּקְּנוּם, רַבִּי יְהוֹשֻׁעַ בֶּן לֵוִי אָמַר תְּפִלּוֹת כְּנֶגֶד תְּמִידִין תִּקְּנוּם...
>
> תַּנְיָא כְּוָותֵיהּ דְּרַבִּי יוֹסֵי בְּר׳ חֲנִינָא: אַבְרָהָם תִּקֵּן תְּפִלַּת שַׁחֲרִית, שֶׁנֶּאֱמַר: וַיַּשְׁכֵּם אַבְרָהָם בַּבּוֹקֶר אֶל הַמָּקוֹם אֲשֶׁר עָמַד שָׁם. וְאֵין עֲמִידָה אֶלָּא תְּפִלָּה, שֶׁנֶּאֱמַר: וַיַּעֲמֹד פִּינְחָס וַיְפַלֵּל.
>
> יִצְחָק תִּיקֵּן תְּפִלַּת מִנְחָה, שֶׁנֶּאֱמַר: וַיֵּצֵא יִצְחָק לָשׂוּחַ בַּשָּׂדֶה לִפְנוֹת עָרֶב. וְאֵין שִׂיחָה אֶלָּא תְּפִלָּה, שֶׁנֶּאֱמַר: תְּפִלָּה לְעָנִי כִּי יַעֲטֹף וְלִפְנֵי ה׳ יִשְׁפּוֹךְ שִׂיחוֹ.
>
> יַעֲקֹב תִּקֵּן תְּפִלַּת עַרְבִית, שֶׁנֶּאֱמַר: וַיִּפְגַּע בַּמָּקוֹם וַיָּלֶן שָׁם. וְאֵין פְּגִיעָה אֶלָּא תְּפִלָּה, שֶׁנֶּאֱמַר: וְאַתָּה אַל תִּתְפַּלֵּל בְּעַד הָעָם הַזֶּה וְאַל תִּשָּׂא בַעֲדָם רִנָּה וּתְפִלָּה וְאַל תִּפְגַּע בִּי.
>
> It has been stated: R. Yose b. R. Ḥanina said: The *tefillot* were instituted by the Patriarchs. R. Yehoshua b. Levi said: The *tefillot* were instituted to replace the daily sacrifices (*temidin*)....
>
> It has been taught in accordance with Rabbi Yose b. Ḥanina: Abraham instituted the morning *tefilla,* as it says, "And Abraham got up early in the morning to the place where he had stood (*amad*)" [Gen. 19:27]. And standing means prayer, as it says, "And Pinḥas stood and prayed" [Ps. 106:30].
>
> Isaac instituted the afternoon *tefilla,* as it says, "And Isaac

15. Soloveitchik, "Community," pp. 12–13, 18–20.

> went out to meditate (*lasuaḥ*) in the field at eventide" [Gen. 24:63]. And meditation means prayer, as it says, "A prayer of the afflicted when he faints and pours out his meditation before the Lord" [Ps. 102:1].
>
> Jacob instituted the evening prayer, as it says, "And he encountered (*vayifga*) the place and lay down there" [Gen. 28:11]. And encounter means prayer, as it says, "Therefore do not pray for this people, neither lift up prayer nor cry for them, neither encounter Me" [Jer. 7:16].

The Talmud then presents the position that prayer corresponds to the sacrificial service:

> It has also been taught in accordance with R. Yehoshua b. Levi: Why did they say that the morning *tefilla* could be said till midday? Because the regular morning sacrifice could be brought up to midday. R. Yehuda, however, says that it may be said up to the fourth hour, because the regular morning sacrifice may be brought up to the fourth hour. And why did they say that the afternoon *tefilla* can be said up to the evening? Because the regular afternoon offering could be brought up to the evening. R. Yehuda, however, says that it can be said only up to the middle of the afternoon, because the evening offering could be brought only up to the middle of the afternoon. And why did they say that for the evening *tefilla* there is no limit? Because the limbs and the fat that were not consumed by the evening could be brought all night.[16]

It has been suggested that if *tefilla* corresponds to the Patriarchs, it is fundamentally spontaneous. If it corresponds to the sacrifices, it is standardized.

There is something about the personalities of the Patriarchs that inspired them to pray when they did.

Abraham was an innovator, a trailblazer, the quintessential "morning person." He discovers God and introduces the world to monotheism.

16. Berakhot 26b.

Appropriately, he prays at dawn, when the sun rises. This is the reason that, in describing Abraham at prayer, the biblical text uses the language of *amida,* which literally means "standing," but figuratively refers to standing up for a new idea.

Amida is also an allusion to standing up for justice. The source of Abraham's morning prayer stems from his debate with God concerning the city of Sodom. The language of *amida* is used to emphasize the fact that Abraham stands up for what he believes is right, demanding that God act justly. As wicked as the people of Sodom may have been, Abraham still cares about their fate. Note also the supporting text about Pinḥas. Observing people acting immorally, he stood up (*vaya'amod*), demanding justice.[17]

Isaac, a meditator who evaluated and then transmitted his father's ideas, was in many ways a passive figure, content to follow in Abraham's footsteps. Isaac was taken to Mount Moriah to be offered as a sacrifice (the *Akeda*), had a wife chosen for him, and redug the wells his father had discovered. He was a man who reacted rather than acted, contemplated rather than initiated. Therefore, he prays in the afternoon, as the sun sets, an especially suitable time for contemplative thought. This is the reason the language used to describe Isaac's *tefilla* is *siḥa,* as it connotes a dialogue that is thoughtful and meditative.

Consider the context of Isaac's *tefilla*. Having emerged from the near-death experience of the *Akeda,* he longs for companionship and is hopeful that Eliezer, his father's steward, has found a wife suitable for him. Perhaps that was the essence of his *tefilla* that late afternoon, as the sun set. Soon after, his wife-to-be, Rebecca, arrives. Consider also that the supporting text is King David's description of an afflicted person deep in thought (*siḥo*). Perhaps David is alluding to his ongoing struggles against the Philistines and King Saul or his inner struggles concerning Bathsheba and Uriah – struggles that prompt him to engage in serious introspection and self-evaluation.

Isaac's son Jacob was the most tragic of the biblical figures. Hated by his brother, he was separated from his parents for twenty-two years. His beloved wife, Rachel, died young; his favorite son, Joseph,

17. In Numbers 25:7, the text uses the verb *vayakam.*

disappeared and was believed to be dead. Appropriately, Jacob prayed at night, when one is often overcome by fear and a sense of deep loneliness. This is the reason the language used to describe Jacob's *tefilla* is *pegi'a*, which means "bump into" or "encounter," implying a sudden, if not unknown obstacle.

Jacob had just run away from home, managing to escape his brother, Esau, from whom he had taken their father's blessing. Facing the unexpected, with the darkness of night upon him, he begins to offer his *tefilla*. And the supporting text is God's decree to Jeremiah – just prior to the destruction of the First Temple – that interceding or entreating (*tifga*) on behalf of Israel would be to no avail.

In contrast, viewing *tefilla* as a replacement for the sacrifices highlights the standardization of prayer.

At the end of this talmudic passage, R. Yose b. R. Ḥanina concludes:

> תְּפִלּוֹת אָבוֹת תִּקְּנוּם וְאַסְמְכִינְהוּ רַבָּנָן אַקָּרְבָּנוֹת.
>
> The *tefillot* were instituted by the Patriarchs, and the rabbis found a basis for them in the offerings.[18]

From here we see again that prayer is meant to serve as a structure in which personal expression can – and should – flourish.

The balance of spontaneity and structure that emerges as a key element of *tefilla* is a central dynamic of any thriving love relationship. The first words the Torah uses to describe human love are *ezer kenegdo* (Gen. 1:18). *Ezer* literally means "help." In love, this is a reference to our responsibility to share a common vision, a common purpose, with the other. Maimonides refers to this ideal as the highest love:

> אוֹהֵב מַעֲלָה הוּא שֶׁיִּהְיֶה תַּאֲוַת שְׁנֵיהֶם וְכַוָּנָתָם לְדָבָר אֶחָד.
>
> The highest love is that both [parties] share common purposes and goals.[19]

18. Berakhot 26b.
19. See Maimonides, *Peirush HaMishnayot* on Mishna Avot 1:6.

Kenegdo, on the other hand, means "against," or "apart," or "opposite." In love, it speaks of the reality that even in the most intimate relationship, we are each responsible for doing all we can to maintain our own identity – and help the other realize his or hers.[20]

Tefilla, too, is a love encounter of *ezer kenegdo*. We seek to be one with the larger Jewish family, to share in its mission through our actions and prayers. When we do this, we relate to *Knesset Yisrael* as an *ezer*. At the same time, *kenegdo* encourages us to nurture and express our individuality. For the talmudic rabbis, this was also a key function of prayer:

> רַבִּי אֱלִיעֶזֶר אוֹמֵר הָעוֹשֶׂה תְּפִלָּתוֹ קֶבַע [אֵין תְּפִלָּתוֹ תַּחֲנוּנִים]. מַאי קֶבַע? אָמַר רַבִּי יַעֲקֹב בַּר אִידִי אָמַר רַבִּי אוֹשַׁעְיָא: כָּל שֶׁתְּפִלָּתוֹ דּוֹמָה עָלָיו כְּמַשּׂוֹי; וְרַבָּנָן אָמְרִי: כָּל מִי שֶׁאֵינוֹ אוֹמְרָהּ בִּלְשׁוֹן תַּחֲנוּנִים; רַבָּה וְרַב יוֹסֵף דְּאָמְרִי תַּרְוַיְיהוּ: כָּל שֶׁאֵינוֹ יָכוֹל לְחַדֵּשׁ בָּהּ.
>
> R. Eliezer says: He who makes his prayer a fixed task [his prayer is not a genuine supplication]: What is meant by a fixed task? R. Yaakov b. Idi said in the name of R. Oshaya: Anyone whose prayer is like a burden on him. The rabbis say: Whoever does not say it in a manner of supplication. Rabba and R. Yosef both say: Whoever is unable to insert something fresh in it.[21]

According to R. Oshaya, if an individual experiences prayer as a burden, his is not a sincere prayer. The rabbis take this position one step further, arguing that prayer must also be supplicatory. Rabba and R. Yosef then present yet another qualification, insisting that one add something new and unique to the *tefilla*.

While each of these opinions presents a different standard, they all maintain that the individual must fully bring himself or herself to the *tefilla*. This talmudic passage teaches us that even within the standardized prayer service, one is not just permitted but *obligated* to express

20. Here lies what is perhaps the greatest challenge of love. How can a couple share a common goal without becoming clones of one another? The flip side is equally daunting. How can a lover help his or her beloved realize his or her full, unique potential without the two drifting apart?
21. Berakhot 29b.

one's individual feelings. Even within the framework of structured *tefilla*, there is room – indeed, need – for spontaneity.

This is not just a theoretical idea, but a practice that many rabbis used in their own *tefillot*. The Talmud provides examples of the personal *tefillot* added by Rav and by Mar b. Ravina to the standard *tefilla* text:

> רַב בָּתַר צְלוֹתֵיהּ אָמַר הָכִי: יְהִי רָצוֹן מִלְּפָנֶיךָ ה׳ אֱ־לֹהֵינוּ שֶׁתִּתֵּן לָנוּ חַיִּים אֲרוּכִּים, חַיִּים שֶׁל שָׁלוֹם, חַיִּים שֶׁל טוֹבָה, חַיִּים שֶׁל בְּרָכָה, חַיִּים שֶׁל פַּרְנָסָה, חַיִּים שֶׁל חִלּוּץ עֲצָמוֹת, חַיִּים שֶׁיֵּשׁ בָּהֶם יִרְאַת חֵטְא, חַיִּים שֶׁאֵין בָּהֶם בּוּשָׁה וּכְלִימָּה, חַיִּים שֶׁל עוֹשֶׁר וְכָבוֹד, חַיִּים שֶׁתְּהֵא בָּנוּ אַהֲבַת תּוֹרָה וְיִרְאַת שָׁמַיִם, חַיִּים שֶׁתְּמַלֵּא לָנוּ אֶת כָּל מִשְׁאֲלוֹת לִבֵּנוּ לְטוֹבָה.
>
> Rav, on concluding his prayer, added the following: May it be Your will, O Lord our God, to grant us long life, a life of peace, a life of good, a life of blessing, a life of sustenance, a life of bodily vigor, a life in which there is fear of sin, a life free of shame and confusion, a life of riches and honor, a life in which we may be filled with love of Torah and fear of heaven, a life in which You shall fulfill all the desires of our heart for good![22]

> מַר בְּרֵיהּ דְּרָבִינָא כִּי הֲוָה מְסַיֵּים צְלוֹתֵיהּ אָמַר הָכִי אֱ־לֹהַי נְצוֹר לְשׁוֹנִי מֵרַע וְשִׂפְתוֹתַי מִדַּבֵּר מִרְמָה וְלִמְקַלְלַי נַפְשִׁי תִדּוֹם וְנַפְשִׁי כֶּעָפָר לַכֹּל תִּהְיֶה פְּתַח לִבִּי בְּתוֹרָתֶךָ וּבְמִצְוֹתֶיךָ תִּרְדּוֹף נַפְשִׁי וְתַצִּילֵנִי מִפֶּגַע רַע...וְכָל הַחוֹשְׁבִים עָלַי רָעָה מְהֵרָה הָפֵר עֲצָתָם וְקַלְקֵל מַחְשְׁבוֹתָם.
>
> Mar b. Ravina, on concluding his prayer, added the following: My God, keep my tongue from evil and my lips from speaking guile. May my soul be silent to those who curse me, and may my soul be as dust to all. Open my heart to Your Torah, and may my soul pursue Your commandments, and deliver me from evil happenings.... And all those who design evil against me, speedily annul their counsel and frustrate their designs.[23]

---

22. Ibid. 16b.
23. Ibid. 17a. Both these *tefillot* have become part of our fixed service. The former is the Blessing for the New Month and the latter is recited at the end of the silent *Shemoneh Esreh*.

Shemuel, in the Talmud, also details the rights of individuals to offer personal *tefillot* within the defined text:

> R. Yehuda said in the name of Shemuel: The law is that one may make any request in the blessing of "He Who Hears Prayer" (*Shome'a Tefilla*).[24]

Shome'a Tefilla, the last of the blessings of request in the *Amida,* asks that God listen to our voice – שְׁמַע קוֹלֵנוּ. It is a summary blessing; hence, within it, one may add any request. Rav expands on this formula:

> R. Ḥiyya b. Ashi said in the name of Rav: Even though it is said that a person may make any request in "He Who Hears Prayer," if one knows of someone who is sick, he may say so in the blessing of healing, and if one needs livelihood, he may say so in the blessing for proseperity.[25]

For Rav, requests can also be added in two particular blessings. In רְפָאֵנוּ ה׳ וְנֵרָפֵא – "Heal us, Lord, and we shall be healed," one can include a *tefilla* for individuals who seek recovery from illness. In בָּרֵךְ עָלֵינוּ ה׳ אֱ־לֹהֵינוּ אֶת הַשָּׁנָה הַזֹּאת – "for us, Lord our God," one can add wishes for personal sustenance.

Rav broadens the possibilities even further, maintaining that one can introduce a personal *tefilla* within any of the standardized paragraphs of *bakasha*:

> [In the name of] Rav [it was] said, even though it is said that a person may make any request in *Shome'a Tefilla,* one has the right to make a request in any of the blessings according to its theme.[26]

24. Avoda Zara 8a. This and the next few citations from Avoda Zara 8a are not presented in the order in which they appear in the Talmud. I have shifted them around to show how the right to insert personal tefillot broadens until it includes all the *bakashot,* and in fact includes the right at the end of the *Shemoneh Esreh* to introduce tefillot even if they are as long as the Yom Kippur service.
25. Ibid.
26. Ibid.

R. Yehoshua b. Levi declares that at the conclusion of the *Shemoneh Esreh,* one can even introduce *tefillot* as long as the Yom Kippur service itself:

> R. Yehoshua b. Levi said: Even though it is said that a person may make any request in *Shome'a Tefilla,* if one wishes to introduce a personal prayer, even as long as the Yom Kippur service, he may do so at the end.[27]

Rabbi Joseph Karo, author of the *Shulḥan Arukh,* codifies the right to introduce personal *tefilla* as the halakha: "If one wishes to add to one of the middle blessings in the spirit of the blessing, it is permissible."[28]

The Rema adds one caveat: "And when one adds, begin the [standard] blessing and then insert. But one should not add before beginning the [standardized] blessing."[29] Here, the Rema insists that the standard text should be the basis for personal *tefilla.*[30] Yet while he argues that individualization can take place only within the sanctioned communal structure, we must remember that the intent of the fixed text is not to silence the individual's *tefilla* but to encourage it. Structured *tefilla* is meant to inspire spontaneous *tefilla.*[31] From this perspective, *tefilla* is a delicate balance between individual aspiration and communal responsibility.

THE HIGHER-OCTAVE *AMIDA*

This background may give us an understanding of why the silent *Amida* is repeated almost verbatim by the leader of the service. This prayer is fundamentally individual in nature, while its repetition is communal. Unlike the private *Amida,* a *minyan* of ten is needed for the repetition,

27. Ibid.
28. *Shulḥan Arukh, Oraḥ Ḥayyim* 119:1.
29. Ibid.
30. See *Mishna Berura* ad loc., n. 3, who argues that the text ordained by the rabbis comes first, as it is the main thing, while personal requests are less important.
31. See Rabbi Shlomo Riskin, "Structure and Spontaneity in Prayer," *Judaism* 21, no. 3 (summer 1972), p. 331, who writes: "The Prayer Book was not meant to exhaust but, rather, to inspire prayer."

and after each blessing, the congregants answer "Amen," signifying the participation of the community. Some even insist that the congregation remain standing during the repetition. As the *Arukh HaShulḥan* codifies,

> There are those who say that the entire congregation should stand during the repetition of the leader of the service. And this is the proper way to conduct oneself.[32]

While it consists of the same words as the silent *Amida,* the repetition of the *Amida* contains a new motif – that of community.[33] Although individuals have the right to add personal requests to the silent *Amida,* the leader of the service cannot add anything when repeating the *Shemoneh Esreh.*[34] This is because the silent *Amida* is, in many ways, a personal prayer, while the repetition is communal in nature. As Rabbi Shlomo Riskin wrote:

> In the private *Amida,* it is primarily the individual who stands before God, albeit an individual who is deeply concerned for the well-being of every Jew and links his personal aspirations with those of his coreligionists. Nevertheless, it is incumbent upon him to depart from the structured text in order to make of his Divine Dialogue a living personal experience. With the repetition of the *Amida,* the individual members of the congregation join in recognition of historic commitment to an ideal which is so movingly expressed in our prayer book. The *sheli'aḥ tzibbur* [person who leads our service] dare not depart from the structured text, since he symbolizes united Israel, standing before his God.[35]

---

32. *Arukh HaShulḥan, Oraḥ Ḥayyim* 123:9.
33. Note that *Kedusha* is recited only during the repetition, as it requires a *minyan.* Moreover, the concluding prayer *E-lohai Netzor,* recited in the singular at the end of the *Shemoneh Esreh,* is dropped in the repetition.
34. Furthermore, when praying privately, one recites the additional prayer for a fast day (*Aneinu*) within the blessing of *Shema Koleinu.* In contrast, during the repetition, *Aneinu* is added as a distinct blessing.
35. Riskin, "Structure and Spontaneity," pp. 331–332.

With this we may understand the flow of *tefilla* leading up to the *Amida* and its repetition. Before the silent *Amida,* a motif of yearning prevails. The yearning manifests itself in the blessings prior to the *Shemoneh Esreh.* There we speak of the universalistic God (*Yotzer HaMe'orot*), then of the particularistic God (*HaBoḥer BeAmo Yisrael BeAhava*), and finally of the God who promises to be with us no matter the challenge (*Ga'al Yisrael*).[36] We then reach the ultimate moment of connection with God, the pinnacle of prayer, the silent *Amida.*

One may gain an understanding of the emotional flow of the prayer service when considering the story of a mother and daughter who were separated during the time when the Berlin Wall divided the eastern and western parts of the city. In time, the wall came down. When the gates opened, the mother and daughter, who had not seen each other in years, began to run toward one another. As they ran, the mother cried out, "My daughter, my daughter!" and the daughter called out, "Mother, mother!" their cries, growing more and more intense as they approached one another. But the moment they embraced, neither said a word. Their encounter was completely silent.

This is the ultimate *tefilla*: First the words of yearning, like mother and daughter calling out to each other. And then the private embrace with God, the silent *Amida,* whose goal is the most impassioned personal relationship. As Rabbi Jonathan Sacks points out: "The *Amida* is the summit of prayer: in it, we enter the Holy of Holies of religious experience. We say it standing because we are conscious of being in the unmediated presence of God."[37]

It can also be suggested that the silence of the *Amida* adds to the religious intensity of the encounter with God. Sometimes the greatest expression of love takes place in silence.

Of course, the silent *Amida* contains words. Still, relative to other *tefillot,* the *Amida* is silent, as one does not raise one's voice when reciting this prayer. As Rabbi Joseph Karo says:

---

36. See chapter 4 for an analysis of these blessings.
37. Jonathan Sacks, *The Koren Siddur* (Jerusalem: Koren Publishers, 2009), p. 109.

> One should not confine his prayer to his heart, but must pronounce the phrases with his lips and say them quietly, loudly enough to be able to hear them with his ears. [Still] he should not let his voice be heard.[38]

In other words, one's voice should be audible only to oneself. Only God and the person praying hear; they, and they alone, are privy to the give and take.

Rabbi Naftali Tzvi Yehuda Berlin (the Netziv) notes that sometimes sounds can have more impact than words. He offers this insight in commenting that when God tells Moses that the Jews will listen to him (and join him in demanding freedom from Pharaoh), the Torah uses the expression וְשָׁמְעוּ לְקֹלֶךָ – "and they will listen to your voice" (Ex. 3:18). *Kol* (voice), the Netziv proclaims, is not the same as *dibbur* (speech). As he puts it: וְשָׁמְעוּ לְקוֹלֶךָ וְלֹא לִדְבָרֶיךָ – "They will listen to your voice and not to your words."[39] That is, the Jews will hear your sounds of concern and respond accordingly. This is what Dr. Avivah Zornberg calls "the murmuring deep"[40] – the sounds that go beyond words, even beyond silence; the sounds of love, of agony, of concern, of oneness. The sounds that only one very close can understand. Private *tefilla* is the personal, intimate conversation that only the person praying and God can hear.

This intensely private moment is followed by the repetition of the *Shemoneh Esreh*, which reminds us that no matter how personal our needs may be, we are part of a larger peoplehood, its celebrations and challenges. Thus, the repetition is not the prayer of an individual, but a prayer of collective "individuality." The leader of the service becomes the embodiment of all those assembled. Disparate people, coming from different places with different needs, pause, reflect, and join, becoming a collective whole – a "unity of souls."[41]

38. *Shulḥan Arukh, Oraḥ Ḥayyim* 101:2.
39. See Netziv, *Ha'amek Davar,* Exodus 3:18, s.v. *veshamu lekolekha.*
40. See Dr. Avivah Zornberg, *The Murmuring Deep* (New York: Schocken, 2009).
41. Natan Sharansky first used the expression "unity of souls" in a letter he sent from the Soviet Gulag to his wife, Avital. See Natan Sharansky, *Fear No Evil* (New York: Random House, 1988), p. 362.

From this perspective, it may be best to use a term other than "repetition of the *Shemoneh Esreh*" to describe the leader's reading of the *Amida*. Repetition has its value. Winston Churchill purportedly said, "Tell 'em what you're going to tell 'em, tell 'em, and then tell 'em what you told 'em."[42] Still, the term "repetition" is problematic, as congregants may feel there is no need to listen, since the *Shemoneh Esreh* has already been said. Rather, this part of the service should be viewed as a "renewal of the *Shemoneh Esreh*." While the words are nearly the same as the silent one, they are new, as we mentally focus on community rather than the individual.[43]

The silent *Amida*, the *Amida* of the murmuring voice, may be an example of "prayer as reliance" – when the human being stands submissively before God, dependent upon Him. The repetition of the *Amida*, the *Amida* of words, may reflect "prayer as responsibility" – when the human being asserts his or her role in helping God redeem the world.

The Mishna offers a different rationale for the repetition of the *Shemoneh Esreh*:

> Just as the congregational reader [*sheli'aḥ tzibbur*] is under obligation, so every individual is under obligation. Rabban Gamliel, however, said that the congregational reader fulfills the whole congregation's obligation. (Mishna Rosh HaShana 4:5)

Rabbi Obadiah of Bertinoro ad loc., s.v. *keshem*, explains the first view in this way:

> Both the *sheli'aḥ tzibbur* and individuals are obligated to recite the silent *Amida*.... The repetition is offered by the *sheli'aḥ tzibbur* to fulfill the obligation of those who are not versed.

He then explains the position of Rabban Gamliel:

> The *sheli'aḥ tzibbur* can fulfill the obligation of every individual, even those who are versed.... Still, the *sheli'aḥ tzibbur* recites the silent *Amida* so he can prepare himself for the repetition.

According to the first view, the repetition is recited only for the sake of those who are not learned and therefore cannot recite the silent *Amida* on their own. As the leader repeats the *Amida*, they can recite the words with him.

According to Rabban Gamliel, the repetition can fulfill the individual's obligation, with the leader's private rendition serving as preparation for this repetition.

The Talmud concludes that even for Rabban Gamliel, the leader of the service can fulfill the obligations only of those who can't pray at that moment, such as those working in the field (Rosh HaShana 35a).

42. Some suggest that this was said by Dale Carnegie, a motivational speaker of the early twentieth century.
43. The rabbinic term *Ḥazarat HaShatz* – usually translated as the "Reader's Repetition" – can have a different meaning. *Ḥazor* can mean returning to the starting

Prayer is song; prayer of prayers – song of songs. This is the *Shemoneh Esreh*, the *Amida*, what the rabbis call *tefilla*.[44] Using the metaphor of melody, the *Shemoneh Esreh* said aloud by the leader of the service can be called "The Higher-Octave *Amida*." The musical cycle contains seven notes, popularly sung do-re-mi-fa-so-la-ti. There is, however, an eighth note – do. The eighth is the same as the first, except that it is sung one octave higher.[45] Thus, the *Keli Yakar* maintains, **כָּל קִלּוּסוֹ שֶׁל מֹשֶׁה הָיָה בְּאָז** – "All of Moses' songs begin with *Az* (Then),"[46] a Hebrew word with the numerical value of eight, as the songs were all-encompassing, all-inspiring, going beyond the seven-note scale, reaching a higher plane.

The communal *Shemoneh Esreh* represents this next cycle, this higher octave. It is similar to the silent *Amida*, and yet is significantly different. It is higher, as it manifests the yearnings, the hopes, the aspirations, the angst and dreams not only of the individual, but of the whole Community of Israel.[47] The communal *Shemoneh Esreh* rides the back of the silent one,[48] becoming the prayer of the higher octave, "The Higher-Octave *Amida*."[49]

---

point, not to "repeat" but to begin anew by reciting the communal *Amida*.

Rabbi Joseph B. Soloveitchik often distinguished between *tefilla betzibbur*, praying the silent *Amida* with the community, and *tefillat hatzibbur*, the leader's recitation of the *Amida* on behalf of the community. See, for example, Rabbi Hershel Schachter, *Nefesh HaRav* (Brooklyn, NY: Flatbush Beth Hamedrosh, 1994), p. 123.

44. See, for example, Berakhot 4:1.

45. Technically, the eighth note is the last of the previous octave, or the first of the next.

46. *Keli Yakar*, Leviticus 9:1, s.v. *vayehi bayom hashemini*. See also Rabbi Samson Raphael Hirsch's *Commentary on the Torah*, Leviticus 9:1.

47. The psalmist refers to "the music of the ten-string lyre" as *alei asor* (Ps. 92:4). Homiletically, the term *Shemoneh Esreh* could refer to the eight (*shemoneh*), the higher octave, atop the ten (*esreh*)-string lyre, encompassing not only the silent *Amida*, but the higher-octave communal *Amida*.

48. See *Keli Yakar*, Leviticus 9:1.

49. The repetition of the *Shemoneh Esreh* as "The Higher-Octave *Amida*" was inspired by a talk I heard by Rabbi Ari Hart. I am grateful to him.

Part Three
Spirituality

The Midrash describes the Torah as אֵשׁ שְׁחוֹרָה עַל גַּבֵּי אֵשׁ לְבָנָה *– "black fire on white fire."*[1] *On a simple level, the black fire represents the letters of the Torah, while the white fire is the space between the letters. On a deeper level, the black fire may represent halakha, formal Jewish law, while the white fire may represent the spiritual counterpart of the law. Spirituality is to halakha as heaven is to earth, as soul is to body, giving that which is anchored the ability to soar.*

Rabbi Shneur Zalman of Liadi, the first Lubavitcher Rebbe, echoes this idea in his teaching that every mitzva – whether of thought, word, or deed – reflects a spirituality that emanates from the soul. In his words:

> *Every divine soul possesses three garments. They are the thought, speech, and action of the... mitzvot of the Torah. For when a person fulfills... the commandments... his soul is clothed with the... mitzvot of the Torah.*[2]

---

1. See Rashi, Deuteronomy 33:2, s.v. *eish dat*, quoting Midrash Tanḥuma, Genesis 1. See also Jerusalem Talmud, Shekalim 6:1.
2. Rabbi Shneur Zalman of Liadi, *Liqqutei Amarim* (*Tanya*), trans. Nissan Mindel (Brooklyn, NY: Kehot Publication Society, 1962), 1:4, p. 34.

Often, halakha is seen as constricting one's spirituality – we become so involved in the minutiae of halakha that it blocks our connection to God. The very term halakha, however, comes from the word halakh *(go), as it is a system that enables the finite human being to go toward the infinite God. We must remember that halakha is the "garment," shaping the spiritual moment, helping us encounter God Himself.*[3]

It is within this framework that we begin our discussion about spirituality in general, and more specifically about bringing spirituality into prayer. First, we will present the halakhic aspects of kavana *(intent) in prayer. We will then delve into* kavana's *inner spiritual realms with the goal of seeing how the laws and spiritual dimensions of* tefilla *enhance each other. Finally, we will discuss how spirituality can be brought into the synagogue, the central place of prayer.*

3. Our analysis of spirituality will offer an understanding of how the word "spiritual" complements such terms as "observant" and "religious." The word "observant" is commonly used to denote one who follows ritual, especially ritual that governs one's relationship with God, i.e., Shabbat and the dietary laws. The word "religious" refers to a person's sense of interpersonal ethics. It follows that one could be observant without being religious, and vice versa. In fact, one could be observant and religious but not spiritual, as observance and ritual may be bereft of God. Spirituality, however, means that in all one does, one powerfully feels the presence of God. The goal of the halakhic person is to be all three – religious, observant, and spiritual – merging these dimensions into one personality.

Chapter Seven

Kavana

A rabbi was once informed that a crazed woman was in the *beit midrash* (the study hall, which is sometimes used as a small prayer room). "She is standing in front of the Ark, the Ark is open, and she is babbling and gesturing wildly," he was told. "She seems to be mentally imbalanced. Perhaps you can go in and help her."

The rabbi went in. As he sat quietly in the back, he could see that the woman was deeply immersed in *tefilla*. The rabbi overheard some of her words as she swayed and cried out: "Dear God, I know I was here just last week, but I am back because I need your help. My daughter is still not well. Please, please, in my hour of need, do not forsake me, do not leave me!"

Understanding the privacy of her *tefilla*, the rabbi left the woman alone. Upon his return, he was asked, "So what did you do with the babbling crazy lady?" The rabbi responded, "This morning I got up, put on my prayer shawl, donned my *tefillin* and *davened*. But this woman wasn't *davening*, she was talking to God. That's a whole different world."[1]

---

1. I first heard this story from Rabbi Kenneth Hain.

As mentioned, the Talmud considers Hannah the paradigm of prayer (Berakhot 30b; 31a). Yet in the book of Samuel, the high priest mistakes her fervent prayer for drunkenness. Interestingly, the word for "drunk" in Hebrew – שִׁכּוֹר (*shikkor*) – is an anagram for the word כָּשֵׁר (*kasher*, or kosher). Sometimes the line between "drunkenness" and appropriate spiritual intensity is very thin. See I Samuel 1:13–17.

UNDERSTANDING THE WORDS

Tefilla is not about superficially reciting words, it's about internalizing them so that one can communicate powerfully with God. The halakhic term for internalization is *kavana*. *Kavana* is associated not only with *tefilla*, but with Jewish ritual in general. The term comes from the root K-V-N, which means "direction." An important goal of religious ritual is to direct one's intention to the ritual's deeper meaning.

In prayer, the first level of *kavana* is to understand the literal meaning of the words being recited. The talmudic rabbis discussed the scope of this requirement. Must one maintain such awareness throughout the entirety of the *Shemoneh Esreh*? And if one doesn't maintain such awareness, is one's prayer invalid?

One view quoted in the Talmud is that while it is optimal to have *kavana* throughout the *Shemoneh Esreh*, it would be sufficient *bedi'avad* (*ex post facto*) if one had *kavana* only while reciting the first paragraph (the paragraph of *Avoteinu*):

> When one recites the *tefilla* [i.e., the *Shemoneh Esreh*], he must say all the blessings attentively, and if he cannot say all attentively, he should say one attentively. R. Ḥiyya said in the name of R. Safra, who had it from a member of the school of rabbis: This one should be the blessing of the Patriarchs (*Avoteinu*).[2]

Maimonides accordingly concludes:

> One who has prayed but did not sustain *kavana* should repeat the prayer with *kavana*. But if one had *kavana* for the first blessing, he need not [pray] again.[3]

Concurring with Maimonides, the *Shulḥan Arukh* states:

2. Berakhot 34b.
3. Maimonides, *Code*, Laws of Prayer 10:1.

> One who is praying [the *Shemoneh Esreh*] should sustain *kavana* for all the blessings. And if he can't have proper *kavana* for all the blessings, he should minimally have *kavana* in *Avoteinu*.[4]

The Rema adds:

> And today we do not repeat [the *Shemoneh Esreh*] for lack of *kavana*. Because even if one repeats the prayer, it is virtually certain that he will still not have *kavana*. Under these circumstances, why repeat the prayer?[5]

It is clear that over time the level of *kavana* declined.[6] Although the Rema concludes that one should not repeat the *Shemoneh Esreh* if *kavana* is lacking, optimally one should have *kavana* throughout *Shemoneh Esreh*; minimally, during *Avoteinu*.

---

4. *Shulḥan Arukh, Oraḥ Ḥayyim* 101:1.
5. Rema, ibid.
6. This applies to the *Shema* as well. Mishna Berakhot 2:5 (Berakhot 16a) states: "A bridegroom is exempt from reciting the *Shema* on the first night [of his marriage]." This is because the bridegroom, intent on performing his marital duty, lacks the proper concentration (*kavana*) to recite the *Shema*.

   A thousand years later, *Tosafot*, Berakhot 17b, s.v. *Rav Shisha*, states that people no longer pray with such concentration even under normal circumstances, so the bridegroom should read the *Shema* on his wedding night. In fact, say the *Tosafot*, were he not to recite the *Shema*, he would appear arrogant. In the words of the *Tosafot*:

   > Since we no longer pray with proper *kavana*, even a bridegroom should read the *Shema* [on his wedding night]. In fact, if he were not to recite the *Shema*, he would appear to be arrogant, as if trying to create the impression that he normally prays with proper *kavana*.

   Here again, *kavana* is crucial in the recitation of the *Shema*, but the decline in *kavana* over the course of history is readily apparent.

   The Mishna does not speak of the bride, because women are exempt from reciting the *Shema* (see Berakhot 20a). With the passage of time, women were obligated to accept the yoke of the Kingdom of Heaven and recite the *Shema*. See *Mishna Berura, Oraḥ Ḥayyim* 106:4. See also *Arukh HaShulḥan, Oraḥ Ḥayyim* 70:1; Rabbi David Auerbach, *Sefer Halikhot Beitah: Otzar Dinim uMinhagim al Mitzvot HaIsha BeYisrael* (Jerusalem: Mekhon Sha'arei Ziv, 5743 [1983]), p. 27, halakha 1.

TO FULFILL THE MITZVA

The second component of *kavana* is recognizing that one is praying to fulfill the mitzva of prayer. The *Shulḥan Arukh* states:

> There are opinions that mitzvot do not require *kavana* [referring to the *kavana* that one is fulfilling the mitzva], and there are those who say that they do require *kavana*, and this is the law.[7]

While the *Magen Avraham* suggests that this halakha applies only to biblical commandments, not rabbinic ones,[8] the Vilna Gaon applies it to both.[9] The *Ḥayyei Adam* maintains that if one studies the *Shema* (Deut. 6:4–9), it is clear that there is no intent to fulfill the mitzva of *reciting* it. However, if one recites the *Shema* in the context of a prayer service, even if there is no active intent to fulfill the mitzva of *Shema*, its recitation within the service is sufficient for this type of *kavana*. It is viewed as a kind of passive *kavana*, which is deemed adequate.[10]

Yet the *Mishna Berura* declares:

> All this is *ex post facto*. Optimally, it is certain that one should be careful to have the intention before every mitzva to fulfill the obligation of performing the mitzva.[11]

Other authorities distinguish between commandments of action and commandments of speech. Rabbi Jonah Gerondi states:

> Even those who rule that mitzvot do not require intention rule so only where the mitzva is the performance of some act, since

7. *Shulḥan Arukh, Oraḥ Ḥayyim* 60:4. See Eiruvin 95b, Pesaḥim 114b, and Rosh HaShana 28b, where this issue is debated.
8. *Magen Avraham* on *Shulḥan Arukh, Oraḥ Ḥayyim* 60:3, in the name of Radbaz.
9. Gra on *Shulḥan Arukh, Oraḥ Ḥayyim* 489, quoted in *Mishna Berura* on *Oraḥ Ḥayyim* 60:10.
10. See *Ḥayyei Adam*, Laws of Caution, mitzva 68:9, and *Ḥayyei Adam* quoted in *Mishna Berura* op cit. This principle seems to apply to biblical law. In rabbinic law, the mitzva is considered fulfilled without "active" or even "passive" *kavana*.
11. *Mishna Berura, Oraḥ Ḥayyim* 60:10.

> here the act takes the place of the intention, i.e., the taking of the lulav, where it is concluded that once the lulav is lifted, one has fulfilled his obligation.[12] This ruling applies to similar situations [which involve action].
>
> However, mitzvot that depend on speech alone [like prayer] certainly require intent, since the recital is to be performed with the heart. If, in these cases, the worshipper has no intent, since he performs no overt act, he has not performed any mitzva whatever.[13]

In contemporary times, Professor Yeshayahu Leibowitz articulated the importance of intending to fulfill the mitzva. For Professor Leibowitz, praying for any reason other than its being a mitzva commanded by God dilutes the very meaning and purpose of prayer:

> The sole meaning of prayer as a religious institution is the service of God by the man who accepts the yoke of the Kingdom of Heaven. His acceptance becomes real through his assumption of the burden of Torah and mitzvot. Only the prayer that one prays as the observance of a mitzva is *religiously* significant. The spontaneous prayer ("when he is overwhelmed and pours out his complaint before God") a man prays of his own accord is, of course, halakhically permissible, but, like the performance of any act that has not been prescribed, its religious value is limited. As a religious act it is even faulty, since he who prays to satisfy his needs sets himself up as an end, as though God were a means for promotion of his welfare. As in the case of any mitzva, prayer – especially prayer – is religiously significant only if it is performed because it is a mitzva. Its religious value is minimal when it is performed out of free inclination.[14]

---

12. Sukka 42a.
13. Rabbeinu Yona, *Berakhot*, end ch. 1, s.v. *omnam*. See *Beit Yosef* on *Tur Shulḥan Arukh, Oraḥ Ḥayyim* 589, s.v. *vetzarikh sheyekhaven*. See also *Ḥayyei Adam*, Laws of Caution, mitzva 68:9.
14. This paragraph first appeared in Hebrew, in *De'ot* (1960), and was reprinted in *Yahadut, Am Yehudi, uMedinat Yisrael* (Jerusalem/Tel Aviv: Schocken, 1975), pp. 409–410.

IN THE PRESENCE OF GOD

A third element of *kavana* is recognizing that one is praying in the presence of God. *Ḥiddushei Rabbeinu Ḥayyim HaLevi* analyzes this form of *kavana* by noting a contradiction in Maimonides. Maimonides first states:

> What is meant by *kavana* of the heart? Any *tefilla* [referring to the *Shemoneh Esreh*] which lacks *kavana* is not considered *tefilla*. If one prays without *kavana*, he must repeat the *tefilla* with *kavana*. If his thoughts are confused and his heart burdened, he is forbidden to pray until his mind is calmed [i.e., he regains his composure]. Therefore, if one returns from a journey and is tired or distressed, he should not pray until his mind is calm. Our sages have said one should wait three days, until his mind rests and is cleared, and [only] afterward should he pray.[15]

He then writes:

> One who prayed [the *Shemoneh Esreh*] but did not have *kavana* should repeat the prayer with proper *kavana*. But if one had *kavana* in the first blessing [*Avoteinu*], he need not repeat [the prayer].[16]

The contradiction is obvious. Maimonides first declares that *kavana* is necessary throughout the *Shemoneh Esreh*. Without *kavana*, one should

---

The English translation is based on Yeshayahu Leibowitz, *Judaism, Human Values and the Jewish State*, ed. Eliezer Goldmann, trans. Goldmann et al. (Cambridge: Harvard University Press, 1992), p. 31. This translation is not word for word, but it poetically expresses Professor Leibowitz's message.

Leibowitz's approach to prayer is much in sync with his generic approach to mitzvot. For him, the mitzva has nothing to do with yielding personal benefit to its practitioner. Rather, it is observed for only one purpose – to fulfill the will of God.

15. Maimonides, *Code*, Laws of Prayer 4:15. See Berakhot 30b. See also Eruvin 65a: "The father of Samuel, after having returned from a journey, did not pray for three days." The same talmudic passage adds: "Said R. Ḥiyya b. Ashi in the name of Rav: Anyone whose mind is not calm should not pray."

See *Kesef Mishneh* on Maimonides, *Code*, Laws of Prayer 4:15, s.v. *lefikhakh* and *matza dato*.

16. Maimonides, *Code*, Laws of Prayer 10:1, based on Berakhot 34b.

not pray, even if it means waiting three days for the proper devotion required for *tefilla*. Maimonides then proclaims that *kavana* during the blessing of *Avoteinu* is sufficient.

In resolving the contradiction, Rabbi Ḥayyim HaLevi Soloveitchik of Brisk maintains that Maimonides distinguishes between two types of *kavana*: the *kavana* of *peirush hamilot*, understanding the words being said, and the *kavana* of *da lifnei mi ata omed*, recognizing that one is praying in the presence of God:

> It seems that there are two kinds of *kavana* in prayer. The first is the *kavana* of the meaning of the words. This is the foundation of *kavana*.
>
> The second is the *kavana* wherein one realizes that he or she stands before God....
>
> It seems that this [second] aspect of *kavana* is integral to the act of prayer. If his heart does not turn from other things, and he does not see himself as standing before God and praying, then this is not an act of prayer. He is like one who is busy with other matters and not involved in the mitzva act (*mitasek*). Therefore, lack of this kind of *kavana* prevents proper prayer throughout the *Shemoneh Esreh*. For when he is involved in other things, he is judged as not having prayed at all, as if he skipped those words. Certainly, since this [lack of *kavana*] affects the very essence of prayer; it prevents proper prayer in any of the *Shemoneh Esreh*.
>
> When one has *kavana* and realizes what he is doing and knows that he stands in prayer, yet he does not know the meaning of the words, then this is a matter only concerning prayer – an added law of *kavana*. It is this aspect that is the subject of the Gemara in Berakhot: "When one recites the *tefilla*, he must say all the blessings attentively, and if he cannot say all attentively, he should say one attentively. R. Ḥiyya said in the name of R. Safra who had it from a member of the school of rabbis: This one should be the blessing *Avoteinu*."[17]

17. *Ḥiddushei Rabbeinu Ḥayyim HaLevi*, second comment. The translation here is based on Rabbi David Derovan's, published by the National Commission on Torah

The *kavana* of understanding the words is necessary throughout the *Shemoneh Esreh*, but *ex post facto*, knowing the meaning of *Avoteinu* is enough. However, awareness of being in the presence of God is, for Rabbi Ḥayyim Soloveitchik, even more fundamental than the *kavana* of understanding the words. Without this consciousness, it is as if the words were not recited: "he is judged as not having prayed at all." This awareness is necessary throughout the *tefilla*.

Kavana is therefore crucial to the prayer experience, intrinsic to the very essence of *tefilla*. To borrow from the terminology of Rabbi Joseph B. Soloveitchik, there exists the *pe'ula*, the action of prayer, and the *kiyyum*, the fulfillment of prayer. In *tefilla*, *pe'ula* relates to the enunciation of the words; *kiyyum*, to the *kavana*, the inner intent while praying. In the case of prayer, *pe'ula* is intrinsically bound up with *kiyyum*. Without *kavana*, prayer is devoid of substance; it is body without soul. Explicating the position of Maimonides, Rabbi Soloveitchik says:

> Thus, for Maimonides, "service of the heart" (*avoda shebalev*) encompasses man's whole being, and vocalizing the words of prayer is not enough. The heart must do its share. Of course, "service" involves external acts and performance.... But the act of prayer (*ma'aseh*) cannot in itself exhaust all that is implied in the concept of "service of the heart," which encompasses all of man's being, wherever he is and whatever opportunities are available to him, both his joys and sorrows, his grief as well as his rejoicing.... The act of prayer is merely the performance (*pe'ula*) of the precept, while its fulfillment (*kiyyum*) remains within the realm of the heart.
>
> The best proof of this is the fact that even those sages who argued that "intention" was not a necessary component in the observance of the commandments admitted that conscious intent is a prerequisite for prayer, for its very fulfillment must come from the heart.[18]

Education, Stone-Saperstein Center for Jewish Education, Yeshiva University, in the *Halakha Yomit* prepared for the Yeshiva University High School Seminar, February 12–16, 1976.

The source in Berakhot is 34b.

18. Peli, *On Repentance*, pp. 82–83. Rabbi Soloveitchik made his observation based on

Chapter Eight

Pathway

I had known Mark for several years. During the course of his life, he suffered from an illness and soon began to seriously decline. He had reached his forties, and his life was in jeopardy. I went to visit him in his home and found him lying in his bed, absolutely still, a tracheotomy tube in his throat, his feet extending just beyond his blanket. It was the eve of Passover.

"Which holiday do you like best?" he haltingly asked me.

"Rosh HaShana is a favorite," I replied, "as it celebrates the creation of the world."

"For me," Mark responded, "every morning I wake up is Rosh HaShana."

And then, he started to sing *Dayeinu,* the Seder song in which we thank God for everything He has given us. As I joined in singing the verses of *Dayeinu,* Mark, with a twinkle in his eyes, softly called out, "Amen."

I leaned over and kissed his forehead and said, "Thank you for saving my soul."

As I stepped away to leave, Mark whispered, "Every moment, every moment."

Desperately ill, Mark was saying: "Hold on to every moment, live it to its fullest while feeling the presence of God."

Maimonides, *Code,* Laws of Repentance 10:3.

CONSCIOUSNESS OF MOMENT

My working definition of spirituality is rather simple. Spirituality means having consciousness of the moment while recognizing God's role in that moment. In other words, spirituality is being in the moment while feeling God's presence.[1] In this sense, spirituality is a form of encounter, both with our own consciousness and with the Creator of all life.

One of the most important concepts in the Torah is found at the end of Deuteronomy, when God declares:

> הַעִדֹתִי בָכֶם הַיּוֹם אֶת הַשָּׁמַיִם וְאֶת הָאָרֶץ הַחַיִּים וְהַמָּוֶת נָתַתִּי לְפָנֶיךָ הַבְּרָכָה וְהַקְּלָלָה וּבָחַרְתָּ בַּחַיִּים לְמַעַן תִּחְיֶה אַתָּה וְזַרְעֶךָ.
>
> I call heaven and earth as witnesses today that I have set before you life and death, the blessing and the curse; therefore choose life, that you may live, you and your seed. (Deut. 30:19)

In many belief systems, the goal is to limit physical pleasure in this world so one can merit true life in the next world. Rabbi Soloveitchik makes this point in describing *homo religiosus*, the universal religious person:

> The longing of *homo religiosus* for a supernal world that extends beyond the bounds of concrete reality has been embodied in many doctrines of asceticism, renunciation, and self-affliction. At such moments, *homo religiosus* is of the opinion that sufferings and torments, fasting and seclusion are the means which convey eternal felicity to man and bring him under the wings of the supernal. The individual who forgoes worldly pleasure and renounces temporal life will merit, according to this view, eternal life and a lofty, exalted existence.[2]

---

1. As we continue analyzing spirituality, other aspects of the term will be explored.
2. Rabbi Joseph B. Soloveitchik, *Halakhic Man* (Philadelphia: Jewish Publication Society, 1983), trans. Lawrence Kaplan, p. 15.

In contrast, Judaism maintains that it is this world that counts most. Judaism places the highest value on life as we know it. As such, choosing life means engaging with the world – the world of doing, acting, fixing, repairing, and redeeming. For Rabbi Soloveitchik, this is the credo of "halakhic man":

> The halakha is not at all concerned with a transcendent world. The World to Come is a tranquil, quiet world that is wholly good, wholly everlasting, and wholly eternal, wherein a man will receive the reward for the commandments which he performed in this world. However, the receiving of a reward is not a religious act; therefore, halakhic man prefers the real world to a transcendent existence because here, in this world, man is given the opportunity to create, act, accomplish, while there, in the World to Come, he is powerless to change anything.[3]

The verse from Deuteronomy that implores us to choose life includes the mandate that we do so *hayom*, today. The Torah portion in which this verse appears is read on the Shabbat before Rosh HaShana. On the High Holy Days, we end the service with the prayer *Hayom*, repeating that refrain over and over. On these awesome days, we remind ourselves that the challenge of life is to live every day fully, to be conscious of each moment as it unfolds.

We live in a world of memory and anticipation. So absorbed are human beings in remembering the past and being concerned about the future that the moment is fleeting and rarely experienced. We sing about "yesterday" and "tomorrow" but rarely about "today." Even when we are experiencing important events, we are often too excited or worried about what is yet to happen; in the process of waiting for the next moment, we fail to experience the power of the present.[4]

3. Ibid., p. 32.
4. Of course, memory is central in Judaism. Another name for Rosh HaShana is *Yom HaZikaron*, the Day of Remembrance. My intention is not to minimize the importance of the past (or future) as much as to draw our attention to the present, which provides the true pathway to spirituality.

The Talmud records an account of Alexander the Great asking the sages of Israel the following question: מָה יַעֲבִיד אִינִישׁ וְיִחְיֶה – "What should a person do to live?" The sages respond, יָמִית עַצְמוֹ – "Let him kill himself [i.e., mortify himself with study and hard work]."[5] Commenting on this passage, Rabbi Ahron Soloveichik suggests that Alexander the Great was asking, "What is the secret to life?" In Rabbi Soloveichik's reading, the sages respond, "Let every individual imagine that death is imminent," that the moment being experienced is one's last. In this way, Rabbi Soloveichik explains, the sages inspired us to live life more fully.[6]

Rabbi Soloveichik's teaching reminds us of the story of the rabbi who told a student who had strayed, "Fear not. If you repent, even at the last moment of life, all is forgiven." The student was at first relieved. After thinking about it, however, he became alarmed, and asked his teacher, "But how do you know which moment is the last you will live?" "That's my point," the rabbi said. "Live every moment as if it were your last."

The rabbi's intent was clearly not to burden his student with fear of death, but to encourage him to live every moment in a qualitative way – never taking life for granted. This idea is echoed in the words of Abraham Ibn Ezra:

> אָדָם דוֹאֵג עַל אִיבּוּד דָּמָיו וְאֵינוֹ דוֹאֵג עַל אִיבּוּד יָמָיו, דָּמָיו חוֹזְרִים יָמָיו אֵינָם חוֹזְרִים.
>
> A person is concerned about loss of money and not loss of days. Money can be replenished; days cannot.[7]

This is the message of Thornton Wilder's famous play *Our Town*, about a young woman who dies at a young age. After her death, the woman, named Emily, is given the opportunity to revisit any day of her life. In one magnificent scene, she is allowed to view her twelfth birthday. The

5. Tamid 32a.
6. I heard this interpretation in a class given by Rabbi Soloveichik.
7. Rabbi Menashe Klein attributes this quote to Ibn Ezra. See Klein, Responsa 12:155. The actual ending of the quote reads, דָּמָיו אֵינָם עוֹזְרִים, יָמָיו אֵינָם חוֹזְרִים – "Money doesn't help; days can never be recouped."

dead Emily calls out to her living family, but cannot be heard. The poignant narrative reads:

> **Mrs. Webb:** Well, now, dear, a very happy birthday to my girl and many happy returns. There are some surprises waiting for you on the kitchen table....
>
> But birthday or no birthday, I want you to eat your breakfast good and slow. I want you to grow up and be a good, strong girl....
> **Emily** (*with mounting urgency*): Oh, Mama, just look at me one minute as though you really saw me. Mama, fourteen years have gone by. I'm dead. You're a grandmother, Mama. I married George Gibbs, Mama. Wally's dead, too. Mama, his appendix burst on the camping trip to North Conway. We felt just terrible about it – don't you remember? But, just for a moment now, we're all together. Mama, just for a moment, we're happy. Let's look at one another....
> **Mrs. Webb:** Your father has a surprise for you... don't know what it is myself. Shh – here he comes.
> **Mr. Webb:** Where's my girl? Where's my birthday girl?
> **Emily:** I can't. I can't go on. It goes so fast. We don't have time to look at one another. (*She breaks down sobbing*). I didn't realize. So all that was going on and we never noticed. Take me back – up the hill – to my grave. But first: wait! One more look.
>
> Good-by, Good-by, world. Good-by, Grover's Corners... Mama and Papa. Good-by to clocks ticking... and Mama's sunflowers. And food and coffee. And new ironed dresses and hot baths... and sleeping and waking up. Oh, earth, you're too wonderful for anybody to realize you.
>
> Do any human beings ever realize life while they live it? – every, every minute?[8]

The idea that spirituality is attained by living every instant of life consciously is hinted at in the very first question God asks Adam. Adam

8. Thornton Wilder, *Our Town: A Play in Three Acts* (New York: Perennial Classics, 1998), pp. 106–108.

has just disobeyed the divine command and eaten from the tree. God appears and asks *Ayeka*? – "Where are you?" (Gen. 3:9).

Commentators throughout the ages have noted that God obviously knew where Adam was. *Ayeka*, however, may be understood as an existential question in which God asks Adam to examine his place in the world. "Where are you?" is a question God asks all of us: Have you done your share to fix and improve yourself and the world?

Perhaps even more, *ayeka* is a kind of mystical question, in which God encourages all of humankind to be aware of its surroundings, to be fully appreciative of all that we are experiencing, to be absolutely immersed in every nuance of life.[9]

Thus, the first step of spirituality is choosing life, in all its minutiae. It is becoming fully conscious of the "I," and, by extension, the moment that the "I" is experiencing. Many believe spirituality is an escape from the world. But in Judaism, spirituality is inextricably connected to experiencing each moment that is occurring on the earthly plane.

Heightened consciousness of moment, however, has its dangers. It can lead one to feel a sense of self-importance, to become totally self-absorbed. This is sometimes referred to as "spiritual narcissism." I sensed this many years ago when visiting a swami who was leading a spiritual retreat. I had gone because I knew many Jews were among his followers, and wanted to see why they found him so attractive. His approach to spirituality was quite alarming. He spoke of how in his spiritual moments he felt all the love of the world compressed into his being, even as he had the capacity to emanate endless love to all of humankind. Here, he crossed the line of responsible spiritual leadership, as spirituality for this swami was an extolling of self – all was centered upon him.

The corrective to the pitfalls of spiritual narcissism is the second

---

9. One of the most important mandates in the Torah is *imitatio Dei*. Created in the image of God, human beings are asked to imitate the Divine. In this vein, it can be suggested that just as God lives in "the absolute now," so, too, should every human being.

Rabbi Israel Lipschitz, in his *Tiferet Yisrael* commentary on Mishna Avot 3:99, argues that God created time and is therefore above it, and cannot be constricted by it. For God, there is no past or future. There is only the present. While we lack this divine timelessness, we can learn from God the concept of being fully in the present.

half of our definition. Spirituality is not only having consciousness of the moment, but recognizing God's indispensable role in inspiring and sustaining the moment being experienced. The human being may be in the moment, but it is God who generates it, nourishes it, and supports it throughout. The human being is a key player, but it is God who is in the center. Whatever the human being experiences, it ought to be with the humble recognition that everything comes from God.

In the same breath, heightened consciousness can also lead to an opposite feeling – one of self-abnegation. There are spiritual movements that focus so completely on the moment that it eclipses all else, leading one to feel a sense of nothingness, a negation of being. Total consciousness of the moment can yield a sense of worthlessness in the face of all that is unfolding, as a young woman who plays in a symphony orchestra recently explained to me. She said her spirituality surfaces when listening to the orchestra. That moment, she said, "is so awesome, everything stands still; I lose my sense of self."

Here again, the corrective may be the constant recognition of God's presence, reminding us that we are created in God's image – we are godly, with inherent, inestimable value. The human being is not negated by the experience, but plays a central role in its unfolding. Rather than being diminished by the moment, one emerges from it in full blossom, like a flower whose petals extend outward and upward. Through the experience, the human being attains full beauty.

Thus, experiencing God's presence may be the pathway to living in the moment with both humility and self-worth. Reb Simḥa Bunim of Peshischa made this point by carrying a note in each of his pockets. One read, וְאָנֹכִי עָפָר וָאֵפֶר – "I am but dust and ashes" (Gen. 18:27). The other read, בִּשְׁבִילִי נִבְרָא הָעוֹלָם – "The world was created for me" (Mishna Sanhedrin 4:5). The key, for Reb Simḥa, was knowing when to reach for the first note and when to reach for the second. These two approaches are reflected in Chabad's concept of בִּיטּוּל הַיֵּשׁ, the nullification of self,[10] and Slobodka's notion of וַתְּחַסְּרֵהוּ מְּעַט מֵאֱ־לֹהִים, which posits that the human being is just a little

10. See J. Immanuel Schochet, *The Mystical Tradition* (Brooklyn: Kehot Publication Society, 1990), pp. 50–52.

less than God (Ps. 8:6).[11] Like Reb Simḥa, our spiritual challenge lies in learning how to synthesize these two ideas.

In certain ways, spirituality is counterintuitive. As we've pointed out, while spirituality involves consciousness of moment, it is not the human being who is its key player, but God. And while God is the key player, the human being fills a central role in the moment as it evolves.

The counterintuitiveness of spirituality is most glaring when recognizing that as important as the moment may be, one must be prepared to let it go. In December 1943, Rabbi Milton Steinberg suffered a heart attack. After weeks of recuperating indoors, he was permitted outside. He reflected on that experience:

> As I crossed the threshold, sunlight greeted me…so long as I live, I shall never forget that moment…the golden glow of sunlight. It touched me with friendship, warmth and blessing. In that instant, I looked to see whether anyone else showed on his face the joy I felt. But as far as I could detect, none gave it heed. And then I remembered how often, I, too, had been indifferent to sunlight, preoccupied with petty concerns, I had disregarded it. And I said to myself – how precious is the sunlight, but alas, how careless of it are men…. I was reminded to spend life wisely, not to squander it.[12]

Yet Rabbi Steinberg, who would have us open our eyes to the world's wonders and hold them close, attaches great importance to knowing when one moment has ended and another has begun. In his words:

> Nothing can be more grotesque and more undignified than a futile attempt to hold on. Let us think of the men and women who cannot grow old gracefully because they cling too hard to a youth which is escaping them. Of parents who cannot let their

11. See Hillel Goldberg, *The Fire Within: The Living Heritage of the Musar Movement* (New York: Mesorah Publications, 1987), p. 163.
12. See Rabbi Milton Steinberg, *A Believing Jew: The Selected Writings of Milton Steinberg*, comp. Edith A. Steinberg, ed. Maurice Samuel (New York: Harcourt, Brace and Company, 1951), pp. 311–313.

> children go free to live their own lives. This then is the great truth of human existence. One must not hold life too precious. One must always be prepared to let it go.[13]

How is this accomplished? How can one be in the moment while recognizing the inevitability that nothing lasts forever?[14] Feeling the presence of God may be the pathway to realizing this balance. When taking into account that God created the world, it follows that everything in it is infinitely precious. So we ought to hold it, embrace it, warmly, tightly. However, when considering that whatever is in the world ultimately belongs to God, it is easier to let go, because these things do not belong to us. While we are blessed to enjoy them for a limited time, we know they are on loan. In Rabbi Steinberg's words:

> And when God takes from us we know it will not be lost. The beauty of the world, its sunrise and sunset; the shades of a leaf; the ripple of the soft lake water; the music of a symphony orchestra; the smile of a child; the dreams of a loving couple; the wisdom of the older adult will be placed in God's trust who stands behind us all. There is pain in termination, but no anxiety. When these experiences leave us, they will be given to someone more wise, more beautiful, and more blessed.[15]

While Rabbi Steinberg calls his essay "To Hold with Open Arms," it can be suggested that in spirituality one ought not "hold on" to the moment; rather, one should "be in" the moment. "Holding on" even loosely could involve a constant fear that the moment will soon pass, thereby blocking its full experience. "Being" is a healthy, more natural flow, allowing for a graceful and gentle embrace of the moment at hand.

---

13. Ibid., p. 317.
14. Now, of course, there is a difference between an experience *qua* experience and its residual effect. No experience lasts forever. Still, it can be so meaningful that it forever reverberates. One of my primary goals at life-cycle events is that they become an endless reservoir of deeply felt love from which participants can forever draw – in good times and bad.
15. Steinberg, *A Believing Jew*, p. 318.

The idea that what "leave[s] us" is not lost but is "placed in God's trust" becomes more accessible when we consider real life situations that appear to end, while we know that they continue. Colonel Mickey Marcus offers an example:

> I am standing upon that foreshore. A ship at my side spreads her white sails in the morning breeze and starts for the blue ocean. She is an object of beauty and strength, and I stand and watch her until at length she hangs like a speck of white cloud just where the sea and sky come down to mingle with each other. Then someone at my side says, "There! She's gone!" "Gone where?" "Gone from my sight, that's all." She is just as large in mast and hull as ever she was when she left my side; just as able to bear her load of living freight to the place of her destination. Her diminished size is in me, not her. And just at that moment when someone at my side says, "There! She's gone!" there are other eyes watching her coming and other voices ready to take up the glad shout, "Here she comes!"[16]

KEDUSHA: LETTING GOD IN

Central to spirituality is letting God in. The Torah offers a guide to how we can achieve this goal: קְדֹשִׁים תִּהְיוּ כִּי קָדוֹשׁ אֲנִי ה׳ אֱ־לֹהֵיכֶם – "You shall be holy, for I, the Lord your God, am holy" (Lev. 19:2). One wonders why there needs to be a specific command to be holy. Shouldn't the sum total of Torah observance by definition lead one to a holy life?

It is here that Nahmanides makes a bold comment, suggesting that one can keep all the minutiae of the law and yet live an unholy life. In his words:

> The Torah has admonished us against immorality and forbidden foods but permitted relations between husband and wife and the eating of [certain] meat and wine. If so, a man of desire could

16. This quote is commonly attributed to Col. David "Mickey" Marcus, who played a major role in Israel's War of Independence in 1948, in which he was tragically killed.

> consider this to be permission to be passionately addicted to relations with his wife... and be "among winebibbers and gluttonous eaters of flesh" [Prov. 23:20].... And behold he will be despicable within the boundaries of the Torah (וְהִנֵּה יִהְיֶה נָבָל בִּרְשׁוּת הַתּוֹרָה).[17]

For this reason, the Torah says, "You shall be holy," thereby emphasizing the importance of infusing the letter of the law with the spirit of the law – with meaning, with purpose, with holiness, with godly values.[18] *Kedusha* can serve as a window to bringing God into our lives by incorporating His ways into our everyday existence. If one wishes to be close to God, one must imitate Him.

In this spirit, the students of Rabbi Abraham Isaac HaKohen Kook have quoted their teacher as saying, "There is no such thing as the unholy. There is only the holy and the not yet holy."[19] For Rabbi Kook, the way one eats, engages in business, or makes love has the same capacity for holiness as fasting, meditation, or prayer. Every act of life has the potential to be suffused with *kedusha* – with godly spirituality.

---

17. Nahmanides, Leviticus 19:2, s.v. *kedoshim tiheyu.*
18. Rashi interprets "You shall be holy" to mean "Separate from forbidden relations." In other words, for Rashi, *kedusha* is an expression of being apart.

    As we've pointed out, Nahmanides notes that even if one abstains from that which is forbidden, he or she can still be acting improperly. He goes on to say: "Therefore, after listing matters altogether prohibited, the Torah in general terms commands us to practice moderation even in matters that are permitted."

    Both Rashi and Nahmanides see *kedusha* as reactive, as a form of separation. For Rashi, it separates from the forbidden. For Nahmanides, it separates from the permissible.

    Our perspective presents *kedusha* as a proactive process impressing the law with its spirit, suffusing it with godliness. It involves not separating from the permissible, but sanctifying the permissible.

    One of the great challenges of halakha is to synthesize law with *kedusha*. As we've pointed out, the Hebrew term for Jewish law, halakha, means "go," as it serves as a pathway to infuse all our actions with holiness and godliness. The Torah emphasizes this point when God declares, וְשָׁמְרוּ דֶּרֶךְ ה׳ לַעֲשׂוֹת צְדָקָה וּמִשְׁפָּט – "And they will safeguard the way of the Lord by doing what is just and right" (Gen. 18:19).
19. This quote is commonly attributed to Rabbi Kook, as it represents his philosophy. See Rabbi Norman Lamm, "Two Versions of Synthesis," in Lamm, *Faith and Doubt*, pp. 68–81.

A story: A Hasid living in Minsk decided to seek the heavenly world that he had been told was in Pinsk. Overnight, he slept in an open field, having carefully left his shoes pointing in the direction of Pinsk. As he slept, a scoundrel came by and turned his shoes around. The next morning, the Hasid continued in the direction his shoes were pointing. When he reached his destination, he noticed that all the streets, homes, and people looked familiar. He was puzzled, but delighted to have found heaven on earth.

From a homiletical perspective, the word קָדוֹשׁ (*holy*) can be seen as a compound of ק and דש. The ק represents the name of God, an abbreviated form of הַקָּדוֹשׁ בָּרוּךְ הוּא, the Holy One, Blessed Be He. דש means threshing. קדש means not only incorporating God's ways into our lives, but bringing God Himself into everything, to encounter God as a threshing force in all we do – in the moment being experienced. As Martin Buber writes:

> "God dwells where man lets Him in!" The hallowing of man means this "letting in." Basically the holy in our world is what is open to God, as the profane is what is closed off from Him, and hallowing is the event of opening out.[20]

The nexus of moment and God yields an experience of the Divine that is simultaneously broad and narrow. Consciousness of moment is temporal, fleeting in comparison to the supernal, eternal God. The moment, no matter its import, is infinitesimal, stirring one to sense the infinite endlessness of God, the *Ein Sof* (Infinite) who knows no boundaries. As Rabbi Moses Cordovero, the sixteenth-century kabbalist, writes:

> A simple person thinks that God is an old man with white hair, sitting on a wondrous throne of fire that glitters with countless sparks, as the Bible states, "The Ancient of Days sat, the hair on His head like clean fleece, His throne – flames of fire" [Dan. 7:9].... Imagining this and similar fantasies, the fool cor-

20. Martin Buber, *Hasidism and Modern Man* (New York: Horizon Press, 1958), pp. 28–29.

> porealizes God. He falls into one of the traps that destroy faith. His awe of God is limited by his imagination.
>
> If you are enlightened, you know God's Oneness; you know that the Divine is devoid of bodily categories – these can never be applied to God.... Then you wonder, astonished: Who am I? I am a mustard seed in the middle of the sphere of the moon, which itself is but a mustard seed within the next sphere. So it is with that sphere and all it contains in relation to the next sphere. So it is with all the spheres – one inside the other – and all of them are mustard seeds within the further expanses. And all of these are but mustard seeds within further expanses.
>
> Your awe is invigorated; the love in your soul expands.[21]

On the other hand, consciousness of moment may inspire an opposite feeling, in which one senses that God is nowhere else but in the moment being experienced. In that time, at that place, the infinite God is compressed into the finite. In the words of Moses Cordovero:

> The essence of divinity is found in every single thing – nothing but it exists. Since it causes everything to be, nothing can live by anything else. It enlivens them; its existence exists in each existent.
>
> Do not attribute duality to God. Let God be solely God. If you suppose that *Ein Sof* emanates until a certain point, and that from that point on is outside of it, you have dualized. Perish the thought! Realize, rather, that *Ein Sof* exists in each existent. Do not say, "This is a stone and not God." Perish the thought! Rather, all existence is God, and the stone is a thing pervaded by divinity.[22]

---

21. Rabbi Moses Cordovero, *Ohr Ne'erav*, ed. Yehuda Z. Brandwein (Jerusalem: Yeshivat Qol Yehudah, 1965), 2:2, pp. 18–19. Translation from Daniel C. Matt, *The Essential Kabbalah: The Heart of Jewish Mysticism* (San Francisco: Harper San Francisco, 1995), p. 22.
22. Moses Cordovero, *Shiur Koma* (Modena Manuscript, fol. 206b), commenting on Zohar 3:141b. Quoted by Bracha Sack, *BeSha'arei HaKabbala shel R. Moshe Cordovero* (Beersheba: Ben-Gurion University of the Negev Press, 1995) p. 62. Translation from Matt, *Essential Kabbalah*, p. 24. Many thanks to Professor Matt for bringing these sources to my attention.

These contrasting feelings about God ought to exist in dialectic. People often think in absolutes: If A is right, B is wrong, and vice versa. Thus, there are such categories as heaven and earth, good and evil, particularism and universalism, this world and the next world – each separate and distinct from the other. Dialectic means something very different. It suggests that antithetical concepts can impact each other. Like a thick rope being pulled at each end – causing tension throughout its length – so, too, is the world of opposite ideas. As each pulls at the other, it is the tension between the two that creates true and profound creativity. In our case, a sophisticated awareness of God is sensing that He is simultaneously transcendent and immanent; without and within; beyond and near; there and here – all at once. Consciousness of moment gains meaning when we sense God in all of these complexities and recognize that our divine experience is a drop in the ocean, and yet the ocean is compressed into that experience. This paradox transforms the experience into a moment of holiness, a moment of *kedusha*, a moment of spirituality.

Perhaps the phrase that best reflects our definition of spirituality, of being in the moment while feeling the presence of God – His transcendence and immanence – is what God tells Moses: עֲלֵה אֵלַי הָהָרָה וֶהְיֵה שָׁם – "Come up to Me, to the mountain, and be there (*veheyeh sham*)" (Ex. 24:12). Aren't the last words, "and be there," superfluous? If Moses is on the mountain, then by definition isn't he there?

The word *heyeh*, however, stresses the importance of presence. One can have an experience without integrating it into one's being. God is telling Moses – go atop the mountain and really *be* there; immerse yourself fully in the moment.

Not coincidentally, the word *veheyeh* (וֶהְיֵה) is an anagram of God's holiest name, the Tetragrammaton, Y-H-V-H. God is saying to Moses, "Be there, really be there, while fully feeling My presence."[23]

And so it should be in all of our spiritual moments.

23. See chapter 4, where a similar argument is made in the discussion of the *Shema*.

SPIRITUALITY IN MARRIAGE AND IN MOURNING

Rituals, especially those associated with life-cycle events, provide us with opportunities to cultivate an awareness of the moment and to feel God's nearness. At life-cycle celebrations, I have found it a good idea to have those directly involved, together with family and friends, offer personal reflections about what the experience means to them. Especially during rites of passage, the challenge is to have time "stand still," to ponder the religious significance and spiritual power of the moment.

Consider the rituals of our most joyous and mournful occasions – marriage and death. Under the *ḥuppa,* it can be spiritually uplifting to read words of blessing that the bride and groom have written to each other. The rabbi can then ask for a moment of introspection wherein all present offer their blessings to the couple. During *shiva,* the seven prescribed days of mourning, it can be meaningful for the mourner to offer a personal reflection about the deceased. Others may prefer to share such reflections at the conclusion of *shiva,* or after the month or year of mourning.[24] Alternatively, the *Yizkor* memorial service can be a time to share thoughts of loved ones who are gone.

The idea that the foundation of spirituality involves living in the moment makes many people uncomfortable. We are, by and large, not happy coming face to face with who we are: our physical beings, our emotions, our relationships, our inner essence. When challenged to encounter our inner "I," we often feel vulnerable; it is a place we often do not want to be.

For example, a wedding of spiritual meaning, where aspects of love are touched upon, may conjure up for some the inadequacies of their own marriage. Personal reflections by a mourner may stir deeply buried feelings among friends or family members, forcing them to confront emotions they would rather not face.

Virtually nothing of meaning comes easily. Because spirituality is potentially exhilarating, it is equally daunting. All we can do is be sensitive to the challenges of maintaining consciousness of the moment while

24. The custom in our synagogue (the Bayit) is to encourage people observing a *yahrzeit* (the anniversary of death) or completing the eleven months of reciting *Kaddish* to say a few personal words about the deceased.

carefully forging ahead. This is easier said than done. Halakha may serve to help in this task, with its system of laws that encourage and sometimes compel one to fully experience the moment.

For instance, the mishna we discussed earlier, which declares that a groom is exempt from reciting *Shema* on his wedding night[25] is based on the principle of הָעוֹסֵק בְּמִצְוָה פָּטוּר מִן הַמִּצְוָה – "One who is preoccupied with a mitzva is exempt from performing other mitzvot [at the same time]."[26] Bride and groom should be so immersed in the moment that even if they could find time to say *Shema*, they should not.[27] Here the halakha insists that the new couple not be distracted from full concentration on each other. Similarly, during *shiva*, the mourner is prohibited from learning Torah so that he or she is free to fully experience the emotions that arise upon loss.[28]

Not coincidentally, the rituals at both ends of the life-cycle spectrum – the exhilaration of marriage and pain of mourning – are suffused with symbols and words that convey the constant presence of God.

The *ḥuppa*, suspended over the heads of bride and groom, evokes the image of God hovering over His people like a mother bird gently protecting her fledglings: כְּנֶשֶׁר יָעִיר קִנּוֹ עַל גּוֹזָלָיו יְרַחֵף – "Like an eagle that rouses its nestlings, hovering over its young" (Deut. 32:11). *Raḥaf*, hover, means to protect but not to press; to shield, not crush. Like the mother bird, the *ḥuppa*, symbolic of the Divine Presence, hovers over the couple, providing a sense of protection while allowing bride and groom the space to be themselves.

In a house of mourning, visitors recite the words הַמָּקוֹם יְנַחֵם אֶתְכֶם בְּתוֹךְ שְׁאָר אֲבֵלֵי צִיּוֹן וִירוּשָׁלָיִם – "May God comfort you among the mourners of Zion and Jerusalem."[29] The Hebrew term for God used here is unusual. *HaMakom* literally means "the place," but in this case refers to God's Omnipresence, "The Place." This phrase is uttered by visitors to convey that even in a house of mourning, where the bereaved

25. Brakhot 16a.
26. In chapter 7 we analyzed why today bride and groom do recite *Shema* on their wedding night
27. Mishna Berakhot 2:5.
28. *Shulḥan Arukh, Yoreh De'ah* 384:1.
29. This formula is recited in Ashkenazic houses of mourning.

may feel God has abandoned them, God is present. As Rabbi Joseph B. Soloveitchik teaches:

> Throughout our Torah literature and liturgy, we use numerous different names to refer to Hashem, depending upon which of His attributes is being highlighted. The name used here, הַמָּקוֹם, the Omnipresent, suggests that God is indeed everywhere, even in those places and at those times when we may not readily sense His presence. In fact, it is specifically on those occasions when we may think that God is far away from us and perhaps has even abandoned us entirely that we are reminded, by referring to Him with this particular name, that in truth He is still very much with us in our midst.
>
> We thus find, for example, that a mourner, who certainly feels as though God has turned away from him, is to be consoled with a phrase that uses this name (הַמָּקוֹם יְנַחֵם אֶתְכֶם – "May the Omnipresent console you").
>
> Similarly, when praying on behalf of our brethren who are suffering and in distress, who likewise feel that they have been neglected, we appeal to God using this name (הַמָּקוֹם יְרַחֵם עֲלֵיהֶם – "May the Omnipresent have mercy on them").[30]

PERSONALIZING *TEFILLA*

Our general analysis of spirituality applies to *tefilla*, specifically to each of the halakhic realms of *kavana* as outlined in the previous chapter.

The first level of *kavana*, understanding the words (*peirush hamilot*), is particularly challenging. Words are the garments that mirror

30. *Yom Kippur Maḥzor with Commentary Adapted from the Teachings of Rabbi Joseph B. Soloveitchik*, ed. Dr. Arnold Lustiger and Rabbi Michael Taubes (New York: K'hal Publishing, 2006), pp. 64, 65.

HaMakom may also refer to the very place where the family is sitting *shiva*. The place, the memories, the family may be the greatest comfort to the bereaved. For survivors, *HaMakom* has special meaning, as it refers to the very place of burial, the grave – the kind of resting place denied to virtually all victims of the Holocaust.

our inner feelings, our inner emotions. But words, like garments, have their limitations. Just as the garments we wear can reflect who we are, they can also serve to hide our true personalities.[31] As Rabbi Adin Steinsaltz notes, "Speech is the garment of thought, expressing the thought even as it veils its deeper dimensions."[32]

Ludwig Wittgenstein, the twentieth-century Austrian philosopher, writes starkly about the use of language as a mask:

> Language disguises the thought; so that from the external form of the clothes one cannot infer the form of the thought they clothe, because the external form of the clothes is constructed with quite another object than to let the form of the body be recognized.[33]

One would imagine that the greater the eloquence of an individual, the greater the ability to articulate thoughts. The Israeli poet and writer Ḥayyim Naḥman Bialik, a master of language with perhaps no equal, suggests that no matter one's gift of language, as much as words display, they veil; the inner thought, on some level, always remains hidden:

> הֲרֵי הַדָּבָר בָּרוּר, שֶׁהַלָּשׁוֹן לְכָל צֵירוּפֶיהָ אֵינָהּ מַכְנִיסָה אוֹתָנוּ כְּלָל לִמְחִיצָתָם הַפְּנִימִית, לְמַהוּתָם הַגְּמוּרָה שֶׁל דְּבָרִים, אֶלָּא אַדְּרַבָּא, הִיא עַצְמָהּ חוֹצֶצֶת הַדְּבָרִים.
>
> The matter is clear. Language, in all of its facets, does not allow us to enter its inner chambers, to get at the very essence [of the

31. Perhaps it is no coincidence that the word *beged,* which means clothing, can also be pronounced *bagad,* which means betrayal. Colloquially, it is said that "clothes make the man," but in the same breath, clothes can also hide the person.

    A hasidic observation notes that the א, the first letter of the Hebrew alphabet, marks the beginning of articulation of speech. It is followed by three letters, ב־ג־ד, which together spell *bagad.* This teaches that speech is not a conduit through which one can express his or her thoughts fully. A level of concealment always remains.
32. See Rabbi Adin Steinsaltz, *Opening the Tanya: Discovering the Moral and Mystical Teachings of a Classic Work of Kabbalah* (San Francisco: Jossey-Bass, 2003) p. 121.
33. See Ludwig Wittgenstein, *Tractatus Logico Philosophicus* (New York: Cosimo, 2009) p. 45.

> idea or feeling]. The reverse is the case. [Words] themselves are barriers [concealing what we wish to express].[34]

Words in prayer are not only words, they are holy words. As such, they have an added capacity to express one's inner thoughts. But whatever that capacity, there is a depth of emotion that can never be verbalized; sparks of the soul that forever remain hidden. To compensate for this limitation, prayer requires not only reading and translating,[35] but personalizing – that is, relating the text to one's personal life, with the goal of transforming *tefilla* into a spiritual experience.

Consider, for example, the blessings surrounding the *Shema*. These blessings correspond to the three ways Judaism understands the Divine: as the God of Creation, the God of Revelation, and the God of Redemption. Here, daily *tefilla* serves as a means to articulate basic philosophical tenets concerning God that are central to Judaism.[36]

---

34. Hayyim Nahman Bialik, "*Gillui VeKhissui BaLashon*" (Revelation and Concealment in Language), in *Kol Kitvei H. N. Bialik* (Tel Aviv: Dvir, 5798 [1938]), pp. 191–193. See also Bialik, *Masekhet Gillui VeKhissui BaLashon*, with commentary by Eli Alon and Yariv Ben-Aharon (Oranim: HaMidrasha, 1997), lines 59–60.
35. This involves quite literally going through the liturgy and comprehending its meaning.
36. The trilogy of creation, revelation, and redemption is found in the three portions of the *Shema*. *Shema* itself, which speaks of belief in God, is associated with the existence of God, Creator of the world. *VeHaya* deals with mitzvot, revelation. The portion of *tzitzit* deals with God's role in history, the redemption of the Jews from Egypt as a paradigm for future redemptive moments.

    This trilogy is found elsewhere in *tefilla*. On Shabbat, for example, the *Shemoneh Esreh* prayers said on Friday night, Shabbat morning, and Shabbat afternoon highlight these three themes.

    On Friday night, we celebrate the Shabbat of creation. Hence, in the *Amida* we declare, אַתָּה קִדַּשְׁתָּ אֶת יוֹם הַשְּׁבִיעִי לִשְׁמֶךָ – "You have sanctified the seventh day for Your name's sake." The prayer then quotes the verses from the creation story dealing with Shabbat: וַיְכֻלּוּ הַשָּׁמַיִם וְהָאָרֶץ...וַיְבָרֶךְ אֱ־לֹהִים אֶת יוֹם הַשְּׁבִיעִי וַיְקַדֵּשׁ אֹתוֹ – "And the heavens and the earth were completed, and God blessed the seventh day and sanctified it" (Gen. 2:1–3).

    On Saturday morning, we celebrate the Shabbat of revelation. Thus we say, יִשְׂמַח מֹשֶׁה בְּמַתְּנַת חֶלְקוֹ – "Moses rejoiced in the gift of his portion." The prayer goes on to

And in *tefilla*, they can be expressed in ways that can inspire and touch the soul.[37]

The first blessing said before the *Shema* is בָּרוּךְ אַתָּה ה׳ יוֹצֵר הַמְּאוֹרוֹת – "Blessed are You, Lord, who forms the radiant lights." When reciting this blessing, which deals with the God of nature, who created and perpetually recreates the world, one might meditate on a moment when one felt the presence of God through a powerful nature experience. I had such an experience in Aspen, Colorado, when I stood together with scores of Wexner fellows, Jews from across the denominational spectrum, looking at the majestic Rockies, offering a godly prayer of peace. I thought of the story told about Rabbi Samson Raphael Hirsch, the extraordinary leader of nineteenth-century German Jewry, who, after many decades of ministering to his community, decided to go on vacation. His congregants were stunned that the revered rabbi was finally ready to take a break and inquired why he'd decided to do so. Rabbi Hirsch responded, "I'm getting older. Someday soon I will leave this world. When I get up to heaven, God will ask me all sorts of questions. If and when He asks, 'Shimshon, did you see My Alps?' I want to make sure I have what to say."

The second blessing preceding the *Shema* is בָּרוּךְ אַתָּה ה׳ הַבּוֹחֵר בְּעַמּוֹ יִשְׂרָאֵל בְּאַהֲבָה – "Blessed are You, Lord, who chooses His people Israel with love." When saying this blessing, which deals with Torah

---

quote verses dealing with Shabbat, given soon after revelation, וְשָׁמְרוּ בְנֵי יִשְׂרָאֵל אֶת הַשַּׁבָּת – "And the Children of Israel will observe the Shabbat" (Ex. 31:16, 17). See Shabbat 86b–87a, which records that the Sinaitic revelation occurred on Shabbat.

The afternoon *Minḥa* service celebrates the Shabbat that is yet to be, the Shabbat of redemption. In the *Amida* we call out, אַתָּה אֶחָד וְשִׁמְךָ אֶחָד – "You are One and Your name is One." In the time of redemption, God's name will be accepted as One, and the Jewish people and the world will be redeemed.

The theme of redemption is the centerpiece of the *Havdala* service marking the end of Shabbat and the hope for the week. Elijah the Prophet, harbinger of redemption, is the special guest, and a candle with intertwined wicks is used. While Shabbat begins with two distinct candles, it ends by uniting them – symbolizing the era of redemption, when peace and unity will prevail.

37. In chapter 4, we presented a different approach to these blessings. Also, while our discussion there was more theoretical, here we attempt to offer a pathway to greater spiritual meaning in the morning blessings.

study, one might try to imagine a particular moment when one felt God through the study of Torah.[38] For me, one example is when I met Rabbi Ahron Soloveichik. I had just returned from a year of study in a yeshiva in Israel. I was all of eighteen, and foolishly believed I could learn on my own and had no need for a rebbe. When placed in Rabbi Soloveichik's class, I purposely sat in the back of the room. After all, I thought, what could he teach me? And then, Rav Ahron, as he was affectionately called, walked in. Bent over, with total humility, he slowly made his way to his desk. Something about the way he carried himself profoundly touched me. For me, Rav Ahron was reflecting nothing less than the image of God as He appeared in the lowly burning bush and, later, on one of the lower mountains. The next day, and for months afterward, I sat front and center before Rav Ahron. For years, I considered him *mori verabbi*.

The blessing that follows *Shema* is בָּרוּךְ אַתָּה ה׳ גָּאַל יִשְׂרָאֵל – "Blessed are You, Lord, who redeemed Israel." Here one might think of a powerful redemptive moment, when one truly felt the hand of God. For me, an example was when my nephew, Yoni Weiss, took his oath of enlistment in the Israeli army. Yoni stood there at the Western Wall in Jerusalem with hundreds of other soldiers. Behind him was his family. I glimpsed my father, Yoni's grandfather, shedding a tear. It struck me that in all my years, I had never seen my father cry. Later that evening, I asked him why he was so moved. "I was brought up in the town of Oswiecim, which later became the site of Auschwitz, the notorious death camp," my father said. "During those days the Jewish community was defenseless. We did not have the means to protect ourselves. To see my grandson becoming a full member of *Tzuhal* (the Israeli Defense Force) was overwhelming. Tears flowed as I offered thanksgiving to God for having allowed me to experience a glimpse of redemption."

Lately, I've been thinking about our eldest grandson, Gilad, who lives in Israel together with his family. Gilad is now preparing to enter the army. Often in conversation, I would probe whether Gilad, who just a few years earlier had made *aliya*, was emotionally and spiritually ready for army service. One Friday night as Shabbat began, Gilad and I stood

38. One central phrase of this blessing is וְהָאֵר עֵינֵינוּ בְּתוֹרָתֶךָ – "enlighten our eyes with Your Torah."

together on a hill overlooking Jerusalem. Turning to me, he said, "Look how beautiful Jerusalem is. And it is my merit to do my small share in protecting Jerusalem and all of Israel." I asked Gilad what he hoped to do in the army. He did not hesitate, "I want to be a fighter." "Why?" I asked him. "Why not seek out something easier, like a desk job?" Gilad's eyes mirrored a deep spirituality as he replied, "Sabbi (Grandpa) Avi, Israel has done so much for me. I want to give back." Like my father, tears flowed down my cheeks. I embraced Gilad and thanked God for allowing me to experience this spark of redemption.

And yet, these are tears not only of joy and *naḥat*, but of trepidation. Redemption, even the echo of redemption, comes with a price. Never will I forget the comment my daughter Elana – Gilad's mother – recently made to me. "Abba," she said, "I will be the mother of a soldier for the next twenty-two years." What Elana meant was that Gilad is the first of nine children (seven boys), the youngest just born. I often think of Elana's words during prayer.

"Embodying" is yet another way to give meaning to the words of *tefilla*. As we've pointed out, originally *Birkhot HaShaḥar* – the morning blessings celebrating the renewal of body and soul – were said at different points of rising. While today they are said as a unit during the *tefilla*, we can still embody these blessings, acting them out as they are being said, in order to make their utterance more meaningful. For example, when reciting the blessing for sight, close and then open the eyes. In the blessing the One "who spreads the earth above the waters," be aware of the hardness of the ground. In the blessing the One "who makes firm the steps of the human being," one could actually take a few steps.

At first glance, "embodying" seems to be the opposite of a spiritual concept. After all, spirituality is limited to the sphere of the soul. However, as we have discussed earlier in this chapter, the goal of spirituality is not to negate the body, but to "*kedushify*" it. In prayer, Rabbi Dr. Eliezer Berkovits points out that articulating words audibly or bowing does not conflict with spirituality, but rather helps the whole of the human being – soul and body – to be immersed in *tefilla*. This is the spirit of the psalmist, who sings out כָּל עַצְמוֹתַי תֹּאמַרְנָה ה׳ מִי כָמוֹךָ – "All my bones shall say: Lord, who is like You?" (Ps. 35:10). In the words of Rabbi Berkovits:

> Physical prostration before God is no less essential for prayer than is spiritual concentration. The prayer of man should be human, not angelic....
>
> Contrary to Kant [who limits service of God to the "invisible," to the heart] Judaism teaches that man's true "service of God" must be human. It should be invisible, as man's soul is invisible; and it should be visible, too, because man is visible. It must be "service of the heart," in spirit and in truth as well as of the body. It must be service through the mitzva, the deed in which man's spiritual and material nature have unified. It is a much higher service than that of the spirit alone. It is the religion of the whole man.[39]

Spirituality extends beyond the body to encompass God's entire world – nature itself. Thus, another formula to spiritually elevate words of prayer is to pray in a natural setting. When reciting *Pesukei DeZimra,* which focuses on renewal of nature, one could at times venture outdoors, where the words can be more powerfully felt. As the *Mishna Berura* notes, "When one loses *kavana,* lift the eyes heavenward to awaken *kavana.*"[40] "Lifting one's eyes heavenward" may refer to looking and feeling the glory of God's creation. Meditation outdoors is extolled in hasidic literature. Rabbi Naḥman of Bratslav says it this way:

> Solitude is a superior virtue, greater than all others. At regular intervals, seclude yourself for an hour or more in a room or a field to converse openly with your Creator, [whether] offering arguments or apologies, in words that are grateful, pacifying, and conciliatory, beseeching and imploring Him to bring you close to Him in order to serve Him sincerely.[41]

---

39. Eliezer Berkovits, *God, Man and History,* ed. David Hazony (Jerusalem: Shalem Press, 4th ed. 2004), pp. 124–125. See Immanuel Kant, *Religion Within the Limits of Reason Alone,* trans. Theodore M. Greene and Hoyt H. Hudson (New York: Harper Torchbook, 1960), p. 180.
40. *Mishna Berura, Oraḥ Ḥayyim* 90:8.
41. Rabbi Naḥman of Bratslav, *Likkutei Maharan, Tinyana* 25. Translation from Norman Lamm, *The Religious Thought of Hasidism: Text and Commentary* (Hoboken, NJ: Yeshiva University Press, 1999), pp. 198–199.

Rabbi Naḥman takes it a step further, arguing that an important term for prayer itself, שִׂיחָה (conversation), is associated with the outdoors, specifically with שִׂיחַ הַשָּׂדֶה (shrubs of the field):

> דַע, כְּשֶׁאָדָם מִתְפַּלֵּל בַּשָּׂדֶה, אֲזַי כָּל הָעֲשָׂבִים כּוּלָּן בָּאִין בְּתוֹךְ הַתְּפִילָּה, וּמְסַייְּעִין לוֹ, וְנוֹתְנִין לוֹ כֹּחַ בִּתְפִילָּתוֹ. וְזֶה בְּחִי' שֶׁנִּקְרֵאת הַתְּפִילָּה שִׂיחָה, בְּחִינַת "שִׂיחַ הַשָּׂדֶה"... וְזֶה בְּחִי' "וַיֵּצֵא יִצְחָק לָשׂוּחַ בַּשָּׂדֶה", שֶׁתְּפִילָּתוֹ הָיְתָה עִם סִיּוּעַ וְכֹחַ הַשָּׂדֶה... שֶׁבִּשְׁבִיל זֶה נִקְרֵאת הַתְּפִילָּה שִׂיחָה.
>
> Know that when a person prays in the field, then all vegetation merges into the prayer, helping him, and giving him energy in his tefillot. For this reason, *tefilla* is called *siḥa,* which is associated with *siaḥ hasadeh* [Gen. 2:5] .... And this is the deeper meaning of "And Isaac went out to meditate (*lasuaḥ*) in the field" [Ex. 24:63], that his prayer was with the support and strength of the field.... For this reason, *tefilla* is called *siḥa*.[42]

One of the most meaningful *tefillot* of my youth was *Kabbalat Shabbat,* the service ushering in Shabbat. My parents ran a summer camp in the Catskill Mountains, in upstate New York, and every Shabbat they dressed in white like a bride and groom. The Friday night service was always conducted outdoors as the sun set over the mountains. That setting made the arrival of Shabbat more picturesque; one felt like a beloved going out to greet the Shabbat bride. Just before we began the *Kabbalat Shabbat,* Imma (Mother) would sing the words of Bialik:

> הַחַמָּה מֵרֹאשׁ הָאִילָנוֹת נִסְתַּלְּקָה
> בּוֹאוּ וְנֵצֵא לִקְרַאת שַׁבָּת הַמַּלְכָּה
> הִנֵּה הִיא יוֹרֶדֶת הַקְּדוֹשָׁה הַבְּרוּכָה
> וְעִמָּהּ מַלְאָכִים צְבָא שָׁלוֹם וּמְנוּחָה
> בּוֹאִי, בּוֹאִי הַמַּלְכָּה
> בּוֹאִי בּוֹאִי הַבְּרוּכָה
> שָׁלוֹם עֲלֵיכֶם מַלְאֲכֵי הַשָּׁלוֹם.

---

42. Rabbi Naḥman of Bratslav, *Likkutei Maharan, Tinyana* 11.

The sun has set from the tops of the trees
Come, let us go out to greet the Shabbat bride
She is already descending, the holy, the blessed
And with her angels, a host of peace and rest
Come, come, O Queen
Come, come, O Bride
Welcome to you, ministering angels, angels of peace.[43]

And then we would begin the service: לְכוּ נְרַנְּנָה לַה׳ – "Come, let us sing for joy to the Lord." Shabbat was upon us.

PREPARING FOR *TEFILLA*

Kavana latzeit ba, intention for the mitzva to be fulfilled, involves focusing prior to the formal beginning of *tefilla*. On a purely halakhic level, it is the conscious intent to fulfill God's command that is required before performing a mitzva: לְקַיֵּם בָּזֶה כַּאֲשֶׁר צִוָּה ה׳ – "the intention to thereby fulfill a command of God." [44] In the words of the *Sefat Emet*: עֲשִׂיַּת הַצִּווּי יוֹתֵר מְקוּבָּל מִטַּעַם הַמִּצְוָה – "Doing the mitzva as a commandment [from God] is more important than understanding its meaning."[45] The *Sefat Emet*'s words are long preceded by the Mishna:

> The pious people of early times used to wait an hour before praying in order to focus their thoughts upon their Father in heaven.[46]

---

43. Ḥayyim Naḥman Bialik, "Shabbat HaMalka," in *Kol Kitvei H. N. Bialik* (Tel Aviv: Dvir, 5798 [1938]), pp. 71–72.
44. *Mishna Berura, Shulḥan Arukh, Oraḥ Ḥayyim* 60:7.
45. *Sefat Emet,* Leviticus, first comment on *Aḥarei Mot,* s.v. *BeRashi.*
46. Mishna Berakhot 5:1 (Berakhot 30b). Some suggest that "the pious people of early times" refers to the *vatikin,* people of exceptional piety. See Berakhot 9b and 26a.
    See *Tosefot* Yom Tov, Mishna Berakhot 5:1, s.v. *sha'a aḥat,* and *Tiferet Yisrael* ad loc., Yakhin, n. 2, where *sha'a* is defined as *sha'a davka* (an actual hour), not just a short interval. *Magen Avraham* on *Shulḥan Arukh, Oraḥ Ḥayyim* 93:1, understands *sha'a* as one-twelfth of the day. This period of meditation refers to the pious; others would wait just a few moments, gathering their thoughts prior to prayer. See also *Shulḥan Arukh, Oraḥ Ḥayyim* 90:20.

Some understand this passage to mean that before *tefilla*, one should wait a while, and in that time – pray.[47] Thus, the preparatory period is a time to pray that we will be able to properly pray when *tefilla* formally begins.[48]

The Mishna may refer to actual prayers within *tefilla* – words preparing us for other words. The best example of this phenomenon is *Pesukei DeZimra*, said in the early part of the service. Some suggest that its recitation is based on a talmudic statement: "R. Simlai expounded: One should always first recount the praise of the Holy One, Blessed Be He, and then pray."[49] From this perspective, *Pesukei DeZimra* is a preparatory service leading up to *Barekhu*, the call to prayer, when the central part of the service commences. While *Pesukei DeZimra* literally means "verses of song," it can have another meaning. The term *zimra* may come from the root Z-M-R, prune. Just as one prunes a tree to prepare it for future growth, so, too, do these songs serve as preparatory prayers, setting the mood and arousing the sensitivities so that one may have complete *kavana* during the basic *tefillot*, beginning with *Barekhu*.[50]

Pesukei DeZimra has three themes.[51] It begins with the *Barukh SheAmar* prayer, in which we speak of a universal God who cares for humankind:

בָּרוּךְ שֶׁאָמַר וְהָיָה הָעוֹלָם,
בָּרוּךְ הוּא. בָּרוּךְ עֹשֶׂה בְרֵאשִׁית.

> Blessed be He who spoke and the world came into being.
> Blessed be He. Blessed be He who creates the universe.

One of the central prayers of *Pesukei DeZimra* is *Ashrei*, which is more particularistic:

47. Recalling the popular Hebrew adage לִפְנֵי הַתְּפִילָּה אֲנִי מִתְפַּלֵּל שֶׁבִּזְמַן הַתְּפִילָּה אֲנִי אֶתְפַּלֵּל – "Before I pray, I pray that when I pray, I'll pray."
48. In other words, the term "*umitpallelim*" in Mishna Berakhot 5:1 refers not to the prayer per se, but prayer before the formal *tefilla* begins.
49. Berakhot 32a.
50. See Rabbi Isaac Aboab, *Menorat HaMa'or*, which offers this understanding of *Pesukei DeZimra*, linking *zimra* to *zomer*.
51. Here we are expanding on the theme of *Pesukei DeZimra* as discussed in chapter 4.

קָרוֹב ה׳ לְכָל קֹרְאָיו, לְכֹל אֲשֶׁר יִקְרָאֻהוּ בֶאֱמֶת.
רְצוֹן יְרֵאָיו יַעֲשֶׂה, וְאֶת שַׁוְעָתָם יִשְׁמַע וְיוֹשִׁיעֵם.

> The Lord is close to all who call on Him, to all who call on Him in truth.
> He fulfills the will of those who revere Him; He hears their cry and saves them. (Ps. 145: 18–19)

The last section includes *Az Yashir,* the song Moses and Miriam sang after crossing the sea, focusing on the God of redemption (Ex. 15:1–21):

אָז יָשִׁיר מֹשֶׁה וּבְנֵי יִשְׂרָאֵל אֶת הַשִּׁירָה הַזֹּאת לַה׳.

> Then Moses and the Israelites sang this song to the Lord. (Ex. 15:1)[52]

These three themes prepare us for the formal beginning of the service, starting with *Barekhu* – the call to prayer. *Barekhu* is followed by *Birkhot Shema,* which surround the *Shema* itself. As we've discussed, they include the three blessings of *Shema,* which deal with universalistic, particularistic, and redemptive themes.

My sense is that the mishnaic phrase שׁוֹהִין שָׁעָה אַחַת וּמִתְפַּלְּלִין – "to wait an hour before praying" suggests a pause for a short, quiet period before prayer. In a world that moves so quickly, we need time to go into neutral before beginning *tefilla.* Transitions take time; they evolve. In *tefilla,* too, we need to first slow down, as magically laid out in this poem:

Slow me down, Lord,
    Ease the pounding of my heart
    By the quieting of my mind.
    Steady my hurried pace
    With a vision of the eternal reach of time….

52. *Az Yashir* is the paradigmatic text of redemption. In the prayer service it is preceded by וַיְבָרֶךְ דָּוִיד אֶת ה׳ – "and David blessed the Lord" (1 Chr. 29:10–13) for having allowed him to successfully collect money for the building of the First Temple by his son Solomon; and by אַתָּה הוּא ה׳ לְבַדֶּךָ – "You alone are the Lord" (Neh. 9:6–11), wherein Ezra and Nehemiah celebrate the building of the Second Temple. Both these events are of enormous redemptive import.

Break the tensions of my nerves
With the soothing music
Of singing streams....
To look at a flower
To chat with a friend
Or make a new one;
To watch a spider build a web;
To smile at a child;
Or to read a few lines from a good book.
Remind me each day
That the race is not always to the swift
That there is more to life
Than increasing its speed....
Slow me down, Lord,
And inspire me to send my own roots deep
Into the soil of life's enduring values
That I may grow toward the stars
Of my greater destiny.[53]

Rabbi Kalonymus Kalman Shapira suggests a method through which this can be accomplished. Specifically, one should first remove extraneous clutter. Before we can proactively pray, we must empty and calm our minds, hearts, and souls, so that we are open to a spiritual message. He describes this preparatory phase in this way:

> A dream is considered to be one-sixtieth of prophecy.... For the essence of a human being naturally resists divine inspiration. When a person's mind and thoughts are wakeful, it is difficult to receive divine inspiration. But when a person sleeps, and one's mind is quieted, then one relinquishes one's thoughts and divine inspiration can descend from above. And that is the meaning of "a dream is one-sixtieth of prophecy"....
>
> Therefore, the ultimate prayer state is a sleeplike condition, in which one's perpetual thoughts and desires are quieted. For

53. Wilfred A. Peterson, *Slow Me Down, Lord!*

> thoughts become so intertwined with each other that a person can find it difficult to separate oneself from them.
>
> If a person sits quietly with his thoughts for a good while… then he will slowly feel that his mind has slowly emptied itself, and his thoughts are quieted. At that point one should begin to say a phrase, such as "God is true" (ה׳ אֱ־לוֹהִים אֱמֶת), in order to connect the mind – now emptied of other thoughts – with a single thought that is holy.[54]

The *Sefat Emet* suggests that stillness of mind meets thoughts of holiness when the prayer *Az Yashir* transitions into *Shema*.[55] *Az Yashir* deals with the Exodus from Egypt, which on a deeper level involves leaving the world of vanity and idolatry. Only when freed from these distractions is one calmed and ready for the *Shema*, which is not only our declaration of belief, but God's call to Israel to listen to His words as declared at Sinai – "I am the Lord your God" (Ex. 20:2). At this moment, silence gives way to the sounds of one of the holiest prayers – *Shema Yisrael* – so holy it goes beyond words, echoing Revelation. For the *Sefat Emet*, emptying the mind of clutter is the precursor not only to contemplating and verbalizing holy thoughts, but to hearing the sounds of Sinai. In his words:

> וְזֶה עִיקַּר הַגָּלוּת גַּם עַתָּה מָה שֶׁאֵינֶנּוּ יְכוֹלִים לְהִתְפַּנּוֹת וְלִשְׁכּוֹחַ הֶבְלֵי עוֹלָם לִהְיוֹת הַלֵּב פָּנוּי לִשְׁמוֹעַ דְּבַר ה׳ בְּלִי מַחֲשָׁבָה זָרָה.
>
> וְלָכֵן מַקְדִּימִין יְצִיאַת מִצְרַיִם לִקְרִיאַת שְׁמַע שֶׁעַל יְדֵי גְּאוּלַּת מִצְרַיִם יְכוֹלִין לְהִיפָּנוֹת מִמַּחֲשָׁבָה זָרָה לִהְיוֹת מוּכָן לִשְׁמוֹעַ דְּבַר ה׳.
>
> This is the essence of exile today… our inability to empty ourselves, to forget this world's vanities so that we empty the heart to hear God's word without any distracting thought….

54. Rabbi Kalonymus Kalman Shapira of Piaseczno, *Derekh HaMelekh* (Jerusalem: Va'ad Ḥasidei Piaseczno, 5755 [1995]), pp. 449–450. Thanks to Aryeh Ben-David for bringing this source to my attention. With slight changes, the English translation is his.

55. Here again, *Az Yashir* is a preamble prayer.

> That is why we mention the Exodus [in the Song of the Sea] before the *Shema*. By being redeemed from Egypt, we are emptied of all distractions and become ready to hear God's word.[56]

Specific mechanics may help one attain this level of *kedusha*. While meditation is sometimes viewed as something for people who are spiritually "up in the clouds," it can be a very grounding practice, a helpful tool in preparing for prayer. Rabbi Hyim Shafner shares this simple preparatory exercise:

> While sitting in a chair, straighten the upper body, taking a deep breath in through the nose. Let the breath out through your mouth. Feel your body relaxing and becoming more focused. Take another slow, deep breath through the nose, and as you let it out evenly through your mouth, allow your shoulders to relax, your shoulder blades to descend down your back, and your upper body to become a bit straighter.
>
> Take a few more deep breaths, feeling your stomach go out as you draw air into your lungs and your stomach go in as you exhale. Hear the sound of the breath exiting your mouth on its way out. Close your eyes and take five more slow breaths, feeling your stomach go in and out, hearing the sound of your breath as you inhale and exhale. (You can switch to breathing out through your nose instead of your mouth if this is more comfortable.) Continue to breathe in this way with your eyes closed, and let your attention come to the center of your field of vision, creating calm and focus. Now bring the attention to Whom You Stand Before as you approach your *tefilla*. You may now open your eyes to pray.[57]

56. *Sefat Emet*, Exodus, *Va'era* 5659, s.v. *Bapasuk hein Benei Yisrael*; translation from Green, *Language of Truth*, pp. 90–91. For further discussion of this commentary, see chapter 4.
57. Rabbi Shafner's technique was written at my request, specifically for this book. He points out that this preparatory exercise is "by no means set in stone and should be tweaked to fit the individual's *kavana* needs. It can be practiced alone or in a synagogue or *minyan*, as long as the practitioner feels safe enough to freely close

As hard as one may try to prepare, one may still feel that God is distant. But the effort is sometimes more important than the result. If, after such exercises, one senses that God is still far away, know that He may be near. Rabbi Jaacob Joseph of Polonnoye boldly suggests that feeling God's concealment may be the pathway to feeling God's presence:

> דְּשָׁמַעְתִּי מִמּוֹרִי שֶׁאִם יֵדַע הָאָדָם שֶׁהקב"ה מִסְתַּתֵּר שָׁם אֵין זֶה הַסְתָּרָה... וְאַחַר שֶׁיֵּדַע אָדָם כְּלָל זֶה שֶׁהוּא כְּלָל גָּדוֹל שֶׁאֵין שׁוּם מָסָךְ מַבְדִּיל בֵּינוֹ לְבֵין אֱלֹהָיו בִּשְׁעַת תּוֹרָה וּתְפִילָּה גַּם שֶׁיַּעֲלוּ לְפָנָיו כַּמָּה מַחֲשָׁבוֹת זָרוֹת שֶׁהֵם לְבוּשִׁין וְכִסּוּיִין שֶׁהקב"ה מִסְתַּתֵּר שָׁם מִכָּל מָקוֹם אַחַר שֶׁיֵּדַע אָדָם שֶׁהקב"ה מִסְתַּתֵּר שָׁם אֵין זֶה הַסְתָּרָה.
>
> I heard from my master [the Baal Shem Tov, the founder of Hasidism] that if a person realizes that the Blessed Holy One is hidden, this concealment actually ceases to exist.... If a person is aware of this important principle, that there can be no barrier separating him from his God while he is praying and studying, then even though he may have many extraneous thoughts – which are merely the garments and covering in which the Blessed Holy

---

the eyes and focus without being made to feel self-conscious. As one becomes more adept at *kavana* focusing, more time can be taken. This exercise lasts about five minutes."

For a longer, more intensive pre-*tefilla* meditation, Rabbi Shafner suggests that the following be added to the previous preparation:

> Continue breathing and as you do, begin to equalize the amount of time spent on each of the four steps of each breath: (1) the in-breath, (2) having the air within you, (3) the out-breath, and (4) having no breath within you. As your breathing becomes more even and equalized, focus on one letter of the Divine Name with each step of the breath. The *yod* is the first letter in the four-letter name of God. A *yod* shape is the beginning of every letter, the potential; focus on this letter during the first stage of the breath, which is the lack of breath within you.The *heh*, the second letter in the four-letter name of God, is the focus during the in-breath (which makes the sound of a *heh*). The *vav* (a connector letter) is the third letter of the Divine Name and is the focus while the breath resides within you, connecting the in-breath to the out-breath.The last letter of the name of God, *heh*, is the focus during the out-breath, and, like the in-breath, its sound is "hehhhy." Continue breathing in this manner, focusing on the Divine Name. Try to see each letter in your mind's eye as you progress through the four stages of each breath.

> One hides – still, when one knows that the Blessed Holy One is concealed there, then there is no concealment.[58]

These spiritual approaches to preparatory *kavana* have a common denominator – silence. It is the silence of slowing down, of removing the clutter, of meditation, of concealment. In each, silence is not merely an absence of words, but is above words, transitioning from awestruck speechlessness to verbiage – connecting us to God. In the words of Dr. Michael Fishbane:

> There are two kinds of silence. One of these is natural silence, and is characterized by the absence of noise. It is a modulation, a diminishment, a negative valence. The other kind of silence is spiritual, and is characterized by potentiality and anticipation. We sense this every time we watch a conductor or an ensemble gesture slightly just prior to the production of sound; and we also sense it during moments of self-collection and focus before something of significance is said to another person. With respect to music, anticipatory silence helps prepare the self to hear sound sounding; for it focuses attention on the transition from silence to sound. With respect to deliberate speech, silence conveys the ethical potential of words; for it sharpens the transition from inwardness to worldly expression. Prayer may also stand at this juncture of silence and speech.[59]

Spirituality requires incubation – a gradual development until it reaches full blossom. Most often, the spiritual moment does not happen in an instant – it swells slowly, gaining momentum, and then, gushing like a wellspring, it reaches higher and higher. It is often a silence that is pregnant with words – waiting, waiting to burst forth. The greater the build-up, the more intense the spiritual experience. As Rabbi Joseph

58. *Toledot Yaakov Yosef, Bereshit* 1, s.v. *deshamati.*

59. Dr. Michael Fishbane, *Sacred Attunement: A Jewish Theology* (Chicago: University of Chicago Press, 2008), p. 133.

B. Soloveitchik pointed out, אֵין קְדוּשָּׁה בְּלִי הֲכָנָה – "There is no holiness without preparation."[60]

STANDING BEFORE GOD

Not only is awareness of God required before a mitzva's performance, but, as already noted, Rabbi Ḥayyim HaLevi Soloveitchik of Brisk adds that during *tefilla*, it is important to recognize that one stands before God.[61]

There is a mystical teaching that Hebrew letters all contain sparks of the Divine. Nahmanides insists that the words of the Torah encompass the names of God:

> יֵשׁ בְּיָדֵינוּ קַבָּלָה שֶׁל אֱמֶת,
> כִּי כָּל הַתּוֹרָה כּוּלָּהּ שְׁמוֹתָיו שֶׁל הקב״ה,
> שֶׁהַתֵּיבוֹת מִתְחַלְּקוֹת לְשֵׁמוֹת בְּעִנְיָן אַחֵר.
>
> We have a mystical tradition
> that the whole Torah is comprised of names of the Holy One, Blessed Be He, whose letters have been rearranged into other words.[62]

Perhaps then, the very words of the liturgy, too, resonate with the spirit of God. Their mere recitation reverberates with echoes of the Divine.[63] Spiritually, *tefilla* is a conversation with God. As Rabbi Joseph B. Soloveitchik has pointed out, *tefilla* and prophecy are two sides of the same essential conversation. The only difference is who initiates that dialogue – the human being or God. In Rabbi Soloveitchik's words:

60. This quote is commonly attributed to Rabbi Soloveitchik.
61. *Ḥiddushei Rabbeinu Ḥayyim HaLevi*, second comment. Although Rav Ḥayyim makes this an imperative in *tefilla*, it is sound advice for all mitzvot.
62. Nahmanides, introduction to his commentary on the Torah.
63. For this reason, it may be preferable to pray in Hebrew. Not only is it the language that unites Jews, its very letters and words are godly. See, however, *Shulḥan Arukh, Oraḥ Ḥayyim* 101:4, that one may pray in any language one wishes. See also *Mishna Berura* ad loc., n. 13.

> The prayer community was born the very instant the prophetic community expired, and, when it did come into the spiritual world of the Jew of old, it did not supersede the prophetic community but rather perpetuated it. Prayer is the continuation of prophecy, and the fellowship of prayerful men is ipso facto the fellowship of prophets. The difference between prayer and prophecy is…related not to the substance of the dialogue but rather to the order in which it is conducted. While within the prophetic community God takes the initiative – He speaks and man listens – in the prayer community the initiative belongs to man: he does the speaking and God, the listening. The word of prophecy is God's and is accepted by man. The word of prayer is man's and God accepts it.[64]

Understanding *tefilla* as dialogue can inspire us to a more nuanced awareness of our relationship with the Divine. Consider the biblical narrative wherein Moses asks to see God's glory: הַרְאֵנִי נָא אֶת כְּבֹדֶךָ (Ex. 33:18). God responds that He will pass by and Moses will be able to see Him from the back, as God cannot be seen frontally: וְרָאִיתָ אֶת אֲחֹרָי וּפָנַי לֹא יֵרָאוּ – "and thou shalt see My back; but My face shall not be seen" (Ex. 33:23).[65] And yet, when Moses dies, the Torah describes his uniqueness in this way: וְלֹא קָם נָבִיא עוֹד בְּיִשְׂרָאֵל כְּמֹשֶׁה אֲשֶׁר יְדָעוֹ ה׳ פָּנִים אֶל פָּנִים – "Never again did there arise in Israel a prophet like Moses, whom the Lord singled out, face to face" (Deut. 34:10). Which is it? Did Moses have a "face-to-face" relationship with God or not?

It can be suggested that the latter text deals with everyday life – where God and Moses knew each other "face to face." But the former text deals with prayer. After all, as God passes by, He declares the Thirteen Attributes of Mercy, ה׳ ה׳ אֵ־ל רַחוּם וְחַנּוּן – "The Lord, the Lord is a

---

64. Rabbi Joseph B. Soloveitchik, *The Lonely Man of Faith* (New York: Doubleday, 1992), p. 55.

65. This image has been understood in different ways. Perhaps it means we can understand God's ways only in hindsight, after the fact – not as events unfold. Or perhaps it teaches that we can gain a glimpse of God only by experiencing His characteristics rather than perceiving His very Being.

God of mercy and supplication" (Ex. 34:6).[66] These attributes form the core of the *Seliḥot* – the penitential service, and the conceptual base for *tefilla*, as in prayer one stands before God at His mercy.[67]

Prayer, unlike most everyday activities, is the most intimate of moments, when a human being stands as if naked before God; exposed, open, vulnerable. Ironically, it is precisely when one most powerfully feels God's presence that one feels His hiddenness. You shall see Me from behind, God proclaims, but My face cannot be seen.[68]

We may gain a glimpse of the encounter with the Divine when considering the human one. A verse in the book of Proverbs points us in the right direction:

כַּמַּיִם הַפָּנִים לַפָּנִים
כֵּן לֵב הָאָדָם לָאָדָם.

As face answers to face in water,
So does one man's heart to another. (Proverbs 27:19)

Rashi explains:

הַמַּיִם הַלָּלוּ שֶׁאָדָם צוֹפֶה בָּהֶן וְרוֹאֶה בָּהֶם פָּנִים כְּפָנָיו –
אִם הוּא שׂוֹחֵק הֵם שׂוֹחֲקוֹת
וְאִם הוּא עוֹקֵם הֵם עֲקוּמוֹת,
כֵּן לֵב הָאָדָם לָאָדָם הָאַחֵר –
אִם הוּא אוֹהֵב אֶת זֶה גַּם זֶה הוּא אוֹהֲבוֹ
וְאִם הוּא שׂוֹנֵא אֶת זֶה גַּם הוּא שׂוֹנְאוֹ.

66. See Michael Higger, *Pirkei Rebbi Eliezer* (New York: Horev, 5704–5708 [1944–48]), ch. 45, who suggests that as God passes, Moses calls out, "The Lord, the Lord":

    And when the Holy One, Blessed Be He, passed by... and [Moses] saw the back of the Indwelling... Moses started to call out in a loud voice, "The Lord, the Lord is a God of mercy and supplication."

67. Elsewhere in the Torah, the expression פָּנִים אֶל פָּנִים or פָּנִים בְּפָנִים (face to face) does not refer to prayer. See, for example, Genesis 32:31 and Deuteronomy 5:4.

68. Could it be that the Orthodox custom of the cantor leading the service with his back to the congregation emerges from this narrative?

    Additionally, it is not uncommon in the deepest moments of prayer that one closes the eyes, as *tefilla* is an intense love encounter transcending what one can physically see.

> Like water upon which one gazes and sees his reflection.
> If he is pleasant and gracious, the reflection is such,
> and if he is pained and angry, the reflection is such.
> So, too, is one's heart in sync with one's fellow person.
> If one loves the other, the other loves him;
> if he hates the other, the other hates him.[69]

Rashi's comment teaches us that as water reflects one's face, so too is a friend's heart a mirror of one's own. The more honest and real we are with the other, the more likely the other will be honest and real with us. The gateway to knowing the other is the revealing of self.

Herein may lie the secret to feeling God's presence. Intimacy involves taking off masks and revealing the inner self. To the degree we open up to God, God opens up to us. As Rabbi David Aaron writes:

> If you want to encounter Hashem's essence, then you have to be willing to expose your own essence to Hashem. Hashem can only reflect what you're presenting. If you present yourself with genuineness, with authenticity – your beauty in truth – then you reveal your essence and the essence of Hashem will be revealed to you. You have to be real to see the Real.[70]

But no person can be totally "real." Even if we are prepared to reveal everything about ourselves, there are always aspects that remain hidden.[71] Rabbi Shlomo Carlebach once quipped, "If you think you know [yourself or others], then you know you don't know." As aspects of our being remain hidden, so, too, God.[72] Rabbi Soloveitchik describes this simultaneous closeness and distance:

---

69. Rashi, Yevamot 117a, s.v. *verabbanan kamayim.*
70. Rabbi David Aaron, *Seeing God* (New York: Tarcher/Putnam, 2001) p. 150.
71. In the non-permissive school of sexual behavior, there is the concept of מְגַלֶּה טֶפַח וּמְכַסֶּה טְפָחַיִים – "reveal a handbreadth while concealing two" (Nedarim 20b). This may be not only a physical teaching but a metaphysical one. As revealed as one may be, in moments of intimacy – one is concealed; as connected as one may be, the ultimate moment of love has elements of profound inwardness and separation.
72. For me, revealing our essence in order to receive the essence of God is impossible.

> The Jew observes God's coming closer to the world and, at the same time, separating Himself from it, and there is no distinguishing one from the other. At the very time that His glory fills the universe, the glory conceals itself in the shadows, and He is blessed from His place.[73]

Conversely, even in separation, even in concealment, even in hiddenness, one can be conscious of God. Even when far, God may be close. This occurs when one has a profoundly intense sense of God. It is much like love. If love is deep, even when there is a falling out, even when there is disappointment, even when lover and beloved feel distant, they know, they just know in their hearts and souls, that their love is real.

Rabbi Yitzḥak Hutner formulates this idea in his discussion of a phrase found in the liturgy, וְיַחֵד לְבָבֵנוּ לְאַהֲבָה וּלְיִרְאָה אֶת שְׁמֶךָ – "Unite our hearts to love and revere Your name."[74] He wonders what "uniting our hearts" adds to the love and reverence of God:

> בְּמַצָּב שֶׁהַלֵּב מְיוּחָד הוּא לְאַהֲבָה וּלְיִרְאָה, הֲרֵי אֲפִילוּ בְּשָׁעָה שֶׁאֵין הִתְעוֹרְרוּת הָאַהֲבָה אוֹ הַיִּרְאָה חָיָה בִּלְבָבוֹ, וְהוּא עוֹשֶׂה מַעֲשֶׂה מִבְּלִי שׁוּם כַּוָּנָה שֶׁל אַהֲבָה אוֹ כַּוָּנָה שֶׁל יִרְאָה, מִכָּל מָקוֹם כֵּיוָן שֶׁהַלֵּב מְיוּחָד הוּא לְאַהֲבָה וּלְיִרְאָה,...כָּל מַעֲשֶׂה טוֹב, וְקִיּוּם מִצְוָה, הֲרֵי הוּא מְמִילָא מַעֲשֶׂה שֶׁל אַהֲבָה, וּמַעֲשֶׂה שֶׁל יִרְאָה.
>
> In a situation where the heart is designated for love or awe, then even at a time when there is no awakening of love or awe alive in one's heart, and one does and acts without intention of love or intention of awe, because the heart is designated for love and awe…every good action or fulfillment of a commandment is nonetheless an act of love, or an act of awe.[75]

First, as we have suggested, human essence is so deep it can never be fully revealed. Second, God by definition can never be fully known. For this reason, I use the language of feeling the "presence" rather than the "essence" of God. As intimate as presence is, it is a step removed.

73. Joseph B. Soloveitchik, *And From There You Shall Seek*, trans. Naomi Goldblum (New Jersey: KTAV Publishing House, 2009), p. 72.
74. This is found in the second blessing before the morning *Shema*.
75. Rabbi Yitzḥak Hutner, *Paḥad Yitzḥak*, Shavuot, no. 35, middle of second paragraph.

The Talmud describes the intense bond between God and the human being, drawing close while remaining apart, when it portrays them reaching out from their heavenly and earthly abodes – reaching, reaching, but never quite touching. The Talmud describes this image:

> תַּנְיָא, רַבִּי יוֹסֵי אוֹמֵר: מֵעוֹלָם לֹא יָרְדָה שְׁכִינָה לְמַטָּה, וְלֹא עָלוּ מֹשֶׁה וְאֵלִיָּהוּ לַמָּרוֹם, שֶׁנֶּאֱמַר: הַשָּׁמַיִם שָׁמַיִם לַה׳ וְהָאָרֶץ נָתַן לִבְנֵי אָדָם.
>
> וְלֹא יָרְדָה שְׁכִינָה לְמַטָּה?! וְהָכְתִיב: וַיֵּרֶד ה׳ עַל הַר סִינַי! לְמַעְלָה מֵעֲשָׂרָה טְפָחִים. וְהָכְתִיב: וְעָמְדוּ רַגְלָיו בַּיּוֹם הַהוּא עַל הַר הַזֵּיתִים! לְמַעְלָה מֵעֲשָׂרָה טְפָחִים.
>
> וְלֹא עָלוּ מֹשֶׁה וְאֵלִיָּהוּ לַמָּרוֹם?! וְהָכְתִיב: וּמֹשֶׁה עָלָה אֶל הָאֱ־לֹהִים! לְמַטָּה מֵעֲשָׂרָה. וְהָכְתִיב: וַיַּעַל אֵלִיָּהוּ בַּסְּעָרָה הַשָּׁמָיִם! לְמַטָּה מֵעֲשָׂרָה.
>
> It has been taught, R. Yose stated, Neither did the *Shekhina* ever descend to earth, nor did Moses or Elijah ever ascend to heaven, as it is written, "The heavens are the heavens of the Lord, but the earth has He given to the sons of human beings" [Ps. 115:16].
>
> But did not the *Shekhina* descend to earth? Is it not in fact written, "And the Lord came down upon Mount Sinai" [Ex. 19:20]? That was ten handbreadths above [the summit]. But is it not written, "And His feet shall stand in that day upon the Mount of Olives" [Zach. 14:4]? That will be ten handbreadths above.
>
> But did not Moses and Elijah ascend to heaven? Is it not in fact written, "And Moses went up unto God" [Ex. 19:3]? [That was] to a level lower than ten [handbreadths from heaven]. But is it not written, "And Elijah went up by a whirlwind into heaven" [II Kings 2:11]? [That was] to a level lower than ten.[76]

In the liminal space between the reach, in that silent, surreal vacuum, where God is there but not quite there, the encounter of spiritual prayer takes place.

Many thanks to Rabbi Steven Exler for this translation.

76. Sukka 5a.

OFFERING FAREWELL

While there is no specific halakhic category of *kavana* after prayer, spirituality plays a primary role in the way one bids farewell to the *tefilla* experience.[77] As the Talmud declares:

> R. Yehoshua b. Levi said: One who prays should tarry an hour after prayer, as it says, "The righteous shall surely praise Your name; the upright shall dwell in Your presence" [Ps. 140:14].[78]

By its very definition, spirituality has no borders – it is overflowing. In this vein, *tefilla* can be compared to climbing a mountain. One ascends until reaching the summit and then – allowing for decompression – slowly descends the other side. An example is the closing of the *Amida*. After the request blessings (*bakashot*) crescendo with the hope that Israel will be redeemed, the zenith of spirituality has been reached – the return to Zion. Being at the peak, it is difficult to quickly halt and exit. What is necessary are some words that can ease the pain of departure, slowly, slowly escorting the petitioner from the *Amida*. Hence we recite the soft, longing blessing of *retzeh*:

רְצֵה ה׳ אֱ־לֹהֵינוּ בְּעַמְּךָ יִשְׂרָאֵל וּבִתְפִלָּתָם,
וְהָשֵׁב אֶת הָעֲבוֹדָה לִדְבִיר בֵּיתֶךָ...
וְתֶחֱזֶינָה עֵינֵינוּ בְּשׁוּבְךָ לְצִיּוֹן בְּרַחֲמִים.
בָּרוּךְ אַתָּה ה׳ הַמַּחֲזִיר שְׁכִינָתוֹ לְצִיּוֹן.

> Find favor, Lord our God, in Your people Israel and their prayer.
> Restore the service to Your most holy House...
> And may our eyes witness Your return to Zion with compassion.
> Blessed are You, Lord, who restores His presence to Zion.

---

77. Of course, a blessing is recited after eating as well as after the conclusion of one's *aliya* (being called to the Torah). And when leaving the *beit midrash*, words of parting are suggested (see Berakhot 28b). Still, to my knowledge, there is no specific halakhic category of *kavana* linked to the aftereffects of *tefilla*.

78. Berakhot 32b.

This blessing is not a formal request, but a sweet, gentle way of summarizing the hope, while gradually moving out to recite the remaining exit blessings of thanksgiving (*Modim*) and hope for peace (*Sim Shalom*).

The final paragraph of the *Amida*, אֱ־לֹהַי נְצוֹר לְשׁוֹנִי מֵרָע וּשְׂפָתַי מִדַּבֵּר מִרְמָה – "My God, guard my tongue from evil and my lips from deceitful speech," is the last of the "afterglow" *tefillot*. Having uttered so many words, we offer the prayer that our language was proper, and that this appropriateness extend itself to all vicissitudes of life.

We are then ready to depart by taking three steps backward and then forward, as if we are leaving the inner sanctum of the *Amida* and then returning to the flow of the broader *tefilla*. If praying publicly we stand silently, awaiting the onset of the repetition.

In private prayer, too, it is a good time to stand still, silent, internalizing the awesomeness of the moment, the encounter with God. Like emanations from the sun, the rays of *tefilla* continue to glow even after the words are exhausted. Like the ripples of a pond after a stone has been cast in, the silent reverberations, like concentric circles, continue on, perhaps affecting the world forever.

Prior to *tefilla*, there is the silence of anticipation, during *tefilla* there is the silence of meaning, after *tefilla* – after the final words – there is the silence of beyond. It's that moment after completing a riveting book, or after a gripping movie or powerful personal experience. One is still, absolutely still, taking in the moment, digesting it, integrating it, feeling the warmth of its emanations, which hopefully remain forever.

Knowing how to say goodbye is difficult. How does one say goodbye to a beloved friend, to an intense experience, to life itself? Sometimes I feel we have made far greater inroads in learning how to greet than in bringing moments to a close.

And yet, that moment is one of the holiest. Rabbi Hutner notes that when entering into the covenant of Israel at a circumcision, two blessings are recited. The first, עַל הַמִּילָה, concerns itself with the circumcision itself. The second, recited by the father, is לְהַכְנִיסוֹ בִּבְרִיתוֹ שֶׁל אַבְרָהָם אָבִינוּ – "to bring him [our son] into the covenant of Abraham our father." Rabbi Hutner asks, why the need for the second blessing? He concludes that whereas the former deals with the external circumcision, the second deals with the parents' inward absorbing of its significance. In his words:

> וְאַף עַל פִּי שֶׁמִּצַּד הֱיוֹתָהּ שֶׁל מִצְוָה זוֹ, מִצְוָה שֶׁיֵּשׁ בָּהּ תּוֹרַת בְּרִית, אֵין כָּאן שׁוּם הוֹסָפָה בְּמַעֲשֵׂה קִיּוּם־הַמִּצְוָה, מִכָּל מָקוֹם, אִם חוֹבַת אֵיבָרִים אֵין כָּאן, חוֹבַת דַּעַת יֵשׁ כָּאן. דְּהַיְינוּ חוֹבַת־דַּעַת שֶׁל הַכְנָסָה לַבְּרִית.
>
> Even though from the perspective of its being a commandment with covenantal content, there is no corresponding additional action in fulfilling the commandment, nonetheless, while no additional physical action is required, an additional mindset is necessary – the mindset of entry into the covenant.[79]

A teaching of significant import emerges from this comment. While the circumcision ends with the completion of the act, the second blessing, which deals with its internalization – i.e., the awareness and consciousness of one's covenantal relationship with God – continues on long afterward.

On a spiritual plane, this applies to *tefilla* as well. As we've already noted, for Rabbi Judah HaLevi, there is a correspondence between the morning, afternoon, and evening services and the three daily meals. He adds the following:

> וּמִתְמֶדֶת עָלָיו בִּרְכַּת הַתְּפִלָּה עַד עֵת תְּפִלָּה אַחֶרֶת, כְּהִתְמַדַּת כֹּחַ סְעוּדַת הַיּוֹם עַד שֶׁיִּסְעוֹד בַּלַּיְלָה. וְכָל אֲשֶׁר תִּרְחַק עֵת הַתְּפִלָּה מֵהַנֶּפֶשׁ הִיא הוֹלֶכֶת וְקוֹדֶרֶת בְּמָה שֶׁפּוֹגֵעַ אוֹתָהּ מֵעִסְקֵי הָעוֹלָם.
>
> The blessing of one prayer lasts until the time of the next, just as the strength derived from the midday meal lasts till supper. The further his soul is removed from the time of prayer, the more it is darkened by coming in contact with the worldly matters.[80]

Here, the *Book of Kuzari* is suggesting that the spiritual uplift of *tefilla* continues beyond the service. This may be the basis of the halakha that one should leave the prayer experience slowly, as the Talmud proclaims, "R. Ḥuna said: One who leaves the synagogue should not do so with long

79. Hutner, *Paḥad Yitzḥak*, Shavuot, no. 37, middle of second paragraph. Translation by Rabbi Steven Exler.
80. HaLevi, *Kuzari*, p. 123 (3:5).

strides."[81] Not coincidentally, it is customary to leave a synagogue while walking backward, eyes riveted on the place of prayer, even on the prayer moment, as if taking it with us. Rabbi Shlomo Carlebach describes this phenomenon by relating it to life itself:

> Do you know the way you walk back from the holy Wall? You don't turn around and walk away. When you meet the czar of Russia, you don't turn around and walk away, you walk backward. And I want to bless you, when your children grow up and they walk out of your house, and they build their own houses, sad enough, a lot of children turn around and they don't build a Jewish house anymore. I want to bless you; your children should walk away backward.[82]

One of the sweetest rituals is the tradition of welcoming Shabbat with the singing of *Shalom Aleikhem*. We sit around the Shabbat table greeting and blessing the Shabbat angels, even as we ask that they bless us. And then, something remarkable: We conclude by bidding the angels farewell (*tzetkhem leshalom*).[83] There was a time, when our children were younger, that they refused to sing the words of farewell. With the language of innocence, they argued, "We've just said hello to the angels, why now say goodbye?" Our children were not the only ones struggling with bidding farewell. It is told that the saintly Rabbi Abraham Isaac HaKohen Kook, one of the greatest rabbis of his time, would rise from his Shabbat table as he sang *tzetkhem leshalom* – "go in peace." He would slowly walk to the door, escorting the angels out. Opening the door, he would look out as he longingly, silently, waved his hand in a farewell gesture.

After I shared Rabbi Kook's custom of waving goodbye to the angels on Friday night, Daniella Grunfeld, a wonderful congregant, told me that when her children were younger, she would accompany them

81. Berakhot 6b. Some have even argued that the prayer *Adon Olam*, normally said at the beginning of the service, also concludes the service as a way of holding on to the moment by anticipating its starting anew.
82. This teaching is taken from Rabbi Carlebach's audio tapes.
83. In some Sephardic circles, *tzetkhem leshalom* is omitted.

to their school bus. As they boarded, she'd wave goodbye. But instead of doing so in the normal fashion, she reversed her fingers, motioning toward herself as if imploring her children to stay near. Even as she said goodbye, she was declaring: I love you, come closer, come closer.

As *tefilla* ends, we and God do the same.

A touching example of a deeply spiritual farewell *tefilla* is that of Matt Fenster. Matt died a very young man, of terrible cancer. Even as he was dying, he dedicated his last months to doing good. He became a paragon of acknowledging God for the blessings we receive, whatever one's lot in life. The following is Matt's commentary on Psalm 23:

מִזְמוֹר לְדָוִד ה׳ רֹעִי לֹא אֶחְסָר.

God is my shepherd, I shall not lack.
I never have lacked.

בִּנְאוֹת דֶּשֶׁא יַרְבִּיצֵנִי עַל מֵי מְנֻחוֹת יְנַהֲלֵנִי.

In lush meadows He lays me down,
beside tranquil waters He leads me.
This year I have been able to feel a peace that I had not previously known (in Hebrew, naḥat ruaḥ).

נַפְשִׁי יְשׁוֹבֵב

He restores my soul
which I believe is eternal.

יַנְחֵנִי בְמַעְגְּלֵי צֶדֶק לְמַעַן שְׁמוֹ.

He leads me on paths of justice for His name's sake.
I can only hope that I have followed these paths more often than I have shunned them.

גַּם כִּי אֵלֵךְ בְּגֵיא צַלְמָוֶת לֹא אִירָא רָע כִּי אַתָּה עִמָּדִי.

Though I walk in the valley of the shadow of death,
I will fear no evil, for You are with me.
Throughout this ordeal, I have never been afraid. Perhaps it is because I am a person of faith? Or maybe I am too simpleminded to recognize the magnitude of the loss that I am facing?

שִׁבְטְךָ וּמִשְׁעַנְתֶּךָ הֵמָּה יְנַחֲמֻנִי.

Your rod and Your staff, they comfort me.
I interpret God's "rod" and "staff" to be my family and friends, respectively.

תַּעֲרֹךְ לְפָנַי שֻׁלְחָן נֶגֶד צֹרְרָי

You prepare a table before me in view of my tormentors
I think about the tables in my life... my childhood dinner table... breakfast before school with my kids at a café table... the Seder table... the table from which I read the Torah in synagogue.

דִּשַּׁנְתָּ בַשֶּׁמֶן רֹאשִׁי

You have anointed my head with oil
I was brought up to believe I was special and could accomplish anything that I wanted.

כּוֹסִי רְוָיָה.

my cup overflows.
A phrase I have uttered to myself each Friday night before the words of Kiddush.

אַךְ טוֹב וָחֶסֶד יִרְדְּפוּנִי כָּל יְמֵי חַיָּי וְשַׁבְתִּי בְּבֵית ה׳ לְאֹרֶךְ יָמִים.

May only goodness and kindness pursue me all the days of my life, and I shall dwell in the House of God for eternity.
Although I am saddened by what I will miss, the days with which I have been blessed have been full.[84]

84. Matt's writing can be found at www.caringbridge.org/visit/mattfenster. It is printed here with the permission of his wife, Jennifer.

Chapter Nine

Synagogue

The young girl was crying incessantly as she approached the saintly rabbi, who was sitting in his chair in the front of the synagogue. As she came forward, the rabbi tried to calm her and gently asked, "Why so many tears, my dear child?"

The young girl, out of breath from her sobbing, brokenly said, "I was playing hide and seek and I hid – but no one came looking for me."

The rabbi continued to soothe her, assuring her that she was not alone – she was loved by her family and community. As he spoke these reassuring words, the rabbi thought, I've now gained a glimpse into how God must feel. There He is, present everywhere, even here in the synagogue, and yet far too few people are looking for Him.[1]

1. The source of this story is unknown to me.

SYNAGOGUE AS FAMILY

The sad reality is that prayer in synagogue is too often void of spiritual meaning. Spirituality and synagogue seem to be mutually exclusive. At the same time, people are increasingly searching for *devar Hashem,* the word of God.[2] Amos prophesied:

> הִנֵּה יָמִים בָּאִים נְאֻם ה׳ אֱ־לֹהִים וְהִשְׁלַחְתִּי רָעָב בָּאָרֶץ לֹא רָעָב לַלֶּחֶם וְלֹא צָמָא לַמַּיִם כִּי אִם לִשְׁמֹעַ אֵת דִּבְרֵי ה׳.
>
> Behold, days are coming, says the Lord, that I will send a famine to the land – not a famine for bread, or a thirst for water, but for hearing the word of the Lord. (Amos 8:11)

On our campuses, in our schools, and in our synagogues, our holy task is to respond to this yearning by sharing and spreading spirituality with passion, eloquence, and soulfulness. As this book focuses on *tefilla,* we will give special attention to seeking ways to infuse the synagogue – the central place of prayer – with spirituality. The purpose (and hope) of this chapter is to offer a model for achieving this goal.

The synagogue model with which I am most comfortable is what I call "the *bayit*" (literally, the house or the home).[3] The congregation housed in that *bayit* is nothing less than a *mishpaḥa,* family, whose most basic value is the love between its members. When using the model of family for a congregation, I am referring to families that work, families in which there is a powerful bond and endless love.

When I was a very young rabbi driven to impact the Jewish people

---

2. I have often observed that people who doubt or deny God have what I perceive to be a subconscious sense of the Divine. People across the board are searching for meaning in life. (See Viktor E. Frankl, *Man's Search for Meaning* [New York: Pocket Books, 1963].) This search is reflective of the inner godliness we all possess. As God is good, so, too, is there an inner quest to do good (see Soferim 3:17).

   It is not uncommon for those who do not have traditional belief in God to use spiritual language. Often people speak of a "higher consciousness" or a "higher reality" or a "higher spirit," which they sense is part of their endeavor. That "higher consciousness," that "higher reality," that "higher spirit" may reflect God Himself as well as the spirit of God that courses through all of us.

3. The synagogue where I served as rabbi is affectionately called "the Bayit."

and the world, my congregational board members often advised me to slow down and exercise greater caution. Over and over, they urged me to remember that "a synagogue is a business." With years, I've come to understand that there is some truth to this model, as there are elements of the business world that can be incorporated into the synagogue, which, of course, needs funding in order to survive.

Still, with all my heart and soul, I believe this model to be wrong. A synagogue is not a business. The goal of a business is to make money. The goal of a synagogue is to touch souls. This difference trickles down in the way synagogues operate and connect to their congregants and larger community. The model of family is especially conducive to creating such a soulful atmosphere.

The Torah describes Jacob's dream of the ladder, anchored on earth, reaching heavenward, with angels ascending and descending its rungs. Upon rising from this dream, Jacob makes a vow to create what may be the first synagogue in history:

> וַיִּדַּר יַעֲקֹב נֶדֶר לֵאמֹר אִם יִהְיֶה אֱ־לֹהִים עִמָּדִי וּשְׁמָרַנִי בַּדֶּרֶךְ הַזֶּה אֲשֶׁר אָנֹכִי הוֹלֵךְ וְנָתַן לִי לֶחֶם לֶאֱכֹל וּבֶגֶד לִלְבֹּשׁ. וְשַׁבְתִּי בְשָׁלוֹם אֶל בֵּית אָבִי וְהָיָה ה׳ לִי לֵא־לֹהִים. וְהָאֶבֶן הַזֹּאת אֲשֶׁר שַׂמְתִּי מַצֵּבָה יִהְיֶה בֵּית אֱ־לֹהִים וְכֹל אֲשֶׁר תִּתֶּן לִי עַשֵּׂר אֲעַשְּׂרֶנּוּ לָךְ.
>
> And Jacob vowed a vow, saying, "If God will be with me, and will keep me in this way that I go, and will give me bread to eat, and clothing to wear. So that I come back to my father's house in peace, then shall the Lord be my God. And this stone, which I have set up for a pillar, shall be God's house; and of all that You shall give me I will surely give a tenth to You." (Gen. 28:20–22)

Note that Jacob emphasizes the term *bayit* in his plea, וְהָאֶבֶן הַזֹּאת אֲשֶׁר שַׂמְתִּי מַצֵּבָה יִהְיֶה בֵּית אֱ־לֹהִים – "And this stone, which I have set up for a pillar, shall be God's house." It could be suggested that on a deeper level, Jacob is saying, "If You will be with me, God, I will create for You a *bayit*, a house, in which I will nurture and develop a family, the whole family of Israel." As Rabbi David Silber has pointed out, the Genesis narrative is, in some sense, a narrative of exclusion. Of Adam and Eve's children, only Seth's line survives;[4] of Noah's, Shem is the forerunner of Abraham and Sarah;[5] Isaac, and not Ishmael, inherits their father's (Abraham's) covenant; Jacob and not Esau assumes the birthright. It is within this historical and familial context that Jacob dreams his dream and tells God that his family will be one of inclusion. There will be no more choosing one child at the expense of another. If You will be with me, God, says Jacob, I will create for you a *bayit*, a home, in which no one is excluded.[6]

In the family model of synagogue, the rabbi may assume the role of leader of the *mishpaḥa*. For some congregants, this role is a parental figure, for others, a sibling, and for others still, a child or grandchild. In this role, the rabbi, like the family leader, exhibits unconditional love for his congregants. The rabbi may not agree with or respect all of them, but he still loves them.[7]

The Hebrew language has several terms for synagogue: *beit tefilla* (house of prayer), *beit midrash* (house of Torah study), *beit knesset* (house of community), and *beit E-lohim* (house of God). Each of these terms begins with the word *beit*, a form of *bayit*, home. These various names each describe a different role of the synagogue: as a place to pray, study, gather, and commune with God. The message seems to be that all of these activities ought to take place in the model and spirit of family.[8]

---

4. Adam and Eve had three children – Cain, Abel, and Seth. Cain killed Abel, and Cain's family perished during the Deluge. Seth alone survived, and his descendants were Noah and his family.
5. Noah has three children – Shem, Ham, and Japhet. Shem becomes the ancestor of Abraham and Sarah, the father and mother of Judaism.
6. In an important sense, the book of Genesis is about fragmented families that ultimately reunite. It is only when Jacob's children surround him and receive his blessings in the last moments of his life that he fulfills his goal of creating a *bayit* that encompasses all. Only after the family is whole does the book of Genesis end and the book of Exodus, the story of our nationhood, begin.
7. Rabbis, of course, have other roles. A rabbi is a *moreh*, a teacher who imparts the wisdom and teachings of Jewish tradition.
   A rabbi may also serve as a rebbe. A rebbe is one who teaches by example. It is the teaching that comes from the heart and soul, not just the mind. What counts most is not only what the rebbe says, but what the rebbe does.
8. The model of family is conducive to spirituality. In its simplest form, spirituality means having a relationship with God. As God is One, so, too, should human be-

BEIT TEFILLA

As a *beit tefilla,* a synagogue is a place where we reach inward through *tefilla,* traversing beyond the self to touch the Divine. As we've already discussed, *tefilla* emerges from the inner soul, from the inner heart, from where spirituality is generated. The family model is especially conducive to this experience, as it encourages honesty – the revealing of the true self.

Rabbi Isaiah Horowitz, known as the *Shelah HaKadosh,* writes that *tefilla* is a balance between a commitment to our history and personal, heartfelt striving. Yet he emphasizes that above all else is the obligation to experience God on a personal level:

> The root of everything is "And you will know today and take to heart that God is the Lord" [Deut. 4:39]. This means that knowledge needs to be acknowledged in one's heart with wondrous clarity... in addition to accepting belief through one's tradition.
>
> And this is hinted at in the verse "Know the God of your fathers" [1 Chr. 28:9]. That is to say, in addition to the faith in God that tradition has implanted in your heart through historical transmission, you should also know this personally through your own understanding.
>
> This is the message of the verse, "This is my God and I will beautify Him, the God of my father, and I will raise Him up" [Ex. 15:2]. That is to say, when the awareness of God is mine, through my knowledge and awareness, then I can beautify Him [*anvehu* – the language of *ani ve-hu,* I and He].[9] In other words, it is as if God and I were together, because the knowledge has penetrated my heart.
>
> However, when knowledge of God is only through tradition and not through my personal grasping, when it is only the experience of "the God of my father," then "I will raise Him up," because He is above and beyond me, and the inner recesses of my heart are distant from Him.

---

ings strive to be united – a cornerstone of the family unit.

9. See Rashi, Shabbat 133b.

> Therefore it is incumbent upon each person to examine the inner workings of his heart, to know that "the Lord is One and His name is One" [Zach. 14:9].[10]

It is by no means easy for one to "examine the inner workings of his heart" in a synagogue setting. Synagogues are often caught up in institutional bureaucracy, internal politics, and perfunctory observance. Finding spirituality within the synagogue means going deeper within ourselves to learn how to be in touch with God. In *tefilla*, several pathways can facilitate this journey.

Kavana – Setting the Spiritual Tone

A quick sentence (no more than a minute) before a service or before the recitation of a specific prayer can serve as a point of entry for inspiring *tefilla*. As Shabbat enters, for example, one may reflect on a Shabbat theme. Before lifting the Torah, one can contemplate a pressing issue facing Israel or the world and the imperative to respond. As *Ashrei* is about to be recited, we might pause to think of those who are suffering: **סוֹמֵךְ ה׳ לְכָל הַנֹּפְלִים, וְזוֹקֵף לְכָל הַכְּפוּפִים** – "The Lord supports all the fallen ones and straightens all the bent" (Ps. 145:14).

Eikhut HaTefilla – The Quality of Prayer

Every word of *tefilla* is important, as the *Mishna Berura* states, "One should not skip any words or say them quickly [literally, swallow the words]."[11] The *Arukh HaShulḥan* recognizes, however, that in the process of reciting all the prayers, there may be a qualitative loss as one rushes through the words, saying them with little meaning. The author

---

10. Rabbi Isaiah Horowitz, *Likkutei Shelah: BeInyenei Emuna VeDa'at, Torah UMitzvot, Middot VeHanhagot* (Jerusalem: M. Yeshurun, 2003), p. 12. Thanks to Aryeh Ben-David for bringing this source to my attention. With slight changes, the English translation is his.

    When reciting the *Amida*, we begin with the words in which we proclaim that the Lord is "our God and God of our fathers," **אֱ־לֹהֵינוּ וֵא־לֹהֵי אֲבוֹתֵינוּ**, noting our personal connection to God before mentioning His relationship with our ancestors.

11. *Mishna Berura, Shulḥan Arukh, Oraḥ Ḥayyim* 51:20.

therefore codifies that regarding *Pesukei DeZimra,* one may sacrifice quantity for the sake of quality:

> One should not say the songs of praise quickly; rather, every word should be carefully enunciated. If one, however, wishes to keep up with the congregation, which is rushing through the prayers, it is preferable to skip [some of the songs] rather than say them quickly [with the community]. Concerning this it is said: It is better to say a smaller amount with proper intent than a greater amount without intent.[12]

Shira – Song

Song that is participatory and soulful can bring us to new spiritual heights. Song touches us inwardly, expressing our deepest emotions and igniting our inner spark of God. The act of singing together as part of a congregation has the power to connect us upward to God, while simultaneously enabling us to feel a sense of oneness with others.[13]

Hitboddedut – Meditation

Through silence, meditation, and reflection, one can reach deeply inward. For Rabbi Kook, silence is one of the highest forms of holiness:

> הַקְּדוּשָּׁה הָעֶלְיוֹנָה הִיא קְדוּשַּׁת הַדּוּמִיָּה...
> הַחוּצְפָּא דִבְעִיקְבָא דִמְשִׁיחָא בָּא מִתּוֹךְ תְּשׁוּקָה פְּנִימִית,
> מִקְּדוּשַּׁת הַדּוּמִיָּה הָעֶלְיוֹנָה.

12. *Arukh HaShulḥan, Oraḥ Ḥayyim* 51:9. Here *Arukh HaShulḥan* excludes *Barukh SheAmar, Ashrei,* and *Yishtabaḥ,* which must always be said in their entirety. While saying each of the psalms quickly, my custom is to concentrate on a different psalm (between 146 and 150) every weekday. By the end of the week, all have been said with added *kavana.*

13. Song extends to encompass the tri-directionality of *tefilla* discussed in the first part of this book: inward to touch the soul, upward to bridge the great abyss to God, and outward to interface with our fellow person.

    Live music can be uplifting. For Orthodox Jews, this may be possible during the *Havdala* ceremony marking the end of Shabbat or on a weekday morning when *Hallel* is recited (for example, on Rosh Ḥodesh or Ḥanukka).

> The most exalted holiness is the holiness of silence….
> The boldness that will be felt in the Messianic Era comes from an internal yearning,
> which is rooted in the exalted holiness of silence.[14]

Tenua VeRikkud – Movement and Dance

In *tefilla,* one should be comfortable enough to express oneself completely. At particular moments, it is appropriate to dance – sometimes by ourselves, sometimes with others, much as King David did when he returned the Ark to Jerusalem.[15]

Movement, too, helps us attain the emotional and mental state necessary for prayer. This may explain the underlying reason we take three steps back before the *Amida,* then three steps forward.[16] When we take these steps back, we are in effect moving inward, entering our own space, our own consciousness of moment. It is then that we recite, ה׳ שְׂפָתַי תִּפְתָּח וּפִי יַגִּיד תְּהִלָּתֶךָ – "My Lord, open my lips, that my mouth may declare Your praise" (Ps. 51:17). Through the prayer service, there are moments we are called upon to bow, and in the Yom Kippur service, we go so far as to fall on our faces. In almost any congregation, one can see worshippers swaying in prayer. The swaying to and fro associated with *tefilla* has special meaning in the mystical literature. It is viewed by some as connected to movements of intimacy. In the words of Rabbi Israel Baal Shem Tov:

> הַתְּפִלָּה הִיא זִיווּג עִם הַשְּׁכִינָה. וּכְמוֹ שֶׁבִּתְחִילַּת הַזִּיווּג יֵשׁ נִיעְנוּעַ כֵּן צָרִיךְ לְנַעְנֵעַ עַצְמוֹ בַּתְּפִילָּה בְּהַתְחָלָתָהּ. וְאַחַר כָּךְ יָכוֹל לַעֲמוֹד כָּךְ בְּלֹא נִיעְנוּעַ וְיִהְיֶה דָּבוּק לְהַשְּׁכִינָה בִּדְבֵיקוּת גָּדוֹל.

14. Rabbi Abraham Isaac HaKohen Kook, *Arfellei Tohar* (Jerusalem: HaMakhon al Shem HaR. Tz. Y. H. Kook, 5743 [1983]), pp. 16–17.
15. See II Samuel 6:16.
16. For a halakhic discussion of positioning during the *Amida,* see *Shulḥan Arukh, Oraḥ Ḥayyim* 95.

    See Rabbi Saul Berman, "Overview," in Nosson Scherman and Meir Zlotowitz, eds., *The Rabbinical Council of America Edition of the ArtScroll Siddur* (Brooklyn, NY: Mesorah Publications, 1990), pp. xii–xvii, where he offers an analysis of the steps taken before the *Amida.*

> Prayer is union with the Divine Presence. Just as intimacy begins with movement, so must a person accompany the beginning of prayer with the rhythmic swaying of the body. But as one reaches the heights of union with the Presence, the movement of the body ceases.[17]

Tziurim – Illustrations

A picture reflective of the theme of a particular *tefilla* can enhance the prayer experience. For example, Psalm 98, said on Friday evenings (in *Kabbalat Shabbat*), includes the verse בַּחֲצֹצְרוֹת וְקוֹל שׁוֹפָר הָרִיעוּ לִפְנֵי הַמֶּלֶךְ ה׳ – "With trumpets and the sound of the shofar, shout with joy before the Lord, the King" (Ps. 98:6). A striking image of a shofar being sounded at the Western Wall in Jerusalem as the sun sets stirs one to more powerfully feel the meaning of these words. As Rabbi Yehuda Sarna writes:

> The lost art of prayer in our age is the freelance articulation, visualization, or application of routine phrases. To recover it… a visual commentary to the sections of the liturgy [is meaningful]…. These furnish rich, compelling images designed to clarify and to challenge, to focus and to distract, to enliven and to discipline – all essential habits of the imagination.[18]

Ḥamimut HaMakom – Warmth of Place

The physical space of a *beit tefilla* should be intimate. Long sanctuaries with the *bima* (the platform from which the service is led) in the front leave many sitting too far back. A sanctuary with a *bima* in the center, with people sitting as close to each other as possible, is much more

17. *Tzava'at HaRivash* 7b.
There is an opposite approach. Bearing in mind that *tefilla* is a conversation with God, one may consider how he or she would talk to a head of state. Clearly, one would not move to and fro, but would sit or stand still. Similarly, when speaking with God, the Ultimate Leader, one may reach higher levels of *kavana* by remaining absolutely still.
18. Rabbi Jonathan Sacks and Rabbi Yehuda Sarna, *The Koren Shabbat Evening Siddur* (Jerusalem: Koren Publishers, 2011), pp. ix, 48.

conducive to creating a spiritually uplifting *tefilla*. The general rule should be, better to have many people crowded into a small space than few people in a large one.

BEIT MIDRASH

A synagogue can also serve as a *beit midrash,* a house of teaching and learning, where the upward values of Torah are emphasized. The teaching of Torah values, even when those values conflict with contemporary culture, is a primary ingredient of spirituality.[19] Within synagogues, spirituality is possible only when there is a readiness to criticize the ethics and materialism of society at large, and, through teaching and learning, offer a higher, Torah-inspired alternative. Here again, the family model is helpful, as it allows for open and frank discussions of ideas and values even if they go against the norm.

During much of the twentieth century, Jews who felt themselves to be outsiders in America sought to reinforce, if not glorify, American society in their synagogues. Now that Jews feel at home in America, local synagogues have a unique opportunity to restore their spiritual mandate by raising a voice against cultural conformism and seeking a higher distinctiveness that can be a new source of pride.

Do our synagogues encourage excess in bar/bat mitzva or wedding celebrations, or do they strive to infuse life-cycle events with higher spiritual meaning? When we distribute honors institutionally, are they based on wealth alone, or do they demonstrate our admiration for all who live in accordance with a lofty vision of Jewish values? Do we talk about God in synagogue, and is the presence of God felt in *divrei Torah* and *shiurim* (sermons and classes)? Is the goal of the rabbi's *devar Torah* and *shiurim* to say what people want to hear, or are rabbis willing to lovingly challenge their congregants in order to encourage growth and change? A spiritual synagogue should make its congregants not only comfortable, but also uncomfortable.

---

19. I first heard this formulation in a conversation with Rabbi Saul Berman.

BEIT KNESSET

A synagogue is also called a *beit knesset*, a house of gathering. Here lies the outward ingredient of spirituality. Spirituality involves the transcending of self; the readiness to embrace others, especially those in need. The test of spirituality in the synagogue is not how the community receives its most powerful members, but how it welcomes the most vulnerable. Here too, the family model is instructive, as a loving family embraces all of its members regardless of limitation.

Maimonides codifies the importance of reaching outward to give charity to the community's less fortunate members:

> It is better for a person to be liberal with his donations to the poor (*matanot la'evyonim*) than to be lavish with the Purim feast (*seudat Purim*) or in sending portions to friends (*mishloaḥ manot*). For the greatest joy is to bring happiness to the hearts of the poor, the orphans, the widows, and the strangers. For one who brings happiness to the hearts of these unfortunate individuals resembles the Divine Presence, as it says, "[God] revives the spirit of the lowly and the brokenhearted" [Is. 57:15].[20]

One stream of Jewish thought suggests that doing good for others is in some respects on a higher level than charity:

> Acts of kindness are greater than charity. Charity can be accomplished only with money; deeds of loving-kindness can be accomplished through personal involvement as well as with money. Charity can be given only to the poor; loving-kindness can be done for both rich and poor.[21]

In other words, even the poor, who do not have the means to give charity, can perform acts of loving-kindness. And even the rich, who do not

20. Maimonides, *Code*, Laws of Megilla 2:17. Translation by Rabbi Eliyahu Touger.
21. Sukka 49b.

need charity, can be the beneficiaries of good deeds. The wealthy can be lonely. Like all people, they too are vulnerable.[22]

As a *beit knesset*, the centerpiece of a synagogue is being there for others, especially those in emotional or spiritual need. The primary role of a *beit knesset* is to aid and repair the soul, not to pass judgment, condemn, or ostracize. From this perspective, a synagogue can be seen as a kind of hospital. Just as a hospital is dedicated to healing physically, the purpose of a synagogue is to improve our spiritual health. Thus, the synagogue must admit not only those who are healthy, but those who are not, accept not only those parts within us that are whole, but also those parts that are broken.[23] Here again, the model of family is helpful, as everyone who is a member of the family is welcome. In this spirit, synagogues ought to consider providing programs for the most forgotten.

The Physically and Mentally Challenged

Congregations should provide resources for the visually and hearing impaired, and build ramps to the Ark and *bima*.[24] A synagogue that is beautiful is accessible to all. And synagogues should reach out to

---

22. The Talmud includes yet another way that "acts of kindness are greater than charity": צְדָקָה לַחַיִּים, גְּמִילוּת חֲסָדִים בֵּין לַחַיִּים בֵּין לַמֵּתִים – "Charity can be given only to the living; acts of loving-kindness can also be done for the dead." The dead are the most vulnerable, as they can in no way help themselves. Caring for them, i.e., arranging a proper and respectful burial, is therefore called a *ḥesed shel emet*, an act of true kindness.
23. All of us have broken parts. Rabbi Shlomo Carlebach sometimes quipped that half of his synagogue was made up of psychiatrists, and the other half of their patients. After some laughter, he sweetly smiled and said, "And, you know, I don't know who is who."
24. A photograph in my office powerfully beckons to all to become spiritual activists in demanding accessibility for everyone. It is a picture of a man sitting in his wheelchair at the bottom of a flight of steps leading up to the entrance to the synagogue. Emblazoned over its grand doors is a verse from Psalms 118:19, פִּתְחוּ לִי שַׁעֲרֵי צֶדֶק אָבֹא בָם אוֹדֶה יָ־הּ – "Open the gates of righteousness for me; I will enter through them and thank God." The man sits with his back to the doors, unable to enter. We have failed him. Our task is to make sure he can face the doors, and to welcome him as he makes his way on his own.

    See Avraham Weiss, *Spiritual Activism: A Jewish Guide to Leadership and Repairing the World* (Woodstock, VT: Jewish Lights, 2008), pp. 15–17.

"Special Friends," the mentally challenged, who live with their parents or in group homes. Over the years, I've come to recognize that Special Friends play a critical role in the synagogue family, as they carry themselves with an innocence and purity that brings out the best in others. A *beit knesset* embraces all, teaching that Special Friends should not be treated as outcasts; it's not *them* and *us* – it's *we*.

A poignant talmudic story tells us that even great Torah scholars may be guilty of bias, and leaves us with the message that whatever our physical or mental state, we are all God's creations and should be treated with dignity and respect:

> Once R. Elazar b. R. Simon was coming ... from the house of his teacher ... and was feeling elated because he had studied much Torah. There chanced to meet him an exceedingly ugly man, who greeted him, "Peace be upon you, my rabbi." He, however, did not return his salutation but instead said to him, "Good-for-nothing, how ugly you are." ... The man replied ... "Go and tell the craftsman who made me." ... He [R. Elazar] dismounted from the ass and prostrated himself before the man and said to him, "I submit myself to you. Forgive me." The man replied, "I will not forgive you until you go to the craftsman who made me and say to Him, 'How ugly is the vessel you have made.'"[25]

The Elderly

As families are intergenerational, so too should synagogues span all ages.[26] There is a tendency these days to discriminate against the elderly by compartmentalizing and dividing prayer groups by age, thereby separating the young from the old, when, in fact, intergenerational *tefilla* is most

25. Ta'anit 20a–b. Apparently, the man was not satisfied with an apology made to him, as he felt the aggrieved "party" was not he, but God. The Talmud goes on to recount R. Elazar's attempts to obtain forgiveness.
26. Note the biblical term for cornerstone – אֶבֶן – used by Jacob when establishing the first *beit E-lohim*, House of God. אֶבֶן is a compound of אָב and בֵּן, father and son, denoting the importance of intergenerational participation. See Genesis 28:20–22, and the beginning of this chapter.

conducive to spiritual striving. Judaism encourages such interaction with the elderly and grants them status, in the spirit of שְׁאַל אָבִיךָ וְיַגֵּדְךָ זְקֵנֶיךָ וְיֹאמְרוּ לָךְ – "Ask your parents and they will tell you, ask the elderly and they will teach you" (Deut. 32:7).[27] The Midrash speaks with grandeur about older people:

> אָמַר רַבִּי יְהוּדָה בַּר סִימוֹן: אַבְרָהָם תָּבַע זִקְנָה. אָמַר לְפָנָיו: רִבּוֹן הָעוֹלָמִים אָדָם וּבְנוֹ נִכְנָסִין לְמָקוֹם וְאֵין אָדָם יוֹדֵעַ לְמִי מְכַבֵּד, מִתּוֹךְ שֶׁאַתָּה מְעַטְּרוֹ בְּזִקְנָה אָדָם יוֹדֵעַ לְמִי מְכַבֵּד. אָמַר לוֹ הקב"ה: חַיֶּיךָ, דָּבָר טוֹב תָּבַעְתָּ וּמִמְּךָ הוּא מַתְחִיל. מִתְּחִלַּת הַסֵּפֶר וְעַד כָּאן אֵין כְּתִיב זִקְנָה, וְכֵיוָן שֶׁעָמַד אַבְרָהָם נָתַן לוֹ זִקְנָה, וְאַבְרָהָם זָקֵן בָּא בַּיָּמִים.
>
> R. Yehudah b. Simon said: Abraham requested [the appearance of] old age, pleading before Him, "Sovereign of the Universe! When a man and his son enter a town, none know whom to honor! But if You crown him [the father] with [the appearance of] old age, one will know whom to honor." Said the Holy One, Blessed Be He, to him, "As you live, you have asked well, and it will commence with you." Thus from the beginning of the book

27. Rabbi Abraham Joshua Heschel sees the "years of old age" as deeply "formative":

> May I suggest that man's potential for change and growth is much greater than we are willing to admit and that old age be regarded not as the age of stagnation, but as the age of opportunities for inner growth. The years of old age may enable us to attain the high values we have failed to sense, the insights we have missed, the wisdom we have ignored. They are indeed formative years, rich in possibilities to unlearn the follies of a lifetime, to see through inbred self-deceptions, to deepen understanding and compassion, to widen the horizon of honesty, to refine the sense of fairness.

Heschel, speaking at the 1961 White House Conference on Aging, quoted by Rabbi Benjamin Blech, "Judaism and Gerontology," *Tradition* 16, no. 4 (summer 1977), p. 73. Rabbi Blech notes that the verse in the Torah asking that we honor older people underscores the spiritual value of embracing them. There the Torah declares, 'מִפְּנֵי שֵׂיבָה תָּקוּם וְהָדַרְתָּ פְּנֵי זָקֵן וְיָרֵאתָ מֵּאֱ־לֹהֶיךָ אֲנִי ה' – "You shall rise before the aged and show deference to the old; you shall fear your God: I am the Lord" (Lev. 19:32). Why does the verse conclude with the words "I am the Lord"? What is the association between God and honoring the elderly? A hasidic master suggested that in effect, God says, "Please understand, I am the oldest entity in the world. As a consequence, I take special interest in the aged. If you disrespect them, I, the Lord, take it very 'personally.'"

> [of Genesis] until here, old age is not mentioned, but when Abraham arose [the appearance of] old age was granted to him: "And Abraham was old, well stricken in age" [Gen. 24:1].[28]

Note that God grants *zikna* (old age) in response to Abraham's request. And those years are called *atara* (crown), a symbol of dignity and majesty. In contemporary times, people gravitate toward the young, often setting the old aside, segregating them from the rest of the community. In our midrash, as young and old walk together, homage is given to the elderly – they are venerated rather than cast aside. The Talmud reinforces the image of old and young walking hand-in-hand when it declares:

> What was [on] the coin of Abraham our Patriarch?
> An older man and an older woman on the one side,
> And a young man and a young woman on the other.[29]

For me, this means that Abraham, the father of *Am Yisrael*, carried around a message that people of all ages have much to contribute and much to learn from each other. The wisdom of life experience together with youthful energy are both necessary to forge a better destiny for Israel and the world. In a similar spirit, old and young together can lift the prayer experience to extraordinary heights – synthesizing the ancient words of prayer with the yearning for a better tomorrow.

The prayer service draws to a close with a comforting passage from the book of Isaiah that relates to God's unwavering love for the elderly:

וְעַד זִקְנָה אֲנִי הוּא,
וְעַד שֵׂיבָה אֲנִי אֶסְבֹּל,
אֲנִי עָשִׂיתִי וַאֲנִי אֶשָּׂא,
וַאֲנִי אֶסְבֹּל וַאֲמַלֵּט.

> When you grow old, I will still be the same (*Ani Hu*);
> When your hair turns gray, I will still carry you (*esbol*);

28. Genesis Rabba 65:9.
29. Bava Kama 97b.

> I made you, I will bear you,
> I will carry you, and I will rescue you. (Is. 46:4)[30]

We can interpret this passage by understanding its biblical partner text from the book of Exodus. After the Exodus from Egypt and the miraculous crossing of the sea, the Israelites declare: זֶה אֵ־לִי וְאַנְוֵהוּ – "This is my God and I will beautify Him (*anvehu*)" (Ex. 15:12). As noted earlier, the word *anvehu* is a contraction of *ani ve-hu,* I and he. Here, in our *tefilla* from Isaiah, positions are reversed. God tells the elderly: Even when you grow older, I see you as beautiful (*ani hu*). Even as you turn gray, God goes on to say, I will be your *sabal* (related to the word *esbol*), literally, your porter, carrying you, caring for you, being there for you.

The Unaffiliated

The role of a synagogue is to embrace every person who passes through its doors, regardless of affiliation, commitment, or background.[31] All should be welcome: the less knowledgeable and the more knowledgeable, the less observant and the more observant, the less involved and the more involved. Regardless of level of knowledge and observance, every person has something to offer.

This concept became a mainstay of the philosophy of Rabbi Abraham Isaac Kook. The rabbi was roundly criticized for being too open and welcoming and accepting of non-ritually observant Jews. Over and over, Rabbi Kook responded that he and the larger ritually observant community had much to learn from everyone. And so he courageously wrote:

> וּתְתוּקַּן הַנֶּפֶשׁ שֶׁל הַיְּרֵאִים שׁוֹמְרֵי תוֹרָה עַל יְדֵי שְׁלֵמוּת הַנֶּפֶשׁ שֶׁבַּפּוֹשְׁעִים הַטּוֹבִים בְּיַחַשׁ לְעִנְיְנֵי הַכְּלָל, וְתִקְוַת הַגַּשְׁמִיּוֹת וְהָרוּחָנִיּוֹת הַמּוּשָּׂגוֹת בְּהַכָּרָה וְהַרְגָּשָׁה הָאֱנוֹשִׁית.

30. This is part of a compilation of verses beginning with אַל תִּירָא מִפַּחַד פִּתְאֹם – "Have no fear of sudden terror" (Proverbs 3:25), and said after *Aleinu.*
31. A synagogue that is family should metaphysically expand its walls and find ways to embrace the larger community, even those who do not come through its doors.

> The souls of the Torah-observant will be perfected through the wholeness of the souls of the good sinners with regard to matters of Jewish peoplehood, and their physical aspirations and spirituality, which is realized through the recognition of universal sensibilities.[32]

Speaking about the pioneers who built Israel and were predominantly non-ritually observant, Rabbi Kook insisted that they taught the message of caring for all Jews and all people, as well as teaching the importance of working and defending the land.

Rabbi Kook's approach echoes the position of R. Elazar b. Azaria, who parted from Rabban Gamliel by allowing everyone, whatever his status or learning level, into the study hall. The Talmud records that on that day, great advances were made in learning. No doubt, the input of those who were previously excluded contributed to the unlocking of difficult talmudic texts. In the words of the Talmud:

> On the day [R. Elazar b. Azaria was appointed], they removed the doorkeeper [of the study hall], and permission was granted to all students to enter, as opposed to Rabban Gamliel, [who] would proclaim and say that any student whose inside was not as his outside (שֶׁאֵין תּוֹכוֹ כְּבָרוֹ) was not allowed to enter the study hall....
>
> On that day, Tractate Eduyot was taught.... And there was not a [single] law that had [thus far] been left unresolved in the study hall which they did not [then] resolve.[33]

While the term "outreach" is generally understood to mean that only the person reaching out has something to offer, our broader understanding of *beit knesset* suggests that both parties can grow. Those being reached are not viewed as having little to contribute the Jewish community either spiritually or religiously; rather, outreach becomes an experience that offers a great deal to everyone involved. For this reason, a more appropriate term than "outreach," would be "encounter," which describes a

---

32. Kook, *Arfellei Tohar* 21.
33. Berakhot 28a.

mutual interaction in which all parties benefit and acquire deep respect for one another.[34]

Beleaguered Jewry

Beit knesset also means that we encompass the dreams and angst of all of Israel. The Midrash tells the story of a man born with two heads who came before King Solomon. Since he had two heads, the man felt he deserved two portions of the inheritance. His siblings responded that while he had two heads, he had one body, and therefore deserved only one share. This is the way Solomon responded:

> Solomon in his wisdom boiled water, covered one of the heads, and poured water over the second. The pain from the boiling water caused both heads to cry out. Solomon concluded that the two heads were still one person who should be judged as one individual [and receive one share of the inheritance].[35]

---

34. See Avraham Weiss, "Creating a Kiruv Center," *Jewish Action* 55, no. 1 (fall 1994), pp. 71–75.

    The goal of inclusivity may lead rabbis to move off the pulpit and sit near different people during the service. This creates an atmosphere of inclusion and warmth. In this spirit, it is important for rabbis to be the first to the door to welcome newcomers and personally wish everyone well upon leaving the synagogue. It is my custom to hug every man as he leaves, while my wife Toby hugs the women.

    Inclusivity also means that women and men be equally welcome. In Orthodox synagogues, where a partition (*meḥitza*) separates men and women during services, it is important that women be able to see and hear equally. In our synagogue, for example, the *meḥitza* bisects the sanctuary, merging into the walls that surround an elevated *bima* (the platform from which the services are led) in the center of the sanctuary and an elevated Ark against the eastern wall. Both the *bima* and the Ark are therefore placed equally within the men's and women's sections.

    For some people, synagogues – especially ritual as celebrated in synagogues – are barriers to Jewish involvement. In my experience, there are two times during the year when people, no matter how distant, are drawn to synagogue – Yom Kippur and the Passover Seder. A good idea would be to develop free High Holy Day services and free Passover Seders geared especially for these individuals. Such open services and Seders could serve as gateways to greater Jewish involvement.
35. Rabbi Menashe Klein, *Mishneh Halakhot* 16:37. See *Tosafot*, Menaḥot 37a, s.v. *o kum gali*, and *Shita Mekubbetzet* ad loc.

It is the same with the Jewish people. If someone in our national family anywhere in the world is suffering – in effect, has boiling water poured over his or her head – and we feel that scalding, we are one. If not, we are a fragmented nation. The *Mekhilta* makes this point when it compares Israel to a single body:

> מְלַמֵּד שֶׁהֵן כְּגוּף אֶחָד וְנֶפֶשׁ אַחַת...לָקָה אֶחָד מֵהֶן כּוּלָּן מַרְגִּישִׁין וְכֵן הוּא אוֹמֵר: שֶׂה פְזוּרָה יִשְׂרָאֵל, מָה רָחֵל זוֹ לָקָה אֶחָד מֵאֵבָרֶיהָ כּוּלָּן מַרְגִּישִׁין, כָּךְ יִשְׂרָאֵל לָקָה אֶחָד מֵהֶן כּוּלָּן מַרְגִּישִׁין.
>
> [Israel is] like one body and one soul.... If one of them is struck, all of them feel it. And thus Scripture states, "Israel is a scattered sheep" [Jer. 50:17]. Just as with this sheep, if one of its limbs is struck, all of them feel it, likewise with Israel: If one of them is struck, all of them feel it.[36]

The *beit knesset* has long been the venue to rally the community to speak out on behalf of beleaguered Jewry around the world – not only to sympathize with their plight, but to empathize with them, to integrate their pain into our very being as if it were ours. It is not *them* and *us*, but *we*. An example of this phenomenon was the Soviet Jewry movement in the latter half of the twentieth century, wherein synagogues around the world served as the headquarters to encourage and inspire Jews to reach out to Soviet Jewry and declare, "Your pain is our pain, your tears are our tears, and only when you are free will we be free!"

The State of Israel

To this day, the synagogue is the arena in which to raise a voice of moral conscience, of Jewish conscience, on behalf of the State of Israel. It is the venue to engender a proactive relationship with the covenantal mission of Israel as the place where the national destiny of the Jewish people is unfolding. All this is in the spirit of Rabbi Judah HaLevi, who proclaims: לִבִּי בְמִזְרָח, וְאָנֹכִי בְּסוֹף מַעֲרָב – "My heart is in the east, but I am at

36. *Mekhilta de-Rabbi Shimon bar Yoḥai*, trans. W. David Nelson (Philadelphia: Jewish Publication Society, 2006), 19:6, p. 219.

the uttermost of the west."[37] To paraphrase Rabbi Naḥman of Bratslav, wherever I go, I am going to Israel. Even though we may be in the Diaspora, we can be *dorshei Tziyon,* constantly seeking and yearning for Zion.[38]

The Family of Humankind

As stated in chapter 4, an enlightened sense of national identity, rather than being a contradiction to universal consciousness, is in fact a prerequisite for it. Thus, an inclusive *beit knesset* means that we also connect with *mishpeḥot amim,* the "families of humankind" (Ps. 96:7). Synagogues should therefore be places to pray and act not only on behalf of *Am Yisrael,* but also on behalf of all of humankind. Rabbi Kook magically lays out this vision:

> There is one who sings the song of his own life, and in himself he finds everything, his full spiritual satisfaction.
>
> There is another who sings the song of his people. He leaves the circle of his own individual self, because he finds it without sufficient breadth.... He aspires toward the heights, and he attaches himself with a gentle love to the whole community of Israel. Together with her, he sings her songs. He feels grieved in her afflictions and delights in her hopes....
>
> There is another who reaches toward more distant realms, and he goes beyond the boundary of Israel to sing the song of humankind. His spirit extends to the wider vistas of the majesty of the human being in general, and his noble essence....
>
> Then there is one who rises toward wider horizons, until

---

37. Rabbi Judah HaLevi longed for *Eretz Yisrael,* in the east, even as he lived in Spain, which in his lifetime was thought to be the westernmost place on earth.
38. See Rosh HaShana 30a: מִכְּלָל דְּבָעְיָא דְּרִישָׁה – "From this we gather that [Israel] ought to be [constantly] inquired after." See my contribution to *A Dream of Zion: American Jews Reflect on Why Israel Matters to Them,* ed. Rabbi Jeffrey K. Salkin (Woodstock, VT: Jewish Lights, 2007), part 4, pp. 162–165.

    As a way of emphasizing the importance of seeking Zion, some congregations conclude services on Shabbat morning with the singing of Israel's national anthem, *Hatikva.*

> he links himself with all existence, with all God's creatures, with all worlds, and he sings his song with all of them....
>
> And this full comprehensiveness rises to become the song of holiness, the song of God, the song of Israel, in its full strength and beauty, in its full authenticity and greatness. The name "Israel" stands for *shir El,* the song of God. It is a simple song, a twofold song, a threefold song, and a fourfold song.[39]

BEIT E-LOHIM

Optimal *tefilla* is holistic, whole Holistic *tefilla* means synthesizing the whole of the human being – heart, mind, soul, and body – in service of God. The heart inspires prayer; the mind requires study, and the soul stirs the body to act on behalf of community. In holistic *tefilla,* these elements come together, reaching a crescendo when they join in magical symphony.

The term for a synagogue that best expresses this synergy is *beit E-lohim. Beit E-lohim* evokes a place where primary attention is given to sensing and responding to the presence of God. The Jewish conception of God is identified first and foremost with Oneness.[40] As Rabbi Abraham Joshua Heschel has argued:

> How do we identify the Divine?
>
> Divine is a message that discloses unity where we see diversity, which discloses peace when we are involved in discord. God is the One who holds our fitful lives together, who reveals to

39. Rabbi Abraham Isaac Kook, "A Fourfold Song," in Kook, *Orot HaKodesh,* vol. 2, in Kook, *The Lights of Penitence, the Moral Principles, Lights of Holiness, Essays, Letters, and Poems (Classics of Western Spirituality),* trans. Ben Zion Bokser (New York: Paulist Press, 1978), pp. 444–445.

    An example of a universal *beit knesset* program would be a commemoration of Dr. Martin Luther King Jr.'s birthday, where African-Americans and Jews can come together in hope and song. It could become a living example of כִּי בֵיתִי בֵּית תְּפִלָּה יִקָּרֵא לְכָל הָעַמִּים – "For My House shall be a house of prayer for all the peoples" (Is. 56:7) – a glimpse of redemption itself.

40. The very noun *E-lohim* is plural, implying a multiplicity of characteristics that come together in the One God.

> us that what is empirically diverse in color, in interest, in creeds – races, classes, nations – is one in God's eyes and one in essence.
>
> God means: No one is ever alone; the essence of the temporal is the eternal; the moment is an image of eternity in an infinite mosaic.
>
> God means: Togetherness of all beings in holy otherness.[41]

Thus, we must ask ourselves, is our *tefilla* inspired by an experience of oneness, of the coming together of prayer, Torah, and good deeds? Does it strive to express a sense of the Unity of God and the unity of all creation?

Holistic *tefilla* insists that prayer is not a narrow experience, but a broad sweep, which is expansive and far-reaching. It is spiritual, as spirituality is the discovery of the open in the closed, the infinite in the finite, the wide in the narrow. In midrashic terms:

> פִּתְחוּ לִי פֶּתַח כְּחוּדוֹ שֶׁל מַחַט וַאֲנִי אֶפְתַּח לָכֶם כְּפִתְחוֹ שֶׁל אוּלָם.
>
> Open for Me an opening the size of the point of a needle, and I will open for you an opening as wide as can be.[42]

In holistic *tefilla*, movement is neither inward nor upward nor outward, but circular – embracing all directions simultaneously. Thus, spirituality leads to recognizing that the core values of the synagogue – *beit tefilla, beit midrash, beit knesset* – are inextricably bound. They are holistic in nature, as no one value of the synagogue can be separated from another – they unite under the rubric of *beit E-lohim.*[43] How does this occur? How does *tefilla* interface with Torah, how does it interface with good deeds?

---

41. See Rabbi Abraham Joshua Heschel, *Man Is Not Alone* (New York: Farrar, Straus and Giroux, 1951), pp. 101–109.
42. Song of Songs Rabba 5:2.
43. Note that the three terms for a synagogue parallel Mishna Avot 1:2: "The world stands on three things: on the Torah [*beit midrash*], on divine worship [*beit tefilla*], and on acts of loving-kindness [*beit knesset*]."

Meshing *Tefilla* with Torah

Tefilla and Torah are indelibly linked. Consider the psalms that make up a significant portion of the Siddur. The book of Psalms is a book of both prayer and Revelation – *tefilla* and Torah. Historically, the work contains actual prayers of human beings to God.[44] Over the ages, the rabbis viewed Psalms not just as a collection of prayers from humanity to God but as containing revelations and divine truths communicated by God to humanity; Psalms, for them, was an integral part of the Written Torah, and parts of it were formally integrated into the prayer service. For the rabbis, Psalms was a communication both from below to above and from above to below.[45]

The prayer service itself is punctuated with Torah. We have already pointed out that we begin the morning service with the recitation of the Blessings of the Torah followed by sections from the written and oral traditions. The intersection of *tefilla* and Torah may explain the halakha that after reciting the *Shema*, one may fulfill the mitzva of learning Torah.[46] The *Amida* ends with the words שֶׁיִּבָּנֶה בֵּית הַמִּקְדָּשׁ בִּמְהֵרָה בְיָמֵינוּ וְתֵן חֶלְקֵנוּ בְּתוֹרָתֶךָ – "May the Temple be speedily rebuilt in our days, and grant us a share in Your Torah." The Temple (*Beit HaMikdash*) was the central place of sacrifice, the forerunner of prayer. Not coincidentally, after mentioning the *Mikdash*, the liturgy points out the importance of Torah study – thus linking *tefilla* to Torah. And a central part of the prayer services are those times when we read from the Torah scroll.

44. The psalms were written primarily by David. However, according to Bava Batra 14b, the book of Psalms also includes the words of other writers, including Moses. See, for example, Psalm 90, *Tefilla LeMoshe* – "A Prayer of Moses." Rashi posits that the next eleven chapters of Psalms were written by Moses. See Rashi, Psalms 90, s.v. *tefilla leMoshe*.

45. This ambiguity as to whether Psalms is fundamentally *tefilla* or Torah led one major medieval philosopher, Sa'adia Gaon, to refute the idea that this biblical book originated as an actual human prayer to God. For him, God revealed these prayers in the form and guise of human supplication as a rhetorical method of stressing humanity's "relative weakness and reliance upon Him." See Moshe Sokolow, "*Saadiah Gaon's Prolegomenon to Psalms*," *Proceedings of the American Academy for Jewish Research* 51 (1984), p. 148.

46. See Nedarim 8a and Berakhot 11b.

Meshing *Tefilla* with Communal Responsibility

Tefilla is also intensely intertwined with a sense of responsibility to the larger community. In no small measure, prayer spells out the total vision of Judaism and our responsibility to translate that blueprint into reality. As Rabbi Heschel writes:

> At the beginning of all action is an inner vision in which things to be are experienced as real. Prayer, too, is frequently an inner vision, an intense dreaming for God – the reflection of the divine intentions in the soul of man. We dream of a time "when the world will be perfected under the kingship of God, and all the children of flesh will call upon Thy name, when Thou wilt turn unto Thyself all the wicked of the Earth." We anticipate the fulfillment of the hope shared by both God and man.
>
> To pray is to dream in league with God, to envision His holy visions.[47]

This may be the deeper meaning of the talmudic passage mandating that one should pray in a place where there are windows:

> R. Ḥiyya b. Abba said: A person should always pray in a house possessing windows, for it says, "And he [Daniel] had windows open [in his upper story, facing Jerusalem, and three times a day he fell to his knees and prayed]" [Dan. 6:11].[48]

Praying near a window can connect one to what is happening outside. *Tefilla* should not be an insular experience. Rather, it should encourage one to see and empathize with those beyond the windows who are in need.[49]

---

47. Heschel, *Quest for God*, p. 19.
48. Berakhot 31a. See also *Shulḥan Arukh, Oraḥ Ḥayyim* 90:4.
49. Rabbeinu Yona suggests that the windows should face Jerusalem. From this perspective, the purpose of the windows is to direct one's heart to the Holy City. See Rabbeinu Yona, Berakhot 31a (in Rabbeinu Yona 24b), s.v. *bevayit*.

In the end, prayer, Torah, and service interface as they are all transformative. Prayer has the power to alter one's moral plane, and, in so doing, turn the individual into a new person.[50] Torah is often referred to as *Mikra*, a calling, as it is a call to change ourselves, our community, our people, and the world. In the words of the Talmud, תַּלְמוּד מֵבִיא לִידֵי מַעֲשֶׂה – "Study leads to action."[51] And acts of loving-kindness by their very definition impact society, changing the status quo. To be serious about *tefilla*, one must integrate all these values, making it a holistic experience. As Rabbi Saul Berman writes:

> Effective prayer is a vibrant conversation between an individual... and God. But modern Western civilization has...distance[d itself] from God.... To make prayer meaningful for moderns... we need to get God and God's values into the truly vibrant dimensions of our lives...into our productivity and our relationships, into our daily lives as individuals, as communities and as nations.[52]

Rashi, Berakhot 34b, s.v. *ḥalonot*, suggests that the purpose of the windows is to inspire a sense of oneness with the heavens, with God Himself.

The textual source from Daniel, which includes his praying three times daily, may support the suggestion here that windows serve as a link to those in need on the outside. The needs of people change as the day progresses from morning to afternoon to evening. Here we may have another approach to why there are three services. They help sensitize us to others – those who are beyond the windows, whose needs change as the day unfolds.

The idea that *tefilla* intersects with good deeds is the Maimonidean motif of prayer as formulated in chapter 1 of this study. For Maimonides, *ule'ovdo* mandates that we partner with God to redeem the world.

50. See the beginning of chapter 2.
51. Kiddushin 40b. Not coincidentally, after studying Torah with a *minyan*, the *Kaddish DeRabbanan* is said. Having participated in Torah learning, one declares, יִתְגַּדַּל וְיִתְקַדַּשׁ שְׁמֵהּ רַבָּא. Loosely translated, this means that through Torah study, one can implement its teachings, thereby allowing God's principles of ethical monotheism to be magnified and sanctified.
52. Rabbi Saul J. Berman, "Even a New Siddur Can't Close 'God Gap,'" *The Jewish Daily Forward*, August 28, 2009, accessed April 30, 2012, http://forward.com/articles/112469/even-a-new-siddur-can-t-close-god-gap/.

Mission and *Beit E-Lohim*

Tefilla as a holistic experience gives rise to a model of synagogue that is mission-centered. In general, there are two types of synagogues. There are functional synagogues that focus on the services they offer. They include classes and prayer services, and they include the rabbi overseeing what are affectionately referred to as "The Big B's" – birth, *brit, simḥat bat,* bar mitzva, bat mitzva, betrothal, and burial.

And then there are synagogues that focus on a mission. These are the synagogues that cultivate a vision and core values, which give meaning and purpose to the services they provide. In this model, the functional synagogue is influenced and informed by its mission.[53]

There are great differences between a synagogue that is exclusively functional and a synagogue that combines function with mission. By and large, a functional synagogue focuses on the individual. In contrast, the synagogue that links function with mission stresses the importance of creating community. When one prays or studies, it is with a larger sense of involvement in something much bigger.

It follows, then, that a synagogue that is purely functional is one that stresses the "I"; the "I" who asks, how can *I* best be served? In contrast, a synagogue that is both functional and mission-driven stresses the "we"; not how can I be served, but how can I serve others? That's probably why most functional synagogues are generally homogeneous, while those that include mission are heterogeneous.

Functionality by itself engenders a culture of entitlement; with mission, it engenders a culture of contribution. Functionality by itself engenders a culture of taking; with mission, it engenders a culture of giving.

A functional synagogue also stresses what it is doing now, listing the programs and services that it already provides. It sees progress as enriching what it has always done. In contrast, the synagogue of mission focuses not only on what it's doing now, but on what it ought to be

53. Meir Lakein of Jewish Funds for Justice formulates a similar distinction, substituting the word "maintenance" for "functional." He says: "[It's] not that maintenance is bad – if we create good things, we should maintain them – it's just that maintenance is limited, and less than what we were created to do." This comment was part of a talk Lakein gave at Yeshivat Chovevei Torah (YCT) in the fall of 2010.

doing. Not only on where it is, but where it should be. Always reaching, always growing.

Finally, a functional synagogue approaches *tefilla* as an exclusive endeavor – involving prayer and little else. In contrast, mission-centered synagogues interweave the *beit tefilla* with the *beit midrash* and *beit knesset*, forming a *beit E-lohim*. In the end, one should pray with a community inspired by a mission which recognizes that prayer is an inclusive endeavor, a holistic enterprise – meshing God with Torah and good deeds.[54]

BECOMING YOUR PRAYER: THE *TEFILLA* OF TORAH AND GOOD DEEDS

Not only does holistic *tefilla* encompass Torah and good deeds, but Torah and good deeds may be a form of *tefilla*. Rabbi Naḥman of Bratslav writes:

> גַּם טוֹב לַעֲשׂוֹת מֵהַתּוֹרָה תְּפִלָּה. דְּהַיְנוּ כְּשֶׁלּוֹמֵד אוֹ שׁוֹמֵעַ אֵיזֶה מַאֲמַר תּוֹרָה... אֲזַי יַעֲשֶׂה מִזֶּה תְּפִלָּה... וִיבַקֵּשׁ מֵאִתּוֹ יִתְבָּרַךְ שֶׁיְּזַכֵּהוּ לָבֹא לְכָל זֶה.
>
> It is also important that Torah be transformed into *tefilla*, that is, when one learns or hears a thought from the Torah ... he or she should turn it into *tefilla* ... and request of the Blessed One that he merit to fulfill what he has learned.[55]

---

54. Prayer *qua* prayer falls into two categories: functional prayer and mission prayer. Decorum in a synagogue, for example, falls into these respective realms. Functional decorum involves remaining silent because the law demands it, or because one feels totally disconnected from the prayer experience. In contrast, mission decorum involves remaining quiet during prayer as a deep expression of reflective dialogue with God.

    In some circles people tend to synagogue-hop, searching for the fastest or earliest functional *minyan*. This practice may have its benefits. Still, there is a price one pays, as the place of prayer should be the place where one is involved with a community that lives and breathes a mission. The goal ought to be not only to pray with a *minyan*, but to pray with such a community.

    While the term *minyan* is commonly used to refer to a prayer service, my preference is to use the term "*tefilla*." *Minyan*, in Orthodoxy, includes men but does not count women. *Tefilla* transcends gender. Women are not part of the quorum of ten, but *tefilla* describes an experience in which they too are critical participants.
55. Rabbi Naḥman of Bratslav, *Likkutei Maharan, Tinyana* 25, s.v. *gam*.

Rabbi Joseph B. Soloveitchik takes it a step further. Not only should Torah inspire *tefilla*, Torah is *tefilla*. Both involve song, a song to the Lord. In his words:

> One who learns Torah… and engages in the study of Torah, is considered as one who pours forth his speech, as a supplication and request, as a song and melody….
>
> *Tefilla* includes, of course, saying favorable words of praise and song to the Holy One, Blessed Be He…. The learning of

---

In general, parts of the Oral Law are studied at the beginning and end of the prayer service. The learning of the Oral Law is followed by the Rabbis' Kaddish, which is made up of the Mourner's Kaddish plus the following paragraph:

עַל יִשְׂרָאֵל וְעַל רַבָּנָן
וְעַל תַּלְמִידֵיהוֹן וְעַל כָּל תַּלְמִידֵי תַלְמִידֵיהוֹן
וְעַל כָּל מַאן דְּעָסְקִין בְּאוֹרַיְתָא
דִּי בְּאַתְרָא הָדֵין וְדִי בְּכָל אֲתַר וַאֲתַר,
יְהֵא לְהוֹן וּלְכוֹן שְׁלָמָא רַבָּא
חִנָּא וְחִסְדָּא וְרַחֲמֵי וְחַיֵּי אֲרִיכֵי וּמְזוֹנֵי רְוִיחֵי
וּפֻרְקָנָא מִן קֳדָם אֲבוּהוֹן דִּי בִשְׁמַיָּא,
וְאִמְרוּ אָמֵן.

To Israel, to the teachers,
their disciples and their disciples' disciples,
and to all who engage in the study of Torah,
in this place or elsewhere,
may there come to them and you great peace,
grace, kindness, and compassion,
long life, ample sustenance… and deliverance,
from their Father in Heaven –
and say: Amen.

Torah study is beautiful, but it has its dangers. Rabbis are often in bitter conflict; Torah scholars can be unyielding and overbearing; sometimes students of Torah struggle to provide for themselves and their families. The *Kaddish DeRabbanan* is a gentle prayer that the Torah studied be a Torah of "great peace," of "grace, kindness, and compassion," accompanied by "long life, ample sustenance, and deliverance." Appropriately, this paragraph is inserted just prior to the last section of *Kaddish,* which deals with the hope for peace: יְהֵא שְׁלָמָא רַבָּא – "May there be great peace."

Note also that Torah study is not limited to the rabbis, as *Kaddish DeRabbanan* first mentions "Israel," then speaks of "all who engage in the study of Torah." Perhaps for this reason, this *Kaddish* is also called "*Kaddish 'al Yisrael,*'" referring to the first two words of this paragraph. See the end of chapter 1 for further analysis of *Kaddish*.

> Torah can be considered like presenting a song before the Holy One, Blessed Be He. Is there any greater praise than a person who plumbs to the depths of the wisdom of Torah? The study of Torah is considered the most exalted *tefilla* that a Jew can put forth.[56]

For Rabbi Soloveitchik, the study of Torah, like *tefilla*, is the human being singing to God.[57] Perhaps the confluence moves in different directions. In *tefilla*, the human being sings to God. In Torah, God sings to the human being. Together, they harmonize, expressing the ultimate song of unity between heaven and earth.

Song comes from within; it is an expression of the soul. Not only is *tefilla* a "service of the heart" but Torah, too, is the revealing of one's inner purity, one's inner heart and soul. In the words of Rabbi Kalonymus Kalman Shapira of Piaseczno:

> בְּמָה נוֹתְנִים אָנוּ אֶת עַצְמֵנוּ לַתּוֹרָה...בְּלִימּוּד סִתְרֵי תּוֹרָה...
>
> וּמַהוּ לִימּוּד סִתְרֵי תּוֹרָה, לֹא קַבָּלָה וּרְמָזִים בִּלְבַד, כִּי אֵיךְ הֵם סִתְרֵי תּוֹרָה אִם כְּבָר נִדְפָּסִים בִּסְפָרִים קְדוֹשִׁים לְעֵינֵי כֹּל.
>
> אֲבָל לִימּוּד סִתְרֵי אוֹרַיְיתָא הוּא הַמְגַלֶּה בְּלִימּוּדוֹ אֶת נִשְׁמָתוֹ הַמּוּסְתֶּרֶת עַתָּה... וּמִי שֶׁלּוֹמֵד בְּנִשְׁמָתוֹ וּמְגַלָּה אוֹתָהּ, זֶהוּ לִימּוּד סִתְרֵי אוֹרַיְיתָא.

---

56. Rabbi Joseph B. Soloveitchik, *Shiurim LeZekher Abba Mori z"l* (Jerusalem: Akiva Yosef, 5743), vol. 2, pp. 14–15.

Note also the Jerusalem Talmud, Berakhot 8a–b. There, R. Shimon bar Yoḥai posits that one who studies Torah all day is exempt from reciting the *Shema*. In the words of the Jerusalem Talmud, "This [Torah study] is learning, and this [recitation of the *Shema*] is learning. And [the former] learning is not overridden by [the latter] learning."

It seems to me that the *devar Torah* (sermon) a rabbi gives before *Musaf* (the additional Shabbat or holiday service) is a form of *tefilla*. As such, it does not interrupt the service, but is part of its flow.

57. The Bible calls the Torah "a song." See Deuteronomy 31:19: וְעַתָּה כִּתְבוּ לָכֶם אֶת הַשִּׁירָה הַזֹּאת וְלַמְּדָהּ אֶת בְּנֵי יִשְׂרָאֵל – "And now, write this song for yourselves, and teach it to the Children of Israel." While Rashi understands שִׁירָה as referring to the song of *Ha'azinu*, Maimonides insists it refers to the commandment of writing the Torah. See Maimonides, *Sefer HaMitzvot*, positive commandment 18.

> How does one become immersed in Torah?… One does so through the secrets of Torah.
>
> And what does it mean to learn the secrets of the Torah? This cannot refer simply to learning Kabbala or esoteric hints alone, for how can those be considered esoteric aspects of the Torah when they are already printed in holy books that anyone can access?!
>
> Rather, learning the secrets of the Torah is the one who discovers in his learning his own soul, which is currently hidden…. And whoever learns his own soul, and reveals it – that is what we call learning the secrets of the Torah![58]

One of the great Torah scholars of our time who lives this idea is Dr. Avivah Zornberg. Listening to her Torah is not only an intellectual exercise, but a religious experience. Her Torah is holistic; it is a form of *tefilla*, a song that reveals the inner soul. As the psalmist declares, שִׁירוּ לַה׳ שִׁיר חָדָשׁ – "Sing to the Lord a new song" (Ps. 96:1).[59]

Rabbi Kalonymus Kalman HaLevi Epstein adds that good deeds are a prerequisite to pure prayer. For him, the efficacy of *tefilla* depends on one's broader commitment outside the prayer service.

> צָרִיךְ לָזֶה לָבֹא לִתְפִלָּה זַכָּה... לִיגִיעָה יוֹמָם וָלַיְלָה בַּתּוֹרָה וּבְמַעֲשִׂים טוֹבִים עַד שֶׁעַל יְדֵי זֶה יְכוֹלִים לָבֹא בֶּאֱמֶת לֵידַע לְהִתְפַּלֵּל בְּיִרְאָה וּבְאַהֲבָה רַבָּה כַּיָּדוּעַ לַמְּבִינִים.
>
> In order for a person to attain pure prayer… it is necessary for him to engage in much service, to labor long, night and day, in the

58. Shapira, *Derekh HaMelekh*, p. 197. Many thanks to Rabbi Mishael Zion for this translation.
59. Not only do Torah and *tefilla* interface, but so do Torah and good deeds. For this reason, the recitation of Torah blessings in the morning covers the entire day of Torah learning, even if there are intervals between periods of study. All human actions, even those that do not involve Torah study per se, relate to Torah learning in some way, since every aspect of human existence involves the implementation of Torah principles. From this perspective, one never finishes learning Torah as long as one is awake. Reciting the morning Torah blessings is therefore sufficient for the whole day. See *Tosafot*, Berakhot 11b, s.v. *shekvar niftar beAhava Rabba.*

> study of the Torah and in performance of good deeds, so that as a result, he may learn how to truly pray with awe and great love, as those who have discernment know full well.[60]

Good deeds may be not only the precursor to prayer, but a form of prayer itself. This may be the deeper meaning of the prayer וַאֲנִי תְפִלָּתִי לְךָ ה׳ עֵת רָצוֹן אֱ־לֹהִים בְּרָב חַסְדֶּךָ עֲנֵנִי בֶּאֱמֶת יִשְׁעֶךָ – "As for me, may my prayer come to You, Lord, at a time of favor. O God, in Your great love, answer me with Your faithful salvation" (Ps. 69:14).[61] The flow of the verse is that the first two words, וַאֲנִי תְפִלָּתִי, are linked to what follows. My sincere prayer to You, O Lord, hopefully inspires favorable acceptance.

In hasidic thought, however, the first two words form an entity unto itself. That is, one pauses after the first two words, allowing them, so to speak, to stand on their own. "I am my prayer." Quite literally, then, וַאֲנִי תְפִלָּתִי (*va'ani tefillati*) means that ultimate prayer is declaring, as King David said, וַאֲנִי תְפִלָּה – "And I am prayer" (Ps. 109:4). Rabbi Samson Raphael Hirsch adds one word to the translation, "And I am *all* prayer."[62] The way I talk and walk and conduct myself in business; the way I eat and love and interact with others; the way I treat the forlorn, the hungry, the homeless – my very being, my very essence, my every endeavor is *tefilla,* holistic prayer.

The individual who reflected this teaching for me was my father-in-law, the late Zalman Aryeh Hilsenrad. I have memories of the way my father-in-law prayed. Lowering his head, he'd softly say every word. But for me, what made him a paragon of prayer was not only the words he offered, but the way he lived – his good deeds, his kindness, became

60. Rabbi Kalonymus Kalman HaLevi Epstein, *Sefer Ma'or VaShamesh* (Jerusalem: Even Yisrael, 5748 [1988]), *Vayeḥi,* s.v. *beforat Yosef,* p. 143.
61. *Va'ani tefillati* is said daily after *Ma tovu* at the start of the morning service. It is also said on holidays when the Torah is removed from the Ark.
62. Rabbi Samson Raphael Hirsch compares וַאֲנִי תְפִלָּה to King David's exclaiming, אֲנִי שָׁלוֹם – "All my being is peace" (Ps. 120:7).

    Similarly, we have here, "I am all prayer." David says, "The result of all these attacks by my foes is simply that I devote more and more effort to the mustering of my spiritual resources for my endeavors at moral and spiritual self-improvement before God."

    See Hirsch, *The Psalms* (New York: Feldheim, 1966).

his very being. For the last twenty-five years of his life, he organized a charity program wherein almost a thousand Americans adopted poor Israeli families. Every month he'd send the Americans an envelope with an Israeli family's address, reminding them of their responsibility to send a check. His bedroom became his office – a reservoir of boxes, boxes of envelopes that he and his wife, Ida, would laboriously address by hand. He *was tefilla* – holistic prayer.

CREATING A SPIRITUAL CULTURE

To succeed in bringing spirituality into the synagogue, a culture of spirituality must be created. To create such a culture, rabbis and lay leaders must inspire their communities to be committed, invested, grounded, and humble in their quest for spirituality. The endeavor requires adaptive changes wherein the individual is encouraged to find his or her unique way within the framework of community.

Commitment to create a synagogue driven by spirituality is an important first step. But it is not enough. It is critical to translate the commitment into reality by actively investing and developing creative paths to spirituality, such as learning seriously about *tefilla* and finding meaningful ways to integrate spirituality into our lives.

And the spirituality we invest in must be grounded in deference to *tirḥa detzibbura* (burden to the community); it should not be open-ended. Spirituality in the synagogue must have a solid foundation, with a formula that has a beginning, a middle, and an end.

An example of sensitivity to *tirḥa detzibbura* is the manner in which R. Akiva prayed. When praying alone, he allowed himself a lengthier *tefilla*. In public, however, he took into account the needs of the community and was brief. R. Yehuda documented this:

> R. Yehuda said: This was the custom of R. Akiva. When he prayed together with the congregation, he would shorten [his prayer] and finish because of the burden to the community [which would otherwise wait until R. Akiva concluded his *tefilla*].
>
> But when he [R. Akiva] prayed by himself, a person would leave him in one corner and find him [after some time] in another

> corner. And why was this so? Because of R. Akiva's bowings and prostrations.[63]

Most important, spirituality requires humility. Spiritual leadership requires someone whose leadership is so obvious, it appears he or she is not leading. As God balances greatness with humility, so should we. In the words of the Talmud:

> אָמַר רַבִּי יוֹחָנָן: כָּל מָקוֹם שֶׁאַתָּה מוֹצֵא גְּבוּרָתוֹ שֶׁל הַקָּדוֹשׁ בָּרוּךְ הוּא אַתָּה מוֹצֵא עַנְוְותָנוּתוֹ.
>
> R. Yoḥanan said: Wherever you find the greatness of the Holy One, Blessed Be He, there you find His humility.[64]

Humility also means that one should be open to every person (*kol adam*), as everyone has a spiritual message to share.

And humility means the recognition that we are never quite sure we are getting it right; we are never complacent; we are always aspiring to new levels. Spirituality in the synagogue is more a process than the achievement of a goal; it is more a journey than a destination. If we think we have made it, we have failed. King David said it best when he asked: מִי יַעֲלֶה בְהַר ה׳ – "Who will ascend the mountain of the Lord?" (Ps. 24:3). The answer lies in the question – it is the one who is constantly seeking and constantly climbing.

For rabbis to bring spirituality into their synagogues and communities, adaptive rather than technical changes are needed. Giving a class is laudatory, but it is only the beginning. What is needed is to develop a synagogue philosophy that is fully and wholly suffused with spirituality. For this to occur, it is critical that there be a synthesis of emotion and intellect, the heart as well as the mind, the interfacing of spirituality with halakha.

---

63. Berakhot 31a. See Rabbeinu Yona, Berakhot 22b, s.v. *haya mekatzer*, who points out that even in public, R. Akiva recited all the words. However, he said them more quickly – without including personal pleas – so as not to burden the community.
64. Megilla 31a.

Our goal should be not to clone other spiritual models, but to find our own unique voices. There was only one Rabbi Soloveitchik, only one Nehama Leibowitz, only one Rabbi Shlomo Carlebach, only one Rabbi Abraham Joshua Heschel, and only one *mori verabbi* Rabbi Yehuda Amital. We must glean from their spiritual Torah, but express that spirituality in a way that is authentic to each of us as individuals.

As much as we are part of the larger community, spirituality means we must find our own voice, our own song, our own dance. I am reminded of the story told by Dr. Carl A. Hammerschlag, a Yale-trained psychiatrist, who served for many years as a family physician in a Native American hospital in the American Southwest:

> Santiago…had been admitted to the Santa Fe Indian Hospital with congestive heart failure. I didn't know that he was the Pueblo priest and clan chief. I only saw an old man in his seventies lying in a hospital bed with oxygen tubes in his nose.
>
> Suddenly, there was this beautiful smile, and he asked me, "Where did you learn to heal?"
>
> Although I assumed my academic credentials would mean little to the old man, I responded almost by rote, rattling off my medical education, internship, and certification.
>
> Again, the beatific smile and another question, "Do you know how to *dance*?"
>
> Somehow, touched by whimsy at the old man's query, I answered that, sure, I like to dance; and I shuffled a little at his bedside. Santiago chuckled, got out of bed, and, short of breath, began to show me his dance.
>
> "You must be able to dance if you are to heal people," he said.
>
> "And will you teach me your steps?" I asked, indulging the aging priest.
>
> Santiago nodded, "Yes, I can teach you my steps, but you will have to hear your own music."[65]

65. Carl A. Hammerschlag, *The Dancing Healers: A Doctor's Journey of Healing with Native Americans* (San Francisco: Harper & Row, 1988), pp. 9–10.

This is the paradox of spiritual life. Spirituality radiates outward, encompassing all – and yet it comes from within.

Based on the writings of Rabbi Naḥman of Bratslav, Naomi Shemer makes this point in *Da Lekha*, a song she wrote and composed. The first paragraph is personal; the second is communal. Such is the way of spirituality. We can share each other's steps, but the music must emanate from our inner beings. Together, individual and community form a holistic whole – holistic prayer.

דַּע לְךָ שֶׁכָּל רוֹעֶה וְרוֹעֶה
יֵשׁ לוֹ נִיגּוּן מְיוּחָד מִשֶּׁלּוֹ
דַּע לְךָ שֶׁכָּל עֵשֶׂב וָעֵשֶׂב
יֵשׁ לוֹ שִׁירָה מְיוּחֶדֶת מִשֶּׁלּוֹ
וּמִשִּׁירַת הָעֲשָׂבִים
נַעֲשֶׂה נִיגּוּן שֶׁל רוֹעֶה.

כַּמָּה יָפֶה כַּמָּה יָפֶה וְנָאֶה
כְּשֶׁשּׁוֹמְעִים הַשִּׁירָה שֶׁלָּהֶם
טוֹב מְאוֹד לְהִתְפַּלֵּל בֵּינֵיהֶם
וּבְשִׂמְחָה לַעֲבוֹד אֶת ה׳
וּמִשִּׁירַת הָעֲשָׂבִים
מִתְמַלֵּא הַלֵּב וּמִשְׁתּוֹקֵק.

Know this, that each and every shepherd
Has a special tune of his own.
Know this, that each and every blade of grass
Has a special song of its own.
And from the song of the grass
Comes the tune of the shepherd.

How beautiful, how beautiful and pleasant it is
To hear their song.
It is very good to pray among them
And to serve God with joy.
And from the song of the grass
The heart becomes full and yearning.[66]

66. See Rabbi Naḥman of Bratslav, *Likkutei Maharan, Tinyana* 11 and 63. Naomi Shemer's song continues with a third verse yearning for the Land of Israel.

Conclusion

As a youngster, I loved listening to my father's stories. Some I've repeated over and over. To this day, I tell them as if I've just heard them for the first time. My favorite I call *Gib Mir a Nahgel,* Yiddish for "Give Me a Nail."

It's the story of a poor man who came from Europe to America. In time, he married, had a family, became wealthy and well-known. As he stood under the *ḥuppa,* the wedding canopy of his youngest daughter, he began to call out, "*Gib mir a nahgel!*" His guests thought he had gone crazy and tried to calm him. Still, he called out, "*Gib mir a nahgel, gib mir a nahgel!*" Finally, he explained.

Life, he said, is like a wheel, a *galgal haḥozer,* a wheel that forever turns. Sometimes you're up, sometimes you're down. When I came from Europe, I was at rock bottom. But now, as I marry off my youngest child, I am at the top of the world. As much as I'm enjoying the moment, I recognize the inevitability that the wheel will not remain at the top – it will one day descend. So I call out, "*Gib mir a nahgel,*" and let me take it and drive it into the wheel, so that it never moves – so that it remains at its greatest height.

The story speaks to our definition of spirituality, consciousness of the moment and God's role in that moment. This definition, however, does not mean that we do not recognize that nothing lasts forever. Moreover, it doesn't mean that when I'm in the moment, I'm not cognizant of the multiplicity of elements that together make up the experience at hand. Consciousness of moment always has context. Whatever we experience in life, it most often is a rainbow of many colors, meshing, weaving, interconnecting – making up the whole. The nail is engulfed by the wheel.

Yehuda Amichai, the great Israeli poet, captures this life reality:

> A man doesn't have time in his life to have time for everything.
> He doesn't have seasons enough to have a season for every purpose.
> Ecclesiastes was wrong about that.
> A man needs to love and hate at the same moment,
> To laugh and cry with the same eyes.
> With the same hands to throw stones
> And gather them in,
> To make love in war and war in love,
> And to hate and forgive, and remember and forget,
> To arrange and confuse, to eat and digest,
> What history takes years and years to do.
> A man doesn't have time.
> As he loses he seeks,
> As he finds he forgets,
> As he forgets he loves,
> And as he loves he begins to forget.[1]

Jewish law marks this phenomenon when it asks that at the height of joy, a wedding, we break a glass, remembering the shattered Temples and shattered human temples that need fixing. And at the moment of deepest grief, after one has lost a close relative, in agony, in pain, in anguish, we rend our garment, declaring, *Barukh Dayan HaEmet* – "Blessed is the True Judge" – God Himself.

This has been the main theme that I have tried to share in this work. At its core, *tefilla* is not intended to be an experience of separateness,

1. Yehuda Amichai, "A Man in His Life," in Amichai, *The Selected Poetry of Yehuda Amichai*, ed. and trans. Chana Bloch and Stephen Mitchell (New York: Harper & Row, 1986), pp. 158–159.

or apartness. Rather, it is an experience of unity, of blending together different component parts. Its goal is not to disintegrate, but to integrate.

Over the years, all kinds of synagogue communities have evolved. There are "prayer communities," where people gather to pray. There are "learning communities," where people gather to learn. There are "Israel communities" or "social justice communities," where people gather to advocate for Israel and for the world. It is critical, however, to develop "holistic communities," whole communities that bring together *all* of these elements.

This is optimal *tefilla*. It is feeling the presence of God by balancing personal responsibility with reliance upon Him. It is braiding time, venue, and text, for individual and communal prayer. It is the bond between halakhic intent and its spiritual counterparts at home and in the synagogue.

Tefilla is a song, a melody, a word, a sound, silence, murmuring – all coming together. It is a smile, a tear, a hope, a sigh; standing, rising, lifting hands; swaying, dancing, sitting, falling – all coming together. It is a conversation, talking, listening, serious, light, laughing, imploring, demanding, evaluating, and improving – all coming together.

It is reaching inward to stir our soul, outward to embrace our fellow human being, and upward to encounter God. Here, holistic prayer enters a new realm.

Normatively, the holistic concept is a this-worldly idea, synthesizing heart, soul, mind, and body with community, the environment, and the cosmos. In prayer, however, a holistic approach has central aspects of being "other-worldly," as it includes God Himself. As we wear *tefillin*, so does God. As we wrap ourselves in a prayer shawl, so does God. As we pray, so does God.[2] Holistic prayer is the experience not only of the whole but also of the Holy, of the Holy of Holies, of God Himself. It is reaching for God even as He reaches for us. Reaching, reaching, but never quite touching. And in that space between the ultimate Unity above, and the unity we seek below, is the unity of *tefilla* – optimal *tefilla*, spiritual *tefilla*, *tefilla* that is holistic – whole, holy. Holistic prayer.

2. See Berakhot 6a, Rosh HaShana 17b, and Midrash Tehillim 76:3.

May the *tefilla* of Rabbi Judah HaLevi – of God and the human being searching for each other – be forever ingrained in our hearts.

דָּרַשְׁתִּי קִרְבָתְךָ
בְּכָל לִבִּי קְרָאתִיךָ
וּבְצֵאתִי לִקְרָאתְךָ
לִקְרָאתִי מְצָאתִיךָ

I have sought Your nearness,
With all my heart have I called You,
And going out to meet You
I found You coming toward me.[3]

3. Heinrich Brody, ed., *Selected Poems of Yehuda HaLevi*, trans. Nina Salaman (Philadelphia: Jewish Publication Society, 1924), pp. 134–135. Rabbi Heschel quotes the poem in English in *God in Search of Man*, pp. 136–137

Role Models & Acknowledgments

While the study and analysis of *tefilla* have importance, there is a level of learning from others that goes beyond the written word. From my earliest years, I have been blessed to know individuals who have served as models of *tefilla*. They planted within me seeds that, over time, helped shape my own theology of prayer.

The most important of these individuals is my father, Rabbi Dr. Moshe Weiss. My earliest memories of *tefilla* are standing at his side as a five-year old, singing with my brother Mordechai in Abba's children's choir on Rosh HaShana and Yom Kippur. I can still see my father giving us signals indicating when we should repeat a word, hum, sing a particular tune to *vene'emar*, and even sing solo. His *nusaḥ* (the traditional singsong of the verbiage), the ins and outs of the *tefilla*, will forever remain with me. What one learns at an early age remains forever; it is long-term memory that never goes away.

Even more important are the memories of simply looking at my father, a young man then, much younger than I am now, and yet, even as a child, I could discern his depth of feeling as he sang, implored, and led the service.

A few years ago, Abba turned ninety; a young ninety. All my siblings, all his children gathered in Jerusalem for the Shabbat of his birthday. Around the table we sang the *zemirot* (songs) of our youth, some known only to our family. Abba spoke of his life experiences. As usual, not even once did he say a bad word about anyone, even of those with whom he had had disagreement. This is Abba's greatest *midda* (trait). His *tefilla*, ה' שְׂפָתַי תִּפְתָּח – "My Lord, open my lips," is not only to know what to say, but what not to say. This, too, is holistic *tefilla*.

And then there is Imma, who died much too young, almost thirty years ago. My memory of her *tefilla* was sitting with Abba, an *Ivris Ḥayya* (the book used then to learn the Hebrew language) open, reviewing the meaning of the prayers. I can still see her on the other side of the *meḥitza* (partition) as she quietly prayed. She taught me the beauty of a soft word, the enduring quality of an act of kindness, the power of unconditional love. Imma died on Yom Kippur as the sun was setting. When she was found in her room (she was too weak to go to synagogue), her *maḥzor* (Rosh HaShana and Yom Kippur prayer book) was open to the confessional *Al Ḥeit* prayer. That was Imma.

My father-in-law, Zalman Aryeh Hilsenrad, of blessed memory, was a deeply devout Jew. He named his first book, a compilation of articles he wrote for *The Jewish Press*, *My Soul Thirsts*. Years later, he penned a second volume. He called it *My Soul Thirsts... Still*. I will forever remember the way he prayed: his demeanor, his slow and meticulous enunciation of every word, his humble posture as he stood before God.

And Reb Zalman's wife, my mother-in-law, Ida, of blessed memory, prayed in her own way. As I mention in the book, for years she dedicated herself to facilitating a charity founded by her husband – a program wherein hundreds of Americans sent weekly checks to needy families in Israel.

In the various schools I attended as a youngster, I was also taken by different religious personalities. One stands out. As a fifth-grader in Yeshiva Torah Vodaath, I was mesmerized by an older man named Rabbi Chaim Gelb. I can still remember Reb Chaim calling out, "Amen!" Sometimes he'd give me a candy and ask me to recite a blessing so that he could mightily respond, "Amen!" Even then, as a young boy, I sensed his great belief. When the principal of the yeshiva gave Reb Chaim a reproachful glance for answering too loud, Reb Chaim would sometimes break down in tears. He always carried a *tzedaka* (charity) box, urging everyone to throw in a penny to be distributed to the poor.

In rabbinical school, my greatest religious influence was Rabbi Ahron Soloveichik, about whom I write in this work. And in recent years,

I have been deeply impacted by Rabbi Yehuda Amital, about whom I also write. Both men have now left this world, but to me, they will always be *morai verabbotai* – in *tefilla* and all of life

Also in rabbinical school was Rabbi Dovid Lifschutz. He took special interest in his students. A saintly-looking man, he wore a frock coat and a triangular rabbinic hat. He spoke a soft, biblical Hebrew, which added to his righteous, biblical look. And when he prayed, the heavens no doubt opened. Who can forget Reb Dovid on Simḥat Torah (the celebration of ending and beginning the Torah), holding the Torah lovingly as he led his students in the song *VeTaher Libeinu* (Purify Our Hearts). Over and over he'd sing these words, louder and louder, with more and more fervor, his face glowing in religious rapture.

As this work shows, the thoughts of Rabbi Joseph B. Soloveitchik have deeply impacted me. Over the course of my earlier rabbinate, I often met with him to discuss various religious matters. It was Rabbi Soloveitchik who gave verbal consent for the *meḥitza* in our synagogue, which bisects the sanctuary, allowing women to see and hear on the same level as men. And it was Rabbi Soloveitchik to whom I brought Avital Sharansky to hear his insights as she fought for the release of her husband, Natan, from Soviet prison. Finally, for this work, Rabbi Soloveitchik's creative, ingenious thinking on Torah, and how Torah applies to the human condition, has profoundly influenced my life in general and my understanding of *tefilla* in particular.

There are others who have been spiritual role models. Among them are rabbis who have become my mentor-friends much in the spirit of "make yourself a rabbi and acquire a friend." Rabbi Shlomo Riskin has always been that model. Brilliant, bold, dynamic, he is the rabbi's rabbi.

Rabbi Saul (Shalom) Berman has been a cherished teacher and friend. It is with Shalom that I had countless discussions in my years at Stern, and then at Yeshivat Chovevei Torah. So much of my thinking on spirituality has been shaped by him. I am forever grateful to Rabbi Berman for his teaching and friendship.

Rabbi Irving (Yitz) and Blu Greenberg have become dear friends. They are paragons of religious commitment and spiritual striving.

I am blessed with the friendship of Rabbi Marc Angel, a courageous voice in the Modern and Open Orthodox community.

Rabbi Shlomo Carlebach's music, not only his songs but his voice and teachings, have given me some of my deepest religious moments. I feel blessed to have known him – really known him – and learned from him. His melodies offer some of the most profound interpretations of the prayer service.

Stewart Harris, my soul brother, is a man of extraordinary integrity and brilliant common sense. He displays the highest level of spirituality by the way he lives and interacts with people. Stewart is the epitome of *va'ani tefilla* – "and I am my prayer" (Ps. 109:4). Everything he does *is tefilla*. Stewart *is* holistic prayer.

To all these paragons of *tefilla* and many more, I am deeply indebted. If anyone has been moved by parts of this work, it is the words and spirit of these role models, teachers, and inspirations who deserve the credit.

Writing a book – especially a book of this nature – is a loving but complex task. In my case, it required the assistance of many people whom I've met through the institutions I've been blessed to be deeply involved with.

I have been blessed with the most exceptional and loving synagogue-family, the Hebrew Institute of Riverdale (HIR), affectionately known as "the Bayit." My experiences there have framed this book. As one of its spiritual leaders, I have encountered many individuals whose *tefilla* inspired me. Hillel Jaffe, our *gabbai*, has organized our services with dignity and religious meaning. Bernie Horowitz has been my teacher of constancy. Day in and day out, Bernie has been at services, reading the Torah as I believe no one in the world can. Rabbi Murray Schaum is one of the most spiritual congregants I've ever encountered. I have always looked to him as a paragon of genuine spirituality.

Bernard Glickman, who died too young, was a dear, dear, friend. We traveled the world together speaking out for *Am Yisrael*. Toward the end of his life, we sat near each other in prayer. Bernie was a *tzur Yisrael* – a rock of Israel. But Bernie was also a *tzayyar Yisrael* – an artist of Israel, whose soul reached for God in *tefilla*... in life.

Dr. Elli Kranzler is the rebbe of rebbes of spiritual *tefilla*. Elli's consent to become our *sheli'aḥ tzibbur* has changed my life, and, I believe, is the single most important happening that altered the future of our Bayit, forever setting it on a spiritual path. Elli is not only blessed with the voice of an angel, he is not only knowledgeable in Jewish and general music and song, but he is a grounded student of spirituality. He is the quintessential living image of Jacob's dream of a ladder reaching heavenward but anchored on earth, with angels descending and ascending. That's Elli. He's in another world while in this world; the world of reality and yet the world of angels. I am thankful to Elli for our *ḥavruta* learning of the *Sefat Emet* on Friday mornings, for sitting near me as we pray, and for his guidance and friendship.

Many of my associates in the rabbinate and interns at the Bayit profoundly influenced my spiritual life and have gone on to serve their own communities. Among them are Rabbi Ronald Schwartzberg, Rabbi Louis Sherby, Rabbi Binyamin Hecht, Rabbi Chaim Marder, Rabbi Yosef Kanefsky, Rabbi Barry Gelman, Rabbi Aaron Frank, Rabbi Shmuel Herzfeld, Rabbi Adam Starr, Rabbi Etan Mintz, Rabbi Yisrael Hollender, and Rabbi Uri Topolosky, who served as rabbis at the HIR. Among the interns are Rabbi Michael Eisenberg, Rabbi Yamin Levy, Rabbi Ian Pear, Rabbi Yehuda Sarna, Rabbi Yair Silverman, Rabbi Dovid Kalb, and Rabbi Jeff Fox.

Our associate rabbi, Rabbi Ari Hart, is a paragon of social justice and leader extraordinaire.

No words can properly describe my deep respect and love for Rabbi Steven Exler, who now serves as rabbi of the Bayit. He is perhaps the most remarkable young rabbi I've ever met. On many occasions, I leaned on Rav Steven to glean from his insights relative to this study.

The Bayit has also been blessed with women who have served as spiritual leaders. Among them are Sharona Margolin Halickman, Karen Miller, and Stacey Goldman.

Rabba Sara Hurwitz has now assumed a role as a full member of our clergy. Caring, committed, courageous, Sara has powerfully influenced communities around the world as a spiritual leader extraordinaire. For me, Sara is a heroic figure to whom our community owes endless gratitude.

The Bayit is blessed with the most exceptional lay leadership, to whom I am forever indebted: David Mann, Stanley Langer, Hillel Jaffe, Bernie Horowitz, David Eiseman, Howard Jonas, Steven Pretsfelder, Lewis Bernstein, Ari Hait, Dan Perla, David Schwartz, Ronnie Becher, Dr. Jeffrey Gurock, and David Braunstein.

I am indebted as well to all my students at Yeshivat Chovevei Torah (YCT), its administration, staff, and faculty, led by its unparalleled, brilliant rosh yeshiva, Rabbi Dov Linzer, who has developed a rabbinical school that is graduating some of the most important spiritual leaders in America today.

No words can sufficiently thank the founding chairman of YCT, one of the greatest souls of our time, Howard Jonas, who brought the school from dream into reality. Many thanks as well to its present chairman and brilliant leader, Steven Lieberman.

I am also grateful to the faculty, administration, and, of course, the students of Yeshivat Maharat. Some of my most inspiring moments in recent years have come from teaching these outstanding women. Many thanks to its leaders, to its dean, Rabba Sara Hurwitz, and its rosh yeshiva, Rabbi Jeff Fox.

In the preparation of this work, I'm grateful to Rafi Farber for transcribing my classes from the original tapes. I am also grateful to Rabbi Zev Farber for reviewing the first section of this book in its earlier stage. His insights and suggestions were invaluable. Thanks to Rabbi Jeffrey Saks for reading an earlier version of this manuscript and offering suggestions. Thanks as well to many individuals who commented on different parts of this manuscript. They include Rabbi Nati Helfgot, Rabbi Dov Linzer, and Dr. Daniel Matt.

Special thanks to Rabbi Aaron Frank, cherished colleague and friend, for always being there to lovingly offer his insights and critique of parts of this manuscript.

And to my son, Rabbi Dr. Dov Weiss. At different intervals I've shared different parts of this work with him. Dov's genius in analyzing text, his creativity and integrity of thought, and his loving patience were invaluable.

And many, many thanks to Shuli Boxer Rieser, my executive assistant. I do not type. Shuli painstakingly took my dictations, worked on the footnotes, remained patient as I reviewed and rewrote the manuscript countless times, and offered invaluable insights and suggestions as we made our way through this text.

The CEO of Maggid Books, Matthew Miller, an extraordinarily successful publisher, has in recent years redirected his attention to producing works of Jewish learning. Through his publishing, he has single-handedly touched the lives of hundreds of thousands. Our community owes him a tremendous debt of gratitude. I, too, am forever grateful to him. Thanks also to Matthew's wonderful staff: Rachel Meghnagi and Gila Fine; Sara Sherbill, who expertly edited a first-round transcript of this work, helping turn what was an academic thesis into a book; and those from Maggid Books who did the editing and formatting of the book: Reuben Meghnagi, Aharon Admanit, Sara Daniel, Shoshana Rotem, Judy Lee, Renee Schwartz, and Tomi Mager. I am also grateful to David Sclar for preparing the list of traditional authorities and the bibliography.

My siblings – Tova Reich, master writer and one of the great influences in my life; Rabbi Mordechai Weiss, Jewish educator par excellence; Suri Tov, my rebbe in spiritual striving; and Rabbi Dr. David Weiss, acclaimed author and expert teacher of communal and business leadership – have remained my deepest friends. We have taken different paths in life, but our respect and love for each other is deep. My sense is that the model of family I write about in this work was inspired by my relationship with my siblings. It's based on the principle that love for family transcends differences – it is a love that is unconditional and limitless.

Every day, I am thankful to my parents, Miriam Weiss, of blessed memory, whose gentility and sensitivity I still feel to this day; and, *yibbadel leḥayyim,* Rabbi Moshe Weiss, a *talmid ḥakham* par excellence, who has taught me to stand up for what I believe is right, no matter the consequences.

Aḥaron aḥaron ḥaviv – my inner family. Our daughter Dena and her husband, Dr. Mark Levie – models of pure *ḥesed* – and their children, Ariella, Shira, Talia, and Yair; and our daughter Elana and her husband, Michael Fischberger – models of *menschlichkeit* – and their children, Gilad, Eitan, Rami, Ayelet, Noam, Gavriel, Amiḥai, Avigayil, and Itamar, have brought me so much joy. And of course, our son Dov. I was recently asked whom I consider my rebbe. My answer is Dov. Dov has finished his doctorate in religion at the University of Chicago Divinity School and is an assistant professor of religion at the University of Illinois and a Stroock fellow at Harvard's Center for Jewish Studies.

Ultimately, it is my children who are my teachers and inspirations.

This book is dedicated to my beloved wife, Toby. For more than forty-five years she has been my best friend, my confidante whose love for me has been unconditional. I have often taken positions that have provoked great criticism. Through it all Toby has remained loyal, a great listener and loving critic. Her kindness and gentility are what *tefilla* is all about. For this and more, I am forever grateful.

Judaic Sources[1]

Abarbanel, Isaac (Spain and Italy, 1437–1508). Statesman, philosopher, and Bible commentator.

Amital, Yehuda (1924–2010). Leader of religious Zionism, founder of Yeshivat Har Etzion, and representative of Hesder yeshivot.

Arukh HaShulḥan. Halakhic code by Rabbi Jehiel Michel Epstein (Belarus, 1829–1908).

Beit Yosef. Commentary on *Arba'a Turim* by Rabbi Joseph Karo.

Book of Kuzari. Philosophical work by Rabbi Judah HaLevi (Spain, 1080–1145).

Cordovero, Moses (*Eretz Yisrael*, 1522–1570). A central figure in the development of Kabbala in Safed; brother-in-law of Solomon Alkabetz, who authored the Shabbat hymn *Lekha Dodi*.

Ḥayyei Adam. Work of Jewish law on the *Oraḥ Ḥayyim* section of *Shulḥan Arukh* by Rabbi Abraham Danzig (Poland, 1748–1820).

Ḥiddushei Rabbeinu Ḥayyim HaLevi. Commentary on Maimonides' *Mishneh Torah* by Rabbi Ḥayyim HaLevi Soloveichik (Lithuania, 1853–1918), grandfather of rabbis Joseph B. Soloveitchik and Ahron Soloveichik.

Hirsch, Samson Raphael (Germany, 1808–1888). Philosopher, Bible

1. Many thanks to David Sclar for preparing this section and the bibliography that follows.

commentator, and intellectual founder of contemporary Orthodox Judaism.

Karo, Joseph (Spain and *Eretz Yisrael,* 1488–1575). See *Beit Yosef, Kesef Mishneh,* and *Shulḥan Arukh.*

Keli Yakar. Commentary on the Pentateuch by Rabbi Ephraim of Luntschitz (Poland, 1550–1619).

Kesef Mishneh. Commentary on *Mishneh Torah* by Rabbi Joseph Karo.

Kook, Abraham Isaac HaKohen (1865–1935). Renowned Torah scholar and kabbalist, the first Ashkenazic chief rabbi of modern-day *Eretz Yisrael,* and one of the most important thinkers in religious Zionism.

Likkutei Maharan. Collected teachings of hasidic master Rabbi Naḥman of Bratslav (Ukraine, 1772–1810).

Magen Avraham. Commentary on *Shulḥan Arukh* by Rabbi Abraham Gombiner (Poland, 1636–1683).

Maḥzor Vitry. Halakhic/liturgical work by Rabbi Simḥa ben Samuel of Vitry (France, 11th cent.).

Maimonides. Rabbi Moses ben Maimon (Rambam) (Egypt, 1135–1204). Philosopher, talmudist, and physician; author of *Mishneh Torah, Peirush HaMishnayot, Sefer HaMitzvot* (Book of Commandments), and *Moreh Nevukhim* (Guide for the Perplexed).

Malbim. Rabbi Meir Leibush ben Jehiel Michel Weiser (Ukraine, 1809–1879). Author of a novel commentary on the Bible.

Mekhilta. Midrash halakha on the book of Exodus.

Menorat HaMa'or. Ethical work by Rabbi Isaac Aboab (Spain, 14th cent.).

Meshekh Ḥokhma. Commentary on the Torah by Rabbi Meir Simḥa HaKohen of Dvinsk (Latvia, 1843–1926).

Midrash Rabba. Refers to parts of or to the collective whole of aggadic midrashim on books of the Bible.

Midrash Tanḥuma. The name given to three collections of aggadic midrashim on the Pentateuch.

Mishna Avot (or *Pirkei Avot*). Compilation of ethical teachings and maxims of rabbis from the mishnaic period.

Mishna Berura. Commentary on *Shulḥan Arukh* by Rabbi Israel Meir HaKohen (Lithuania, 1838–1933), also known as the Ḥafetz Ḥayyim.

Mishneh Torah (or *Yad HaḤazaka* and Maimonides' *Code*). Halakhic code compiled by Maimonides.

Nahmanides. Rabbi Moses ben Naḥman (Ramban) (Spain, 1194–1270). Philosopher and talmudist, author of numerous halakhic and talmudic works and of a commentary on the Pentateuch.

Netziv. Naphtali Tzvi Yehuda Berlin (Russia/Poland, 1816–1893). Dean of Volozhin Yeshiva and author of several works, including a commentary on the Torah called *Ha'amek Davar*.

Onkelos. A prominent Roman convert to Judaism, to whom tradition ascribes authorship of the famous Aramaic translation/exposition of the Torah, *Targum Onkelos*.

Obadiah of Bertinoro (Italy, 1465–1515). Scholar and spiritual leader best known for his commentary on the Mishna.

Pirkei DeRebbi Eliezer. An aggadic-midrashic work on Genesis and parts of Exodus and Numbers, ascribed to Rabbi Eliezer ben Hyrcanus (80–118 CE).

Ra'avad. Rabbi Abraham ben David (Provence, c. 1125–1198). Author of commentaries on the Talmud, *Sefer Halakhot* of Rabbi Isaac Alfasi, and Maimonides' *Mishneh Torah*.

Rabbeinu Yona. Rabbi Jonah ben Abraham Gerondi (Spain, 1200–1263). Talmudist, author, and moralist; wrote commentary on Rabbi Isaac Alfasi's glosses on Berakhot.

Radbaz. Rabbi David ben Solomon Ibn Abi Zimra (Egypt, 1479–1530). Author of responsa.

Ralbag. Rabbi Levi ben Gerson (Gersonides) (France, 1288–1344). Philosopher, talmudist, and astronomer.

Rambam. See Maimonides.

Ramban. See Nahmanides.

Rashi. Rabbi Solomon ben Isaac (France, 1040–1105). Foremost commentator on the Bible and Talmud.

Rema. Rabbi Moses Isserles (Poland, 1525–1572). Author of *Mappa*, glosses on *Shulḥan Arukh* reflecting Ashkenazic practice.

Rivash. Rabbi Isaac ben Sheshet Perfet (North Africa, 1326–1408). Author of responsa.

Sa'adia Gaon (Egypt, born 880). Philosopher, talmudist, grammarian, and author of a liturgical handbook.

Sefat Emet. Homilies on the Torah by Yehuda Aryeh Leib Alter (Poland, 1847–1905), rebbe of the Gerrer Hasidim.

Sefer Abudarham. Halakhic commentary on prayer by Rabbi David ben Joseph Abudarham (Spain, 14th cent.).

Sefer HaḤinukh. Exposition of the 613 commandments attributed by some to Rabbi Aaron HaLevi of Barcelona (Spain, 14th cent.).

Sefer HaIkkarim. Religio-philosophical work by Rabbi Joseph Albo (Spain, 1380–1444).

Sefer Ḥaredim. Ethical work by the Safed kabbalist Elazar ben Moshe Azikri (*Eretz Yisrael*, 1533–1600), author of the hymn *Yedid Nefesh*.

Seforno, Obadiah ben Jacob (Italy, c. 1475–1550). Bible commentator, philosopher, and physician.

Sha'arei Teshuva. Anthology of responsa from the Geonic period (Babylonia, 8th-10th cent.).

Shelah (acronym for *Shenei Luḥot HaBrit*). Compilation of rituals, ethics, and mysticism by Rabbi Isaiah Horowitz (Prague, 1565–1630).

Shem Tov Ibn Falaquera (Spain, 1225–c. 1290). Philosopher, poet, and commentator on Maimonides' *Moreh Nevukhim*.

Shulḥan Arukh. Preeminent code of Jewish law, written by Rabbi Joseph Karo; printed with the Rema's glosses reflecting customs of Ashkenazic Jewry. It is divided into four parts, following the outline of the *Arba'a Turim*: *Oraḥ Ḥayyim* – daily prayers, Sabbaths and festivals; *Yoreh De'ah* – dietary laws and other religious observances; *Even HaEzer* – family law and matters of personal status; *Ḥoshen Mishpat* – civil law.

Sifrei. Classical exegesis on books of Numbers and Deuteronomy.

Soloveichik, Ahron (1917–2001). Renowned scholar of Talmud and halakha; younger brother of Rabbi Joseph Ber Soloveitchik.

Soloveitchik, Joseph Ber (1903–1993). Talmudist, halakhist, philosopher, and seminal figure in Modern Orthodox Judaism.

Tanya. Hasidic masterpiece by Rabbi Shneur Zalman of Liadi (Russia, 18th cent.), founder of Chabad Hasidism.

Tiferet Yisrael. Commentary on the Mishna by Rabbi Israel Lipschitz (Poland, 1782–1860).

Toledot Yaakov Yosef. The first book of hasidic literature ever printed (Koretz, 1780), written by Rabbi Jacob Joseph ben Tzvi HaKohen Katz of Polonnoye (Poland, 1710–1784), a disciple of Rabbi Israel Baal Shem Tov.

Tosafot (literally "Additions"). Comments on the Talmud by students of Rashi and members of French and German yeshivas (12th–14th cent.).

Bibliography

Aaron, David. *Seeing God*. New York: Tarcher/Putnam, 2001.

Abudarham, David. *Sefer Abudarham HaShalem*. Jerusalem: Usha, 5723 (1963).

Albo, Joseph. *Sefer HaIkkarim: Book of Principles*. Edited and translated by Isaac Husik. Philadelphia: Jewish Publication Society, 1946.

Amichai, Yehuda. "A Man in His Life." In *The Selected Poetry of Yehuda Amichai*, edited and translated by Chana Bloch and Stephen Mitchell. New York: Harper & Row, 1986.

Amital, Yehuda. *HaMa'alot MiMa'amakim*. Jerusalem: Agudat Yeshivat Har Etzion, 5734 (1974).

———. *Jewish Values in a Changing World*. Alon Shevut, Israel: Yeshivat Har Etzion; New Jersey: KTAV Publishing House, 2005.

———. *VeHaAretz Natan LiVnei Adam*. Alon Shevut, Israel: Mikhlelet Ya'akov Hertzog LeYad Yeshivat Har Etzion, 5765 (2005).

Auerbach, David. *Sefer Halikhot Beita: Otzar Dinim Uminhagim al Mitzvot HaIsha BeYisrael*. Jerusalem: Mekhon Sha'arei Ziv, 5743 (1983).

The Babylonian Talmud. Translated by Maurice Simon, edited by I. Epstein. 30 vols. New York: Traditional Press, 1979-1983.

Berkovits, Eliezer. *God, Man and History*. Edited by David Hazony. Jerusalem: Shalem Press, 2004.

———. *Studies in Torah Judaism – Prayer*. New York: Yeshiva University Press, KTAV Publishing House, 1969.

Berman, Saul. "Overview," *The Rabbinical Council of America Edition of the ArtScroll Siddur*. Brooklyn, NY: Mesorah Publications, 1990.

———. "Even a New Siddur Can't Close 'God Gap,'" *The Jewish Daily Forward*, August 28, 2009. Accessed April 30, 2012. http://forward.com/articles/112469/even-a-new-siddur-can-t-close-god-gap/.

Besdin, Abraham R. *Reflections of the Rav*. Jerusalem: World Zionist Organization, 1979.

Bialik, Ḥayyim Naḥman. "*Gillui VeKhissui BaLashon*." In *Kol Kitvei H. N. Bialik*. Tel Aviv: Dvir, 5798 (1938).

———. *Masekhet Gillui VeKhissui BaLashon*. Commentary by Eli Alon and Yariv Ben-Aharon. Oranim, Israel: HaMidrasha, 1997.

———. "*Shabbat HaMalka*." In *Kol Kitvei H.N. Bialik*. Tel Aviv: Dvir, 5798 (1938).

Blech, Benjamin. "Judaism and Gerontology." *Tradition* 16, no. 4 (summer 1977), pp. 62–78.

Brody, Heinrich, ed. *Selected Poems of Yehuda HaLevi*. Translated by Nina Salaman. Philadelphia: Jewish Publication Society, 1924.

Buber, Martin. *Hasidism and Modern Man*. New York: Horizon Press, 1958.

———. *I and Thou*. Translated by Walter Kaufmann. Touchstone, 1971.

Cassuto, Umberto. A *Commentary on the Book of Exodus*. Translated by Israel Abrahams. Jerusalem: Magnes Press, Hebrew University, 1967.

Cordovero, Moses. *Or Ne'erav*. Edited by Yehuda Z. Brandwein. Jerusalem: Yeshivat Qol Yehudah, 1965.

Dessler, E. E. *Mikhtav MeEliyahu*. 5 vols. Jerusalem: Yotzei LaOr al Yedei Ḥever Talmidav, 5723–5757 (1963–1997).

Drazin, Israel, and Stanley Wagner. *Onkelos on the Torah: Understanding the Bible Text – Genesis*. New York: Gefen Publishing House, 2006.

Epstein, Kalonymus Kalman HaLevi. *Sefer Ma'or VaShamesh*. 3 vols. Jerusalem: Even Yisrael, 5748 (1988).

Fishbane, Michael. *Sacred Attunement: A Jewish Theology*. Chicago: University of Chicago Press, 2008.

Frankl, Viktor E. *Man's Search for Meaning*. New York: Pocket Books, 1963.

Fromm, Erich. *The Art of Loving*. London: Harper &Row, 1956.

Goldberg, Hillel. *The Fire Within: The Living Heritage of the Musar Movement*. New York: Mesorah Publications, 1987.

Green, Arthur. *The Language of Truth: The Torah Commentary of the Sefat Emet*. Philadelphia: Jewish Publication Society, 1998.

Greenberg, Irving. *The Jewish Way*. New York: Summit Books, 1988.

HaKohen, Meir Simḥa. *Meshekh Ḥokhma*. Jerusalem, 5751 (1991).

HaLevi, Judah. *Book of Kuzari*. Translated by Hartwig Hirschfeld. New York: Pardes Publishing House, Inc., 1946.

Hammerschlag, Carl A. *The Dancing Healers: A Doctor's Journey of Healing with Native Americans*. San Francisco: Harper & Row, 1988.

Heinemann, Joseph. *HaTefilla BiTekufat HaTanna'im VeHaAmora'im*. Jerusalem: Hebrew University, 1964.

———. *Prayer in the Talmud: Forms and Patterns*. Translated by Richard S. Sarason. Berlin: De Gruyter Press, 1977.

Heschel, Abraham Joshua. *God in Search of Man*. New York: Farrar, Straus and Giroux, 1955.

———. *Man Is Not Alone*. New York: Farrar, Straus and Giroux, 1951.

———. *Man's Quest for God*. New York: Scribner, 1954.

———. *The Sabbath*. New York: Farrar, Straus and Giroux, 1991.

Higger, Michael. *Pirkei Rebbi Eliezer*. New York: Horev, 5704–5708 (1944–1948).

Hirsch, Samson Raphael. *Horeb*. New York: Soncino Press, 1962.

———. *The Psalms*. New York: Feldheim Publishers, 1966.

Horovitz, Saul. *The Microcosm of Joseph Ibn Ṣaddiq*. Cranbury, NJ: Associated University Presses, 2003.

Horowitz, Isaiah. *Likkutei Shelah: BeInyenei Emuna VeDa'at, Torah uMitzvot, Middot VeHanhagot*. Jerusalem: M. Yeshurun, 2003.

Husik, Isaac. *Medieval Jewish Philosophy*. Philadelphia: Jewish Publication Society, 1958.

Jacobson, B. S. *Meditations on the Siddur*. Tel Aviv: Sinai, 1966.

The Jewish Bible: Tanakh: The Holy Scriptures – The New JPS Translation According to the Traditional Hebrew Text: Torah, Nevi'im, Kethuvim. Edited by Adele Berlin and Mark Zvi Brettler. Philadelphia: Jewish Publication Society, 1985.

Jospe, Raphael. *Torah and Sophia: The Life and Thought of Shem Tov Ibn Falaquera*. Cincinnati: Hebrew Union College Press, 1988.

Kant, Immanuel. *Religion Within the Limits of Reason Alone*. Translated with an introduction and notes by Theodore M. Greene and Hoyt H. Hudson. New York: Harper Torchbook, 1960.

Klein, Menashe. *Mishneh Halakhot*. New York, 1998.

Kook, Abraham Isaac HaKohen. *Arfellei Tohar*. Jerusalem: HaMakhon al Shem HaR. Tz. Y. H. Kook, 5743 (1983).

———. *Iggrot HaRe'iya*. 3 vols. Jerusalem: Mossad Harav Kook, 5722–5725 (1961–1965).

———. *The Lights of Penitence, the Moral Principles, Lights of Holiness, Essays, Letters, and Poems (Classics of Western Spirituality)*. Translated by Ben Zion Bokser. New York: Paulist Press, 1978.

———. *Orot HaTeshuva*. Jerusalem: Yeshivat Or Etzion, 1992.

———. *Seder Tefilla im Peirush Olat Re'iya*. Jerusalem: Aguda LeHotza'at Sifrei HaRe'iya Kook, 5699 (1939).

Lamm, Norman. *Faith and Doubt: Studies in Traditional Jewish Thought*. New York: KTAV Publishing House, 1986.

———. *The Religious Thought of Hasidism: Text and Commentary*. Hoboken, NJ: Yeshiva University Press, 1999.

———. *The Royal Reach: Discourses on the Jewish Tradition and the World Today*. New York: Feldheim Publishers, 1970.

Leibowitz, Nehama. *New Studies in Bereshit (Genesis). Translated by Aryeh Newman*. Jerusalem: Ḥemed Press, 1995.

———. *New Studies in Shemot (Exodus)*. Translated by *Aryeh Newman*. 2 vols. Jerusalem: World Zionist Organization, 1993.

Leibowitz, Yeshayahu. *Judaism, Human Values and the Jewish State*. Edited by Eliezer Goldmann. Cambridge: Harvard University Press, 1992.

Lichtenstein, Aharon. "Imperatives and Advantages of Communal Prayer Studied in Depth," *Hamevaser* 6, no. 5 (28 Adar 5728/March 28, 1968), p. 5.

Luban, Marvin. *The Kaddish: Man's Reply to the Problem of Evil*. New York: Yeshiva University Press, 1969.

Lustiger, Arnold, and Michael Taubes, eds. *Yom Kippur Maḥzor with Commentary Adapted from the Teachings of Rabbi Joseph B. Soloveitchik*. New York: K'hal Publishing, 2006.

Maḥzor Vitry. Edited by S. Hurwitz. Berlin, 1896-1897.

Maimonides. *Mishneh Torah*. Edited according to the Bodleian (Oxford) Codex with introduction, biblical and talmudic references, notes, and English translation by Moses Hyamson. 2 vols. New York: Feldheim Publishers, 1981.

Matt, Daniel C. *The Essential Kabbalah: The Heart of Jewish Mysticism*. New York: HarperCollins, 1995.

Mekhilta de-Rabbi Shimon bar Yoḥai. Translated with a critical introduction and annotation by W. David Nelson. Philadelphia: Jewish Publication Society, 2006.

Midrash Rabbah. Translated and edited by Rabbi Dr. H. Freedman and Maurice Simon. 10 vols. London: Soncino Press, 1939.

Nahmanides. *Commentary on the Torah – Exodus*. Translated and annotated by Charles B. Chavel. New York: Shilo Publishing House, 1973.

Peli, Pinchas H. *On Repentance: The Thought and Oral Discourses of Rabbi Joseph Dov Soloveitchik*. New York: Rowman and Littlefield, 1984.

Pentateuch with Targum Onkelos, Haphtaroth and Rashi's Commentary. Translated by M. Rosenbaum and A. M. Silbermann. New York: Hebrew Publishing Company, 1934.

Powell, John. *The Secret of Staying in Love*. Texas: RCL, 1974.

Riskin, Shlomo. "Structure and Spontaneity in Prayer." *Judaism* 21, no. 3 (summer 1972), pp. 328–332.

Sack, Bracha. *BeSha'arei HaKabbala shel R. Moshe Cordovero*. Beersheba: Ben-Gurion University of the Negev Press, 1995.

Sacks, Jonathan. *The Koren Siddur*. Jerusalem: Koren Publishers, 2009.

Sacks, Jonathan, and Yehuda Sarna. *The Koren Shabbat Evening Siddur*. Jerusalem: Koren Publishers, 2011.

Schachter, Hershel. *Nefesh HaRav*. Brooklyn, NY: Flatbush Beth Hamedrosh, 1994.

Schochet, J. Immanuel. *The Mystical Tradition*. Brooklyn, NY: Kehot Publication Society, 1990.

Schorr, Gedaliah. *Sefer Or Gedalyahu*. 3 vols. Brooklyn, NY, 5745–5746 (1985–1986).

Shneur Zalman of Liadi. *Liqqutei Amarim (Tanya)*. Translated by Nissan Mindel. Brooklyn, NY: Kehot Publication Society, 1962.

Seforno, Obadiah ben Jacob. *Commentary on the Torah*. Translated by Raphael Pelcovitz. Brooklyn, NY: Mesorah Publications, 1987.

Shapira, Kalonymus Kalman. *Derekh HaMelekh*. Jerusalem: Va'ad Ḥasidei Piaseczno, 5755 (1995).

Sharansky, Natan. *Fear No Evil*. New York: Random House, 1988.

Shiyovitz, Ḥayyim A., *Shiurei HaRav Yosef Dov HaLevi Soloveitchik, Zatzal, al Mesekhet Ḥalla*. Jerusalem: Mesora, 2003.

Sokolow, Moshe. "Saadiah Gaon's Prolegomenon to Psalms." *Proceedings of the American Academy for Jewish Research* 51 (1984), pp. 131-174.

Soloveichik, Ahron. "Jew and Jew, Jew and Non-Jew." In *Logic of the Heart, Logic of the Mind: Wisdom and Reflections on Topics of Our Times*. Jerusalem: Genesis Jerusalem Press, 1991.

———. *The Warmth and the Light: Illuminating Approaches to the Weekly Torah Portion*. Jerusalem: Genesis Jerusalem Press, 1992.

Soloveitchik, Joseph B. *And From There You Shall Seek*. Translated by Naomi Goldblum. New Jersey: KTAV Publishing House, 2009.

———. *BeSod HaYaḥid VeHaYaḥad*. Jerusalem: Orot, 1976.

———. "The Community." *Tradition* 17, no. 2 (spring 1978), pp. 7–24.

———. *Halakhic Man*. Translated by Lawrence Kaplan. Philadelphia: Jewish Publication Society, 1983.

———. *Ḥamesh Derashot*. Jerusalem: *Mekhon Tal Orot*, 5734 (1974).

———. *Kol Dodi Dofek: Listen, My Beloved Knocks*. Translated by David Z. Gordon and edited by Jeffrey R. Woolf. New York: Yeshiva University Press, 2006.

———. *The Lonely Man of Faith*. New York: Doubleday, 1992.

———. *The Rav Speaks*. Jerusalem: *Mekhon Tal Orot*, 5743.

———. *Shiurim LeZekher Abba Mari z"l*. 2 vols. Jerusalem: Akiva Yosef, 5743 (1983).

———. *Worship of the Heart*. New York: KTAV Publishing House, 2003.

Soloveitchik, Samuel. "I See Him." *Hamevaser*, March 9, 1967, p. 3.

Steinberg, Milton. *A Believing Jew: The Selected Writings of Milton Steinberg*. Compiled by Edith A. Steinberg and edited by Maurice Samuel. New York: Harcourt, Brace and Company, 1951.

Steinsaltz, Adin. *Opening the Tanya: Discovering the Moral and Mystical Teachings of a Classic Work of Kabbalah.* San Francisco: Jossey-Bass, 2003.

Tillich, Paul. *The Courage to Be*. New Haven and London: Yale University Press, 1952.

Urbach, Ephraim E. "'*Kol HaMekayyeim Nefesh Aḥat*...': Development of the Version, Vicissitudes of Censorship, and Business Manipulations of Printers" [Hebrew]. *Tarbiz* 40 (1971), pp. 268–284.

Uziel, Ben-Tziyon Meir Ḥai. *Derashot Uziel al Masekhet Avot.* Jerusalem: HaVa'ad LeHotza'at Kitvei HaRav, 5751 (1991).

Weiss, Avraham. Contribution to part 4 of *A Dream of Zion: American Jews Reflect on Why Israel Matters to Them,* edited by Rabbi Jeffrey K. Salkin, pp. 162–165. Woodstock, VT: Jewish Lights Publishing, 2007.

———. "Creating a Kiruv Center." *Jewish Action* 55, no. 1 (fall 1994), pp. 71–75.

———. *Spiritual Activism: A Jewish Guide to Leadership and Repairing the World.* Woodstock, VT: Jewish Lights Publishing, 2008.

———. "Tefilah: Feeling the Presence of God." In *Wisdom of Bat Sheva,* edited by Barry S. Wimpfheimer, pp. 207–235. New Jersey: KTAV Publishing House, 2009.

———. *Women at Prayer.* New Jersey: KTAV Publishing House, 1990.

Weiss, Dov. *Confrontation with God in Late Rabbinic Literature.* Chicago: University of Chicago, 2011.

Wilder, Thornton. *Our Town: A Play in Three Acts.* New York: Perennial Classics, 1998.

Wittgenstein, Ludwig. *Tractatus Logico Philosophicus.* New York: Cosimo, 2009.

Wolowelsky, Joel B. "A Quiet Berakha." *Tradition* 29, no. 4 (summer 1995), pp. 61–68.

Zornberg, Avivah. *The Murmuring Deep*. New York: Schocken, 2009.

Index of Daily and Shabbat Prayers

SHAḤARIT

Introductory Prayers
Hareini 16
Modeh Ani 93
Adon Olam 218n
Yigdal 61–62
Al Netilat Yadayim 83
Asher Yatzar 83–85
E-lohai, Neshama 84–85
Birkhot HaTorah 85–86
Priestly Benediction 16n, 86–87
Eilu Devarim 26–27, 87n
Birkhot Hoda'a 87–89
Kaddish DeRabbanan 120n, 245n, 248n

Pesukei DeZimra
Mizmor Shir (Psalm 30) 90
Kaddish Yatom 17n, 31n, 59–60, 120n, 191n
Barukh SheAmar 90, 92, 95, 202
Mizmor LeToda (Psalm 110) 92, 93n
Ashrei (Psalm 145) 93–94, 202–203
Oseh Mishpat LaAshukim (Psalm 146) 27
Hallelujah (Psalm 148) 94

Kol HaNshama (Psalm 150) 81n, 95
VaYevarekh David 95–96, 203n
Az Yashir 54–55, 96–97, 203, 205–206
Yishtabaḥ 96–97
Kaddish 29–31, 60n, 97n

Shema
Yotzer HaMe'orot 61, 99, 100n, 101n, 161, 196
Ahava Rabba 99–100, 101n, 102, 161, 196–197
Shema 100–102, 104, 106, 146, 171n, 172, 192, 195n, 205–206, 249
VeHaya 103–104, 195n
Tzitzit *xiv*n, 103–104, 195n
Emet VeYatziv 80–81
Ga'al Yisrael 104, 106–107, 161, 197

Amida
A-donai Sefatai Tiftaḥ 228
Avoteinu 106–107, 170–171, 174–176, 226n
Ata Gibbor 107
Ata Kadosh 107–108
Ata Ḥonen 55, 108–109
Hashiveinu Avinu 108–109
Selaḥ Lanu 55, 109
Re'eh VeOnyeinu 109
Refa'einu 28, 109–110, 158
Barekh Aleinu 110, 158
Teka BeShofar 27, 112n
Hashiva Shofteinu 111
VeLaMalshinim 55, 112n
Al HaTzaddikim 111–112
VeLiYerushalayim 55, 112
Et Tzemaḥ 112n, 113n
Shema Koleinu 113, 158–159, 160n
Retzeh 115, 215–216
Modim 57–58, 115–116, 216
Sim Shalom 16, 116, 216
E-lohai Netzor 92n, 157, 160n, 216
SheYibbaneh Beit HaMikdash 243

Kedusha 18, 118, 160n

Priestly Benediction 16n

Taḥanun 15n, 46, 50, 57n

Concluding Prayers
Ashrei (Psalm 145) 117
LaMenatze'aḥ (Psalm 20) 117
Uva LeTziyon 117–118
Whole Kaddish 17n, 31n
Aleinu 29n, 118, 120
Al Ken Nekaveh 28, 118
Al Tira 235–236
Daily Psalm 120

MINḤA

Ashrei (Psalm 145) 120, 226
Amida 17n, 120
Aneinu (fast days) 160n

MA'ARIV

VeHu Raḥum 121
Emet Ve'emuna 80–81
Hashkiveinu 121–122

The fonts used in this book are from the Arno family

Maggid Books
The best of contemporary Jewish thought from
Koren Publishers Jerusalem